Individual-based Methods in Forest Ecology and Management

T0178368

Arne Pommerening · Pavel Grabarnik

Individual-based Methods in Forest Ecology and Management

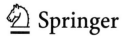 Springer

Arne Pommerening
Department of Forest Ecology
and Management
Swedish University of Agricultural Sciences
Umeå, Sweden

Pavel Grabarnik
Institute of Physicochemical and Biological
Problems in Soil Science
Russian Academy of Sciences
Pushchino, Russia

ISBN 978-3-030-24530-6   ISBN 978-3-030-24528-3   (eBook)
https://doi.org/10.1007/978-3-030-24528-3

This Springer imprint is published by the registered company Springer Nature Switzerland AG
The registered company address is: Gewerbestrasse 11, 6330 Cham, Switzerland

Sic ergo quaeramus tamquam inventuri,
et sic inveniamus tamquam quaesituri.

Let us therefore search as one who expects to
find, and find as one who is determined to
search further.
Augustine of Hippo, *De Trinitate*

Foreword

Forests are vast assemblages of trees, understory plants, large and small animals, and complex biotic soils. The composition, structure, and dynamics of forests result from interacting ecological processes across gradients of space and time. The vast amount of information embodied in a forest is almost incomprehensible.

The early development of forest science and forest management was based on only a very small fraction of the total information residing in forests. Trees were aggregated into stands, and stands were represented by collective traits such as percent species composition and tree sizes. Rates of change in stocking (trees/ha) and stem volume or mass were calculated from information on structural changes of stands between sampling periods. The use of information to characterize stands was sometimes expanded by characterizing variances around mean values, and by characterizing distributions among tree size classes. This level of information supported more than a century of insights into forests and how they change from one period to another, and across sites. Differences in growth rates across sites were classified into site productivity classes, based on information such as heights of dominant trees at a given age. Familiar syntheses of information included site index curves (tree height in relation to age), and tables of stand volumes and yields. In the second half of the last century, computerization of forest science and management greatly expanded the insights that could be gleaned from information present in forests.

Curiously, all of the processes that lead to the amalgamated stand-level characteristics of forests do not happen at the level of stands. Stand growth occurs at the scale of individual trees, and a stand-level representation of forest growth misses many of the information present in tree-level processes. For example, changes in stand-level growth as forests develop over decades result from time trends in the growth of individual trees. A rising (or declining) rate of stand-level growth might result from a synchronous trend among all trees, or from the net outcome of trees showing opposing growth trends. Some of this information was used in classic representation of dominant and suppressed trees, and silvicultural approaches used this information to compare stocking regimes that periodically removed small or large trees.

A major leap in the use of information from trees and forests developed late in the twentieth century as methods of sampling and handling data expanded by orders of magnitude. The quantitative leap in the accounting for growth of thousands of individual trees was joined by spatial information on tree locations. This combination of data on many individuals at defined locations provided a lens for seeing a new dimension of forest information: relationships between individual trees. The growth rate of a given tree could be evaluated not only in terms of environmental factors (such as the supply of soil water and nutrients) but also in relation to competition for resources with neighboring trees. Dominance could be considered in a dynamic sense, accounting for different rates of resource utilization among trees, the efficiencies of using resources to support growth, and how the "story" of each tree's change over time depended on interactions with the stories of neighboring trees.

The examination of individual-tree dynamics in a spatially explicit context enabled scientists in ecology and forestry to explore and test ideas to explain forest structure and dynamics. Advances in science began to explain the processes behind the stand-level patterns that had long been the focus of ecology and forest management. But could analyses of growth of individual trees, and neighborhoods of trees, be harnessed directly to improve forest analysis, planning, and operations? A decade ago, the answer to this question was a nebulous "we hope so, someday". Now the answer is an emphatic "yes".

The forests of our future will not repeat the patterns of forests in the past. Human interactions with forests are now pervasive around the globe. Forest composition is managed directly by fostering some species over others, and indirectly by modifying factors such as populations of tree herbivores. The success of species may now depend on invasions from across the globe, including pathogens that reshape interactions among tree species across landscapes and regions. The changing climate of the twenty-first century will have ecological effects of a magnitude that rivals moving southward by a hundred kilometers or more. The impacts of winds, fires, diseases, and herbivores will have novel impacts under future climates. A retrospective, stand-level view of how forests grew in the past would lack vital information about factors shaping future dynamics of trees and forests. Our ability to envision and explain the forests of our future depends on a foundation of dynamics at the level of trees (and neighborhoods). This book develops the concepts, information, and tools for building such a foundation.

Flagstaff, Arizona   Dan Binkley
May 2019

Preface

Individual-based forest ecology and management, where the focus is on individual plants in the context of their populations, draws on a large body of different quantitative methods that constantly grows and is not well documented in a comprehensive way. This book is intended to serve as a text and reference for undergraduate and postgraduate courses in forest ecology and management. It combines and links the synthesis of important theories and concepts of these two academic fields with new quantitative principles which—although they form a natural and logical unit—so far have not been published together in a single volume.

This book has many boundary encounters in stock. It is about interdisciplinary research situated between ecology, forest science, statistics and computing and facilitates knowledge exchange between different disciplines and research communities. The text attempts to advance forest science in the fields of forest ecology and management through quantitative, individual-based methods and at the same time provides incentives to advance mathematical statistics through a consideration of applications in forest ecology and management.

In a time where firm boundaries between academic fields are rapidly fading, it is an important feature of the book to challenge and re-interpret traditional concepts of forest ecology and management through the findings in tree interaction and forest structure research that we and others have worked on during the last 25 years. Therefore, this book presents a new vision of interdisciplinary, quantitative research and deliberately abandoned the structure of traditional textbooks in forest science and ecology. The text is also instrumental in streamlining the vast amount of localized theories and methods by presenting them in a new, more concise and coherent system.

The book is designed as an English language textbook for a wide range of countries without any particular geographic reference. This textbook stresses the theoretic principles of forest ecology and management and generic quantitative methods which can easily be adapted to different local situations. It is ideal for classes of mixed nationalities with English as the medium of teaching and can therefore be used almost anywhere in the world. Such classes of mixed language and different academic backgrounds are on the increase particularly as part of M.Sc. and Ph.D. courses as well as summer schools.

The book should also appeal as a reference to researchers and is useful as a numerical handbook for practitioners and consultant ecologists or foresters. An effort has been made to prepare the text to be comprehensible also for non-specialists willing to do some limited additional reading.

Chapter 1 introduces individual-based forest ecology and management, explains the vision of this book, and thus sets a common frame.

Chapter 2 synthesizes important ecological theories that form the foundation and the frame of individual-based forest ecology and management.

Chapter 3 reviews important generic concepts and techniques of ecology-based silviculture that are pre-requisites of individual-based forest management.

Chapter 4 is a key part of the book explaining spatial methods of tree interaction research required in individual-based forest ecology and management. The chapter particularly focuses on methods of point process statistics for the analysis of spatial plant patterns.

Chapter 5 serves as an introduction to spatial modelling as a natural continuation of point process statistics outlined in Chap. 4. We introduce here methods of point process modeling, spatial reconstruction, and individual-based models.

Chapter 6 presents tree and forest growth analysis and modelling with a particular focus on relative growth rates. This is an important pre-requisite of individual-based research.

Chapter 7 is dedicated to the analysis of individual human decision making in forests and how the selection of individual trees impacts on forest structure. The chapter outlines theory and concepts of disturbance analysis and the analysis of human tree selection behaviour.

The appendices provide additional background material on forest ecology and management and computational pre-requisites that may not be known to non-specialists.

A book on quantitative forest ecology and management is only complete if explored in practical computer exercises. For this purpose, we integrated quantitative concepts and computations. In our own experience, using computer code in classes greatly enhances the understanding and learning of quantitative concepts, as students acquire both the concepts and programming through their own experimentation at the same time. In this book, we selected the R language but other programming languages would have been suitable as well. Thus, R accompanies the reader throughout the book as a virtual laboratory with a wealth of pre-designed packages and possibilities stimulating self-learning. Finally, the included R code allows the reader to reproduce presented examples and to expand or modify them to be useful for her/his own data analyses. In order to get the most out of this book, it is highly recommended to explore the concepts introduced in the text by using the R software as a virtual laboratory. The code listings are provided directly following mathematical equations so that the code offers another point of access in addition to the sign language of mathematics.

Good research does not unfold without inspiration and intergenerational exchange of ideas. After all, every new generation of researchers naturally stands on the shoulders of the previous generation as Stephen Hawking put it, based on an expression by Isaac Newton and earlier metaphors. In this spirit, the first author gratefully wishes to acknowledge his academic mentors Klaus von Gadow (Göttingen), Hanns H. Höfle (Göttingen), Hans Pretzsch (München), Jean-Philippe Schütz (Zürich), Hubert Sterba (Wien), Dietrich Stoyan (Freiberg), and Günter Wenk (Dresden), who excited him with different aspects of individual-based forest ecology and management at the beginning of his research career and provided him with a thorough scientific education. For the many lively and inspiring discussions, we cannot thank them enough. Their enthusiasm and continuous ready support throughout the years, even from the comfort of their retirement, have been a great asset and a privilege. This work owes a lot to the many fruitful discussions we had. The mutually beneficial knowledge transfer from statistics to ecology and forest science and vice versa has had a significant positive impact on the lives of both authors and with this book we wish to pass on this wonderful experience.

Many good ideas, teaching materials, and computer codes were also developed during (guest) professorships in Austria, China, Denmark, Estonia, Finland, Germany, Ireland, Poland, Spain, Sweden, Switzerland, the UK, and in the US. Discussions with students and colleagues in these countries have had a considerable influence on shaping the text. It is to this international origin that the book owes much of its spirit.

Finally and most importantly, we wish to extend our gratitude to a number of colleagues, friends, and family members who provided helpful suggestions and review comments for various parts of this text including Uta Berger, Harold Burkhart, César Pérez-Cruzado, Roque Rodríguez-Soalleiro, Hongxiang Wang and Zhonghua Zhao. Christopher Guest kindly reviewed Appendix A, and Francis Gwyn Jones and Jens Haufe contributed feedback to Appendix B. Naturally, for all remaining errors or shortcomings in this work, we alone assume responsibility. Discussions with Dan Binkley during his extended Wallenberg visit to Umeå have inspired many reflections on individual-based forest ecology and management and consequently he kindly contributed the foreword to this book.

Umeå, Sweden   Arne Pommerening
Pushchino, Russia   Pavel Grabarnik
May 2019

Acknowledgements A. P. acknowledges the support of the Swedish University of Agricultural Sciences (SLU) and particularly of the SLU Department of Forest Ecology and Management at Umeå while preparing the book manuscript. The contribution of P. G. was funded by the Russian Science Foundation (project no. 18-14-00362).

Contents

Chapter 1
Introduction

Abstract This chapter outlines the vision and principles of individual-based forest ecology and management. For the last 20–30 years there has been a trend in forest ecology and management to interpret the behaviour of forest ecosystems through a bottom-up understanding of interaction processes that start at individual level and eventually lead to important system properties that emerge from individual behaviour. Many publications have demonstrated that the ecological properties of tree populations and woodland communities are much dependent on forest microstructure, which is largely made up by individual woody plants. Also in forest practice the understanding of tree and forest structure is central to management activities. Research results of recent years have shown that the structure of forests to a large degree determines the outcome of forest management, may it be traditional timber production, conservation, recreation, carbon sequestration or mental health therapy to name but a few. All human interventions in forest management and nature conservation are essentially goal-oriented modifications of woodland structure by removing and adding individual trees. Therefore a good understanding of forest patterns helps to predict the likely achievements of forest management.

1.1 Individual-Based Forest Ecology

The term individual-based ecology was coined in the 1990s (Judson 1994) and denotes a strict bottom-up approach, where system properties are derived from the interactions between individuals constituting these systems (Grimm and Railsback 2005). The reasons for this include the complexity, size and slow dynamics of complex ecological systems, which often even prevent the use of controlled experiments (Stillman et al. 2015). Individuals such as trees are understood as building blocks of the system, i.e. the forest, and the properties and behaviour of individuals determine the properties of the system they compose. Individuals grow, reproduce, acquire resources and die and in all these processes they interact with other individuals. To gain and maintain fitness so that they can pass their genes on to future generations, individuals develop adaptive behaviour. This adaptation takes place at individual level whilst ecologists are usually interested in population properties, thus the way to these

© Springer Nature Switzerland AG 2019

A. Pommerening and P. Grabarnik, *Individual-based Methods in Forest Ecology and Management*, https://doi.org/10.1007/978-3-030-24528-3_1

properties is through the individual. Therefore discrete individuals within a population and their individual life cycles are explicitly considered in individual-based ecology. Population-level properties such as persistence, resilience and abundance patterns in space and time are not the sum of the properties of individuals, but they *emerge* from the interactions of adaptive individuals with each other and with their environment. Emergence in this context means that the behaviour underlying demographic rates results from the individuals' behavioural decisions, which are based on fitness-related decision rules (Stillman et al. 2015). As part of this, each individual also contributes to the biotic environment of others (Grimm and Railsback 2005) resulting in complex circular causality.

> Systems are understood and modelled as collections of unique individuals. System properties and dynamics arise from the interactions of individuals with their environment and with each other (Grimm and Railsback 2005).

As other fields of ecology, individual-based ecology is based on theories that are developed from empirical and theoretical ecology and evaluated using a hypothesis-testing approach. Central to these theories are behavioural trends and interactions (Stillman et al. 2015). The standard of accepting theories is how well they reproduce observations of real individuals and systems (Grimm and Railsback 2005). Individual-based ecology is an appropriate conceptual framework when variation and local interactions among individuals, adaptive behaviour or the presence of dynamic or spatially heterogeneous resources are important in determining population processes (Stillman et al. 2015).

Individual-based ecology to a large extent is based on computer experiments and has given rise to a wide range of different models and specific modelling environments, e.g. NetLogo (http://ccl.northwestern.edu/netlogo) (DeAngelis and Mooij 2005) and Jade (http://jade.tilab.com/). In the context of individual-based ecology, pattern-oriented modelling (POM) has been suggested as a new, more detailed way of analysing complex behaviour by using multiple patterns at the same time. POM is the multi-criteria design, selection and calibration of models of complex systems (Grimm and Railsback 2012). A "pattern" is defined as a characteristic, clearly identifiable structure in the data from the system of interest, e.g. the spatial dispersion of trees or the stem-diameter structure. The pattern goes beyond random variation and therefore indicates that there is an underlying process producing this pattern. Such patterns can manifest themselves in spatial and temporal contexts (Janssen et al. 2009). A single pattern observed at a specific scale and hierarchical level is not sufficient to reduce uncertainty in complex systems (Grimm et al. 2005). In traditional forest growth and yield modelling, for example, it was commonly the growth-rate variables, which were of chief importance and other patterns were either ignored or not much considered. By contrast in POM, multiple patterns from the same systems, ideally observed at different hierarchical levels and scales, are used to optimise model complexity and to reduce uncertainty. In forest models, it may therefore be useful to study projected growth rates, size distributions and spatial summary characteristics at the same time. Instead of focussing on the best match between data and model, the approach explores the parameter space and only accepts parameterisations that simultaneously produce simulation results that are close to all the patterns in the observed data. Since several patterns are used, it is less likely that the model is structurally wrong (Janssen et al. 2009). Each pattern used in POM can be considered a filter that helps to reject unacceptable model components or parameterisations. Like any other modelling assumption, the choice of patterns for POM is experimental, i.e. the modeller has to see how well they help to make useful predictions (Grimm and Railsback 2012).

Individual-based ecology and pattern-oriented modelling are comparatively recent developments. As they are gaining in popularity and new results are emerging by the day, it is likely that this field will steadily grow over the next years and decades. Both concepts are central to forest-structure research and vice versa. Therefore many of the methods presented and discussed in this book are about identifying interactions between forest trees. They can be used for analysing and modelling spatial tree relationships and allow to draw conclusions about interaction patterns in forest ecosystems. This is very useful for population and community ecology. At the same time the results from these individual-based analyses prepare and establish the prerequisites for modelling interactions. The common frame and theme of our book is therefore individual-based and interaction-based analysis and modelling and more ecological details are given in Chap. 2.

1.2 Individual-Based Forest Management

It can be argued that forest management was founded on perceived natural competition and facilitation processes. Silvicultural systems (see Sect. 3.7) were, for example, designed to regenerate forest stands naturally thus providing seedlings with sufficient light whilst protecting them against weather extremes (Kimmins 2004; Röhrig et al. 2006). Nurse crops were employed to create artificial shelterwood systems with the aim to protect planted seedlings and species mixtures, which sometimes include nitrogen fixing species thus allowing planted trees to overcome soil nitrogen deficiencies (Pommerening and Murphy 2004). This can be seen as an application of the nurse-plant concept from plant ecology (Keddy 2017). In general these techniques are particularly successful, where there are environmental constraints, e.g. early/late frost events, droughts, nitrogen-poor soils etc. Thinnings (see Sect. 3.6) but also the aforementioned silvicultural systems essentially are strategies to interfere with and to steer interactions towards predefined management objectives. Keddy (2017) argued that disturbances counterbalance competition by giving weaker competitors a chance of survival and since forest management is a type of human disturbance, it is clear that human interference in natural forest development must be a part of this book, too.

The ecological concept of competition has had a profound and long-lasting influence on individual-based forest management, particularly with respect to thinning activities and related applications in near-natural or continuous-cover management types (Pommerening and Murphy 2004; Pommerening and Sánchez Meador 2018). For a long time forest management was dominated by qualitative concepts involving terms such as "light", "moderate" and "heavy" thinnings (for defining thinning intensity) and "thinning from below", "crown" and "schematic thinning" for *global thinning* types. These addressed a forest stand as a population rather than differentiating between individual trees and have not always been helpful in answering the practical question, which trees to mark for thinning and which ones to leave behind. They also created problems for the implementation in simulation models. In Europe and recently also in China, the need to refine such concepts in a more rational and reproducible way but also the advances in ecological research have given rise to the conception of *local thinning* types, which can also be described as individual-based thinning types. Local or individual-based thinning types are a fundamental change in paradigm because they include a strategy to break a large forest stand down into smaller neighbourhood-based units that are easier to perceive and for a forest operator marking trees or for a harvester driver easier to work through one by one. As such local thinning types consequently implement the nearest-neighbour principle outlined in Chap. 4. The basic idea of this bottom-up concept was originally conceived from the insight that the majority of production and profit in each forest stand usually is achieved with a comparatively small number of good-quality trees. Based on this, local thinnings were designed to separate important trees from less important ones and to promote the former only (Röhrig et al. 2006), see Sect. 3.6.1. Only later it dawned on forest managers and conservationists that this concept can be generalised and that importance can be defined in many different ways, e.g. in terms of potential economic value, habitat value, stand stability, spiritual or aesthetic value. This implies that individual-based thinnings can be combined with any silvicultural system and can also be used for conservation or recreation management. Such "trees of importance" or "trees of interest" go by different names in different countries, e.g. frame trees, final crop trees, future trees ("Z-Bäume" in German), elite trees, habitat trees, target or plus trees. In this book, we adopted the British term "frame trees" for the appealing metaphor of a framework of special trees forming the backbone of a forest stand or a tree population. In a way the frame-tree method (used as a synonym of individual-based/local thinning method in this book) also serves as a didactic aid that helps field staff to separate important from unimportant trees regardless of the definition of importance. In our experience, it frequently happens that people unfamiliar with individual-based forest management are at a loss when asked to select trees for thinnings. They simply "cannot see the trees for the wood" and the frame-tree method literally is an eye-opener fostering their observation skills and perception.

Part of the motivation for individual-based forest management is a rationalisation aspect because only those trees are marked whose removal supports frame trees, i.e. the forest operator scans the neighbourhood of frame trees for potential competitors and marks the most urgent cases for thinning. The success of thinnings can also be more easily checked in subsequent years, because only the frame trees need to be assessed. If species diversity is an objective of stand management, it is easy to appoint frame trees in such a way that a long-term species composition is ensured including rare tree species. Also tree harvesting and extraction damage can be minimised as the frame trees are visibly marked (Röhrig et al. 2006).

According to Klädtke (1993) the beginnings of the concept of local thinnings and individual-based forest management goes as far back as 1763 when Duhamel du Monceau mentioned the use of frame trees for oak management in France. The concept was then introduced in Switzerland and Germany around 1840 and developed until now. Schädelin (Switzerland) and Abetz (Germany) are prominent silviculturist, who refined the concept. Numerous variants of the local thinning/frame tree concept are now applied in many European countries, in China and occasionally also in North America (Pommerening and Sánchez Meador 2018), see Chap. 3.

1.3 Fundamental Importance of Tree and Forest Structure

Structure is a fundamental notion referring to patterns and interactions between their components in more or less well-defined systems (Gadow et al. 2012). Typical of biological structures are repetitive patterns which are the result of complex interactions. They can be comparatively simple such as the structure of honey combs or more complex. The fact that structures determine processes and that processes in return modify structures is well known in natural sciences. The patterns we observe and monitor in forests are the traces processes leave behind and they allow us to develop hypotheses that we can test (Gavrikov and Stoyan 1995). However, structure is not only the result of past processes, but also the starting point and often the cause for future developments (Gadow et al. 2012). Forest structure, for example, has a strong influence on tree growth processes. Every individual tree, however, also contributes to changes in forest structure but this is a comparatively slow long-term process (Pretzsch 2009). Also any impact on forests—whether natural or human-induced—is primarily a change of forest structure. In a second step, the modified structure then affects the processes in the forest ecosystem. All data, that are collected in forest ecosystems, have not only a temporal but also a spatial dimension. The properties of the whole system "forest" or "tree population", e.g. forest growth and interactions between trees, to a large degree depend on the structure of this system. This has been known in forest science for a long time and has given rise to traditional terms such as "growing space" and "initial spacing".

In the last decades, new methods were developed in the statistical fields of point process statistics, geostatistics and random set statistics, see Chap. 4. These allow better and more detailed research of the interplay between spatial patterns and ecological processes. Apart from statistics and mathematics also other research fields such as physics and materials science have contributed to structural research. Flocks of birds, insect swarms, herds of buffalo, lichens, stones in an ancient, historical building and even galaxies exhibit specific patterns that can be analysed with similar methods. Structure research is therefore strictly interdisciplinary, often the necessary methods have been developed within the framework of mathematical statistics or of other natural sciences and only later applied to forest research (Gavrikov and Stoyan 1995). Like in chemistry, once we can quantitatively describe the microstructure of a system, we are in a position to predict its properties and even to synthesise it through reconstruction (Pommerening 2006; Pommerening and Stoyan 2008; Nothdurft et al. 2010; Lilleleht et al. 2014 see Sect. 5.1.2).

There is a close relationship between structure and property, which is well known in materials science, physics, geology and the term *structure/property relationships* has been coined in those subject areas (Torquato 2002). According to this term ecological processes not only leave traces as spatial patterns, but the spatial structure of materials or of a forest also determines to a large degree the properties of the system under study. The individual components of a material or the tree species or tree sizes of a forest arranged in various ways may result in very different properties for the material or forest as a whole. This suggests that the complex interactions between the components result in a dependence of the effective properties on nontrivial details of the microstructure.

In forests, properties can be habitat functions, biodiversity, biomass production, recreation and even human health (see Fig. 1.1). This implies that the results of forest management, e.g. forest products, but also natural regeneration responding to human disturbances as part of silvicultural systems (see Sect. 3.7), are examples of such system properties, which are largely determined by its structure.

Competition and survival of trees are such properties as well as the sampling error of forest resource inventories, which is strongly correlated with spatial forest structure. Spatial statistics and inventory research are therefore closely related. Pommerening and Stoyan (2008) and Nothdurft et al. (2010), for example, found that

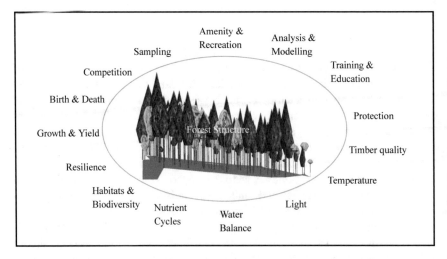

Fig. 1.1 Selection of ecosystem functions, goods and services connected to forest structure. These can be interpreted as structure/property relationships

sampling results can be improved by reconstructing spatial forest structure. Spatial statistics and sampling theory share many overlaps which can be used as synergies (Motz et al. 2010). A proper understanding of (spatial) woodland structure and its temporal evolution also plays a decisive role for forest modelling where the inclusion of spatial measures is often used to generalise models.

Landscape and forest structure determines the occurrence and population dynamics of brown bears, owls and woodpeckers to such a degree that direct conclusions concerning habitat and population development can be made from spatial structure (Letcher et al. 1998; McKelvey et al. 1993; Wiegand 1998). Similar results have been found for other birds, beetles, spiders and other animals living on and in forest trees. Pattern recognition helps to identify distinctive spatial patterns and to link them with the corresponding properties.

Self-organisation: Irreversible processes in non-linear systems, which create complex structures of the total system as a result of interactions between parts of the system (complex interacting systems, see Wolfram 2002; Puettmann et al. 2009).
Structure/property relations: The effective properties of a heterogeneous material depend on the properties of its components (phases) and microstructural information (Torquato 2002).
Pattern recognition: plays an important role in biology, i.e. immune systems and information technology. The basic principle of pattern recognition is to reduce raw data to a useful summary form (Wolfram 2002; Deutsch 1994).

There is even an intriguing mental health example relating to tree structure: Koch (1949) developed a tree-drawing test for detecting schizophrenia. In this psychological examination, patients are required to draw trees. The drawings can then be assessed in a qualitative way (positive, negative or normal). A few studies have attempted to quantify the trees drawn based on structure or morphology, suggesting that the structural differences in the drawings are factors by which schizophrenic individuals and healthy subjects can be distinguished (Kaneda et al. 2010).

Among other things the crown ratio, i.e. crown length to total-tree height (Eq. 2.8), was assessed in those drawings. In pictures of trees drawn by patients in their normal state, the part-to-the-whole proportion most closely approached the golden section.[1] Apparently the constancy in the relation between the whole and its parts makes the image recognisable.

---

[1] A line segment is divided in golden section, the ratio of the whole length to the larger part is equal to the ratio of the larger part to the smaller part. This definition implies that, if the smaller part has unit length and the larger part has length τ, then $(\tau + 1)/\tau = \tau/1$. It follows that $\tau^2 - \tau = 1$, which gives $\tau = 0.5 \cdot (1 + \sqrt{5}) = 1.6180$, to 4 decimal places. This number τ is the golden ratio (Clapham and Nicholson 2005). It arises in a wide range of mathematical and biological contexts.

In upland protection forests, the dispersion of trees and forest structure has an important influence on the ability of forests to intercept stones from rockfall, avalanches and landslides that threaten human settlements (Brauner et al. 2005).

In all these examples the properties of the whole system, the forest, and the interaction between its components, the trees, depend on the microstructure of the system. In materials science, structure/property relationships are employed to predict the properties of a material from known details of the spatial microstructure. In a similar way the projection of forest growth and yield has for a long time been an important objective of tree and stand modelling in forestry (Pretzsch 2009). In this context, forest structural analyses may form the basis for sustainable forest management strategies and pave the way to new ecological theories.

Spatial systems analysis of forest ecosystems is therefore an important branch of ecological statistics integrating research on forest structure, sampling, monitoring and modelling.

Trees fill spatial niches and their morphology reflects the geometry of the niche. The morphology of open-grown trees is very different to the morphology of forest trees. This is the result of a range of complex interactions, one of which is competition. Interaction or interdependence implies that a change in one organism will result in a subsequent change of others (Kimmins 2004, p. 29). Competition for resources is a negative form of plant interaction. It occurs when two or more individuals attempt to utilise the same resource and when that resource is in limited supply (Kimmins 2004; Perry et al. 2008, p. 422 and p. 232, respectively). Competition sets in motion an interaction between individuals leading to a reduction of the performance (e.g. in terms of survival, growth and reproduction) of at least some of the competing individuals (Begon et al. 2006). Trees compete for light, water and nutrients. Competition pressure caused by surrounding trees influences the growth of a tree (see Chap. 2). Too much competition pressure can be lethal and can cause what is referred to as natural mortality or self-thinning. In managed forests, one of the most important tasks of foresters is the management of interaction: Through selective thinning and harvesting more resources are allocated to the remaining trees. Thinnings modify growing space and soon after release a tree puts energy into occupying the newly available space (see Fig. 1.2 and Sect. 3.6). Competition and other interaction processes can be understood as an important part of self-organisation. Forest structure is modified by interactions between individual trees, which to a large degree are influenced by the initial structure.

Wind and snow are important environmental factors that influence tree growth dependent on growing space. This leads to biomechanical optimisation through goal-oriented biomass allocation (see Sect. 2.2). There is also positive interaction between trees that is often referred to as facilitation (Berkowitz et al. 1995; Dickie et al. 2005). Neighbouring trees often support other trees and shelter them from the forces of wind and snow. Also mycorrhizal interactions between different species can have synergy effects in mixed species forest stands (Perry et al. 2008, p. 131ff).

Naturally there is a close link between structure and diversity. Measures of forest structure often are also good diversity indicators and vice versa. The term diversity relates to the variability and unpredictability of living organisms (Gaston and Spicer

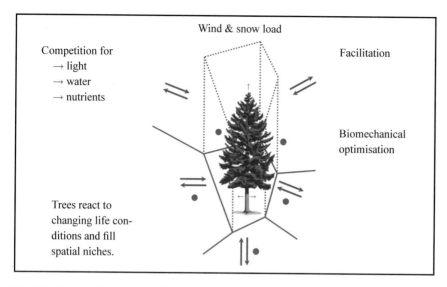

Fig. 1.2 Tree reactions to changing growing space. The red dots symbolise the locations of surrounding trees in a forest

2004; Dale and Fortin 2014). Forest structure and α-diversity can be subdivided into three different aspects, the tree *location, species* and *size* diversity (see Fig. 1.3). These three aspects are useful to describe woodland structure as holistically as possible. When reconstructing forest structure (see Sect. 5.1.2) it helps to include summary characteristics representing all three aspects (Pommerening 2006; Pommerening and Stoyan 2008). In practical applications of the three aspects of forest structure, it is useful to think creatively. The examples in Fig. 1.3 emphasise that almost any tree

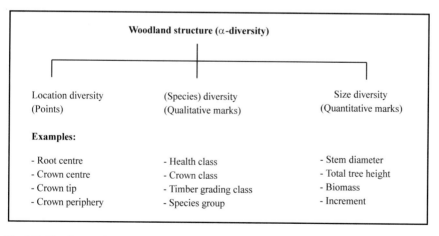

Fig. 1.3 The three major characteristics of forest structure and α-diversity (modified from Pommerening 2002)

characteristic can and should be used to underpin these three basic categories as long as they fulfill the requirements of the corresponding definition. Point process statistics (see Chap. 4) goes a step further in generalisation and distinguishes between *points, qualitative* and *quantitative marks* instead (Illian et al. 2008). These terms and concepts are useful to understand the general nature of structural aspects and clearly highlight the flexibility in defining them.

Tree species and size diversity can be quantified in a non-spatially explicit or in a spatially explicit way. The diversity of tree locations is by definition always spatially explicit. Fichtner et al. (2018) defined the term *individual-based biodiversity effect* as the net effect of all intra- and interspecific interactions within the neighbourhood of a given tree and quantified it in terms of relative volume growth (see Chap. 6).

Another way of subdividing aspects of forest structure is to distinguish between horizontal and vertical elements. A sufficient degree of vertical forest structure is an important habitat requirement for many animal species such as the red squirrel (*Sciurus vulgaris* L.) (Spiecker et al. 2004). Vertical structure is also an important part of the definition of selection forests (Schütz 2001).

Many different concepts of diversity and structural measures have been developed to characterise and to analyse forest structure. They are mathematical expressions of species, dimensional and location diversity of a population and an important pre-requisite for forest structure research (Krebs 1999, p. 440). Such mathematical measures are usually more informative than just the number of species or the mean and variance of tree size.

1.4   Sampling and Quantitative Forest Description

Any data analysis and presentation is preceded by sampling. Usually the object of a quantitative forest description is a forest stand or some other sufficiently homogeneous unit of forest land in terms of environmental conditions, species composition, age/development phase and structure. Data can be gathered in various ways and there is a substantial amount of literature on aspects of forest inventory, see for example Gregoire and Valentine (2008), Kangas and Maltamo (2009) and Mandallaz (2008).

In forest ecology and management, usually the tree community of interest is larger than any feasible sample. Therefore any data collection is generally limited to a sample and also needs to be interpreted as such. Sampling can be achieved in two ways (see Fig. 1.4), by using 1. comparatively *large, sparsely replicated sample plots* (see Appendix B for details) or 2. relatively *small, frequently replicated sample plots*. The decision which of these two methods to use depends on the objective of the study and influences the choice of suitable statistical methods. In point process statistics (Chap. 4), the term *observation window* for sample plot is often used (Illian et al. 2008). All sample plots within a forest unit, e.g. a forest stand, can be interpreted as different realisations of the same unit or stand.

The first option of large, sparsely replicated sample plots can be recommended, if more detailed research is intended, particularly if interactions between trees are the focus of the analysis and if the analyst wishes to use advanced spatial statistics,

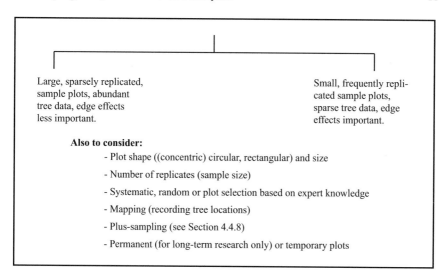

Fig. 1.4 General sampling checklist in forest ecology and management

for example second-order summary characteristics (see Diggle 2014; Illian et al. 2008, and Chap. 4). In such cases, the sample plots should ideally comprise a minimum of 150 trees and the size of the sample plots then depends on stand density (Pommerening and Stoyan 2006; Rajala et al. 2018), whereby the sample size has implications for both the robustness of the estimations of summary characteristics and the power of statistical tests based on them. Particularly when interactions between individuals of many different species are intended to be studied, the sample plot can often not be large enough. If the analysis is not limited to a one-off or snapshot sample, i.e. there is the intention to set up plots for long-term research with regular re-measurements, it is important to ensure that the sample plots contain at least 150 trees *at all times* by anticipating possible losses of trees due to thinnings and natural disturbances. In temperate and boreal forests, one hectare is often a suitable size, however, if whole silvicultural systems (Sect. 3.7) are to be covered by research plots, a minimum size of 3–5 hectares is required (Puettmann et al. 2009, p. 99). The authors stress the increasing importance of large-scale research plots for incorporating greater structural and ecological heterogeneity. Additionally there should be at least two plot replicates in the forest stand or experimental unit that are somewhat representative and typical, i.e. the plot selection calls on the researcher's knowledge and experience. Often to a large extent, the geometry and topography of the experimental unit or forest stand determines the location of the replicated plots. Option one of large, sparsely replicated sample plots in conjunction with mapping (see below) is the most common sampling method in quantitative ecology and permits the use of advanced statistical methods. Details on how to set up such research plots are provided in Appendix B.

The second option of small, frequently replicated sample plots reflects the traditional strategies of forest (stand) inventory and monitoring. To reduce the variability between plots it is often recommended to select sample plots systematically, i.e. the plot centres are located on a systematic grid that does not run in parallel with forest roads, planting rows or extraction racks. The *spatially balanced sampling* method offers an alternative (Stevens and Olsen 2004; Grafström et al. 2012). Small, frequently replicated sample plots should be preferred, if it is the intention to characterise a forest stand or experimental unit only by global, non-spatial general or forestry characteristics such as trees per hectare, mean diameter at breast height or basal area per hectare. Such a design is likely to cover a larger geographic region well.

There are also a number of spatially explicit nearest neighbour summary statistics (NNSS) that can be estimated from such sample data (see Sect. 4.4.7.1). However, if NNSS are used, it is recommended to sample off-plot neighbours as well, to eliminate any edge bias (plus-sampling, see Sect. 4.4.8). The smaller the sample plots, the more important this becomes (Pommerening and Stoyan 2006; Motz et al. 2010). As a general guideline van Laar and Akça (2007, p. 237) suggested that each plot should contain 15–20 trees, 10 trees being the absolute minimum. Obviously the smaller the sample plots, the more limited is research into plant interactions. Motz et al. (2010) described how NNSS can be included in existing forest inventories.

In general, circular and rectangular (including square) plot shapes can be recommended for both sampling options as they simplify the work in the field and are also easier for handling aspects of edge bias in spatially explicit studies. Also with small frequently replicated sample plots, plot and sample size (number of plots) depends on the density and structure of the woodland under consideration. Detailed suggestions are provided in the forest inventory literature (van Laar and Akça 2007; Gregoire and Valentine 2008; Kangas and Maltamo 2009; Mandallaz 2008). Sampling errors can be reduced by always maintaining the same plot size (fixed-area plots) as opposed to using variable plot sizes in the forest stand or the experimental unit under study.

Mapping of trees, i.e. the recording of tree locations, is advisable if spatially-explicit analyses are anticipated or cannot be completely ruled out. NNSS can often also be sampled in-situ in the field, i.e. no explicit mapping is required (Gadow et al. 2012), however, the lack of information on tree locations may limit the subsequent data analysis. Generally, mapping provides more flexibility in the analysis and tree coordinates are useful for relocating trees in re-measurements or for marking trees in marteloscope experiments (Chap. 7).

Diverse, uneven-aged forest stands often contain trees of a wide range of sizes. Trying to sample trees of many sizes in small fixed-sized plots is likely to lead to inadequate sampling of large trees or unnecessarily large and time-consuming measurements of saplings. A useful solution to this problem is to assess circular plots of several different sizes, all centred at the same point (nested plot design), but each concentrating on a specific range of tree diameters (van Laar and Akça 2007, p. 237). This method of concentric circular sample plots leads to a situation where frequently occurring small or medium-sized trees are sampled in small circular plots whilst rare large trees are sampled in large plots (see Fig. 1.5). If this approach is adopted, it

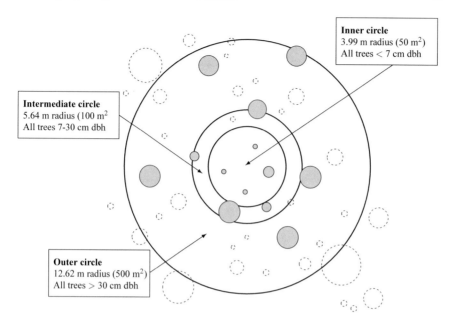

Fig. 1.5 Example of a concentric or nested monitoring plot design. Grey circles represent trees included and dashed circles those that are not included in the sample. All three circular plots are centred on the same sample point, and as plot radius increases progressively larger trees are measured. Another very small circular plot may be used for seedling counts. dbh denotes stem diameter at breast height, i.e. 1.3 m above ground. Modified from Davies et al. (2008)

is important to ensure that correct expansion factors (so-called Horvitz-Thompson weights, see Sect. 4.4.8) are applied when calculating results. The concentric or nested circular sample plot design is often used for permanent sample plots (PSP).

Alternatively angle count sampling (also referred to as variable radius plot sampling, relascope sampling and point sampling) can be used (Bitterlich 1984). Both methods are straightforward to apply and efficient for estimating traditional forestry summary characteristics. However, both sampling with concentric sample plots and angle count sampling may limit the analysis of tree interactions, as only a subset of trees is included in the sample (see Fig. 1.5). In addition it is necessary to take the sampling design into account when estimating summary characteristics from the data and using them for modelling (Ekström et al. 2018). If the analyst intends to monitor changes in forest structure and development by repeated measurements at two or more points in time, it is generally advisable to re-measure trees in the same set of (permanent) sample plots rather than setting up new (temporary) ones for each measurement. This is because the relocation of plots in temporary sampling may mask some of the real changes arising from disturbances and stand development and they do not permit a detailed analysis of changes at plot and tree level (Mandallaz 2008, p. 185ff.).

Table 1.1 A selection of forestry summary characteristics based on Pretzsch (2009) and Wenk et al. (1990)

Summary characteristic	Symbol	Unit
Date of survey	–	–
Tree species	–	–
Age (range)	t, age	Months, years
Length of survey period	–	Months, years
Survey plot area	A	ha
Number of trees for sampling growth rates	n_i	Number
Number of height sample trees	n_h	Number
Number of trees	N	Number per hectares
Top height	h_{100}	m
Top diameter	d_{100}	cm
Top h/d ratio (slenderness)	$\frac{h_{100}}{d_{100}}$	–
Quadratic mean diameter	d_g	cm
Mean height corresponding to d_g	h_g	m
Mean h/d ratio (slenderness)	$\frac{h_g}{d_g}$	–
Basal area	G, BA	$m^2\ ha^{-1}$
Standing volume	V	$m^3\ ha^{-1}$
Cumulative or total volume production	CVP, TVP	$m^3\ ha^{-1}$
Basal area stocking degree	B^o	–
Tree count stocking degree	N^o	–
Volume stocking degree	V^o	–
Biomass	W	$kg\ ha^{-1}$
Periodic annual absolute basal area growth rate	i_G	$m^2\ year^{-1}$
Annual basal area growth percentage	p_G	%
Periodic annual absolute volume growth rate	i_V	$m^3\ year^{-1}$
Annual volume growth percentage	p_V	%
Mean annual absolute volume growth rate	MAI	$m^3\ ha^{-1}\ year^{-1}$

In the analysis, plots can be pooled or analysed separately. For details of these sampling methods, their application and their estimators, the reader is referred to the associated literature (van Laar and Akça 2007; Gregoire and Valentine 2008; Kangas and Maltamo 2009; Mandallaz 2008).

Theory and general statistics of experimental design are well covered by Montgomery (2013) and research questions in individual-based ecology and management may allow the use of some of the techniques described in his book. There is certainly scope for using a wide range of sophisticated summary characteristics in such analyses of the current state of a forest stand. In the subsequent chapters, many of these possibilities are introduced and their calculation is demonstrated by listings of R code.

Table 1.1 gives a selection of summary characteristics which are often used to characterise forest stands in silvicultural and forest growth and yield analyses. Details can be found in literature provided.

Finally, it should be pointed out that some of the large observational sample plots (Zhao et al. 2014) as often used in point process statistics, individual-tree ecology and modelling can also be considered as individual-tree experiments (Pretzsch 2009, p. 143f.). The fundamental idea is to include a wide range of different interaction types reflecting the possibilities listed in Table 2.1 in one or two large plots. Considering a theoretical, quantitative interaction index capable of identifying these different types of interactions, observational plots could be set up in such a way that the index values of all individual trees form a uniform distribution. This implies that all possible interaction types are well represented for one woodland community in one or two plots. Then the data of such sample plots can be used to develop and parametrise an individual-based model (see Sect. 5.2) that allows the analyst to run computer experiments with replicated treatments to study the complex behaviour of individual trees under defined conditions, where the statistical theory of experimental design is given full consideration (Montgomery 2013). This is a successful strategy representing a combination of field trials and computer experiments (Gramelsberger 2010).

1.5 Individual-Based Forest Ecology and Management

In this book, we have integrated three main fields of individual-based forest ecology and management, i.e. *tree/plant interactions*, the *biometry of plant growth* and *human behaviour in forests*, see Fig. 1.6.

In our research vision, individual-based forest ecology and management is part of *quantitative ecology* and particularly of *spatial ecology*, because the analysis and management of individual trees requires information on space and proximity. Therefore the common denominator of the three fields is research on the individual behaviour of plants as well as of humans and how this behaviour contributes to the formation of spatial patterns that evolve through time. The term "behaviour" is used in a very broad sense and also includes growth as well as birth and death processes of plants.

In individual-based forest ecology and management, the main research interest naturally is in tree/plant interactions in space and time and how these interactions affect population dynamics and contribute to shaping the community under study. Research methods and example applications relating to tree/plant interactions are provided in Chaps. 4 and 5.

Fig. 1.6 The three core
fields of individual-based
forest ecology and
management considered in
this book and their
commonalities "individuals"
and "space-time"

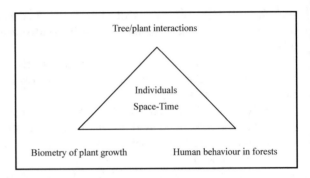

Biometry of plant growth is devoted to the analysis of growth processes that can involve any part of plants and also studies the simultaneous growth of several organs or parts of a plant. Growth analysis greatly contributes to the analysis and modelling of tree/plant interactions, but interactions also help to explain growth processes. Biometry of plant growth is detailed in Chap. 6.

Human behaviour in forests can modify or even steer tree interactions and growth in a particular direction. Here individuals respond to a visual interaction with trees where partly rational but also subconscious, emotional reactions lead to decisions changing forest structure and intertree interactions. Research methods in individual-based forest management and particularly in human behaviour in forests are outlined in Chap. 7.

A complex research area such as individual-based forest ecology and management requires interdisciplinary approaches to be successful. These include methods from ecology, statistics, materials science, plant growth science, computing and psychology and are likely to involve even more fields of natural sciences in the future.

Chapters 2 and 3 facilitate the basic understanding of theories, hypotheses and concepts in forest ecology and management that set the scene for Chaps. 4–7. Additional technical details are given in the three Appendices.

References

Begon M, Harper JL, Townsend CR (2006) Ecology: individuals, populations and communities, 3rd edn. Blackwell Science, Oxford, 1092 p

Berkowitz AR, Canham CD, Kelly VR (1995) Competition vs. facilitation of tree seedling growth and survival in early successional communities. Ecology 76:1156–1168

Bitterlich W (1984) The relascope idea. Relative measurements in forestry. Commonwealth agricultural bureaux. Norwich, 242 p

Brauner M, Weinmeister W, Agner P, Vospernik S, Hoesle B (2005) Forest management decision support for evaluating forest protection effects against rockfall. For Ecol Manag 207:75–85

Clapham C, Nicholson J (2005) Concise dictionary of mathematics, 3rd edn. Oxford University Press, Oxford, 498 p

Dale MRT, Fortin M-J (2014) Spatial analysis. A guide for ecologists, 2nd edn. Cambridge University Press, Cambridge, 438 p

Davies O, Haufe J, Pommerening A (2008) Silvicultural principles of continuous cover forestry—a guide to best practice. Bangor University, Bangor, 111 p

DeAngelis DL, Mooij WM (2005) Individual-based modeling of ecological and evolutionary processes. Annu Rev Ecol Evol Syst 36:147–168

Deutsch A (ed) (1994) Muster des Lebendigen. [Patterns of life.] Friedrich Vieweg & Sohn, Braunschweig, 299 p

Dickie IA, Schnitzer SA, Reich PB, Hobbie SE (2005) Spatially disjunct effects of co-occuring competition and facilitation. Ecol Lett 8:1191–1200

Diggle PJ (2014) Statistical analysis of spatial and spatio-temporal point patterns, 3rd edn. CRC Press, Boca Raton, 267 p

Ekström M, Esseen P-A, Westerlund B, Grafström A, Jonsson BG, Ståhl G (2018) Logistic regression for clustered data from environmental monitoring programs. Ecol Inform 43:165–173

Fichtner F, Härdle W, Bruelheide H, Kunz M, Li Y, Oheimb Gv (2018) Neighbourhood interactions drive overyielding in mixed-species tree communities. Nat Commun 9:1144

Gadow Kv, Zhang CY, Wehenkel C, Pommerening A, Corral-Rivas J, Korol M, Myklush S, Hui GY, Kiviste A, Zhao X H (2012) Forest structure and diversity, 29–83. In: Pukkala T, Gadow Kv (eds) Continuous cover forestry, 2nd edn. Managing forest ecosystems, vol 23. Springer, Dordrecht, 296 p

Gaston KJ, Spicer JI (2004) Biodiversity. An introduction. Blackwell Publishing, Oxford, 191 p

Gavrikov V, Stoyan D (1995) The use of marked point processes in ecological and environmental forest studies. Environ Ecol Stat 2:331–344

Grafström A, Lundström NL, Schelin L (2012) Spatially balanced sampling through the pivotal method. Biometrics 68:514–520

Gramelsberger G (2010) Computerexperimente. Zum Wandel der Wissenschaft im Zeitalter des Computers. [Computer experiments. On the change of science in the computer age.] transcript Verlag, Bielefeld, 313 p

Gregoire TG, Valentine HT (2008) Sampling strategies for natural resources and the environment. Applied environmental statistics. Chapman & Hall/CRC, Boca Raton, 474 p

Grimm V, Railsback SF (2005) Individual-based modeling and ecology. Princeton University Press, Princeton, 448 p

Grimm V, Railsback SF (2012) Pattern-oriented modelling: a "multi-scope" for predictive systems ecology. Philos Trans R Soc Lond B: Biol Sci 367:298–310

Grimm V, Revilla E, Berger U, Jeltsch F, Mooij WM, Railsback SF, Thulke HH, Weiner J, Wiegand T, DeAngelis DL (2005) Pattern-oriented modeling of agent-based complex systems: lessons from ecology. Science 310:987–991

Illian J, Penttinen A, Stoyan H, Stoyan D (2008) Statistical analysis and modelling of spatial point patterns, Wiley, Chichester, 534 p

Janssen MA, Radtke NP, Lee A (2009) Pattern-oriented modeling of commons dilemma experiments. Adapt Behav 17:508–523

Judson O (1994) The rise of the individual-based model in ecology. Trends Ecol Evol 9:9–14

Kaneda A, Yasui-Furukori N, Saito M, Sugawara N, Nakagami T, Furukori H, Kaneko S (2010) Characteristics of the tree-drawing test in chronic schizophrenia. Psychiatry Clin Neurosci 64:141–148

Kangas A, Maltamo M (Eds) (2009) Forest inventory. Methods and applications. Managing forest ecosystems, vol 10. Springer, Dordrecht, 362 p

Keddy PA (2017) Plant ecology. Origins, processes, consequences, 2nd edn. Cambridge University Press, Cambridge, 624 p

Kimmins JP (2004) Forest ecology—a foundation for sustainable management, 3rd edn. Pearson Education Prentice Hall, Upper Saddle River, 700 p

Klädtke J (1993) Konstruktion einer Z-Baum-Ertragstafel am Beispiel der Fichte [Construction of a frame-tree yield table for Norway spruce]. Mitteilungen der Forstlichen Versuchs- und Forschungsanstalt Baden-Württemberg 173. Freiburg, 122 p

Koch K (1949) Der Baumtest: Der Baumzeichenversuch als psychodiagnostisches Hilfsmittel. [The tree test: The tree drawing test as an aid in psychodiagnosis.] Hans Huber, Bern

Krebs CJ (1999) Ecological methodology, 2nd edn. Addison Wesley Longman, New York, 620 p

Letcher BH, Priddy JA, Walters JR, Crowder LB (1998) An individual-based, spatially-explicit simulation model of the population dynamics of the endangered red-cockaded woodpecker, Picoides borealis. Biol Conserv 86:1–14

Lilleleht A, Sims A, Pommerening A (2014) Spatial forest structure reconstruction as a strategy for mitigating edge-bias in circular monitoring plots. For Ecol Manag 316:47–53

Mandallaz D (2008) Sampling techniques for forest inventories. Applied environmental statistics. Chapman & Hall/CRC, Boca Raton, 256 p

McKelvey K, Noon BR, Lamberson RH (1993) Conservation planning for species occupying fragmented landscapes: the case of the northern spotted owl. In: Kareiva PM, Kingsolver JG, Huey RB (eds) Biotic interactions and global change. Sinauer, Sunderland, Massachusetts, USA, pp 424–250

Montgomery DC (2013) Design and analysis of experiments, 8th edn. Wiley, New Delhi, 726 p

Motz K, Sterba H, Pommerening A (2010) Sampling measures of tree diversity. For Ecol Manag 260:1985–1996

Nothdurft A, Saborowski J, Nuske RS, Stoyan D (2010) Density estimation based on k-tree sampling and point pattern reconstruction. Can J For Res 40:953–967

Perry DA, Oren R, Hart SC (2008) Forest ecosystems, 2nd edn. The Johns Hopkins University Press, Baltimore, 632 p

Pommerening A (2002) Approaches to quantifying forest structures. Forestry 75:305–324

Pommerening A (2006) Evaluating structural indices by reversing forest structural analysis. For Ecol Manag 224:266–277

Pommerening A, Murphy ST (2004) A review of the history, definitions and methods of continuous cover forestry with special attention to afforestation and restocking. Forestry 77:27–44

Pommerening A, Stoyan D (2006) Edge-correction needs in estimating indices of spatial forest structure. Can J For Res 36:1723–1739

Pommerening A, Stoyan D (2008) Reconstructing spatial tree point patterns from nearest neighbour summary statistics measured in small subwindows. Can J For Res 38:1110–1122

Pommerening A, Sánchez Meador AJ (2018) Tamm review: tree interactions between myth and reality. For Ecol Manag 428:164–176

Pretzsch H (2009) Forest dynamics, growth and yield. From measurement to model. Springer, Heidelberg, 664 p

Puettmann K, Coates KD, Messier C (2009) A critique of silviculture. Island Press, Washington, 204 p

Rajala T, Olhede SC, Murrell DJ (2018) When do we have the power to detect biological interactions in spatial point patterns? J Ecol 107:711–721

Röhrig E, Bartsch N, Lüpke Bv (2006) Waldbau auf ökologischer Grundlage. [Silviculture on an ecological basis]. Verlag Eugen Ulmer Stuttgart. Stuttgart, 479 p

Schütz JP (2001) Der Plenterwald und weitere Formen strukturierter und gemischter Wälder. [The selection forest and other types of structured and mixed species forests.] Parey Buchverlag, Berlin, 207 p

Spiecker H, Hansen J, Klimo E, Skovsgaard JP, Sterba H, Teuffel Kv (2004) Norway spruce conversion—options, and consequences. European forest institute research report, vol 18. Koninklijke Brill NV, Leiden, 269 p

Stevens DL, Olsen AR (2004) Spatially balanced sampling of natural resources. J Am Stat Assoc 99:262–278

Stillman RA, Railsback SF, Giske J, Berger U, Grimm V (2015) Making predictions in a changing world: the benefits of individual-based ecology. BioScience 65:140–150

Torquato S (2002) Random heterogeneous materials. Microstructure and macroscopic properties. Springer, New York, 701 p

van Laar A, Akça A (2007) Forest mensuration. Managing forest ecosystems, vol 13. Springer, Dordrecht, 383 p

Wenk G, Antanaitis V, Šmelko, Š (1990) Waldertragslehre. [Forest growth and yield science.] Deutscher Landwirtschaftsverlag, Berlin, 448 p

Wiegand T (1998) Die räumliche Populationsdynamik von Braunbären. [The temporal and spatial population dynamics of brown bears.] Munich, 202 p

Wolfram S (2002) A new kind of science. Wolfram Media Inc., Champaign, 1197 p

Zhao X, Corral-Rivas J, Temesgen H, Gadow Kv (2014) Forest observational studies—an essential infrastructure for sustainable use of natural resources. For Ecosyst 1:8

Chapter 2
Theories and Concepts
in Individual-Based Forest Ecology

Abstract Ecology is a comparatively young field of natural sciences. It has gained considerable influence and popularity over the last five to six decades. In ecology, interactions between individuals and environmental factors but also among the individuals of a population play an important role. The understanding of forest ecology is important in itself and prepares the ground for sustainable forest management. A number of conceptual theories have been developed in ecology to explain observed phenomena such as the natural maintenance of species diversity in tropical forest ecosystems. These form the background to individual-based ecology and the quantitative methods described in this book are often used to test them or to develop new ones. Finally tree mechanics offer different insights on interaction processes and tree growth.

2.1 Forest Ecology

Ecology is the science that studies ecosystems and their components, processes and changes over time, i.e. the abundance, dynamics and dispersion of organisms and their interactions with their biotic and abiotic environment. In more general terms, Begon et al. (2006) defined ecology as the scientific study of the distribution and abundance of organisms and the interactions that determine distribution and abundance. An ecosystem or ecological system is composed of living organisms and their abiotic environment. More specifically Judson (1994) defined ecology as a branch of science concerned with the interrelationship of organisms and their environments. The spatial dispersion of ecosystem components and their interactions lead to the capture and storage of energy as biomass and a circulation of nutrients. Ecosystems are typically characterised by their structure, function, complexity, interaction of components and change over time (Kimmins 2004). Forest ecology also includes humans as we will see in Chaps. 3 and 7 (Perry et al. 2008). In this book, apart from individual-based ecology (see Sect. 1.1) we mostly address *population* and *community* ecology. The former is defined as the study of dynamics, structure and distribution of populations, whilst the latter is concerned with interactions among individuals and populations of different species. A population in this context is a group of individuals of the same species living close enough together that they experience the same environmental conditions and interact with one another in some significant fashion (Perry et al. 2008).

Interactions between plants are central to plant community ecology and is one of the fundamental ecological forces that shape dynamics in space and time at all organisation levels (Armas et al. 2004; Seifan and Seifan 2015). Competition, as one possible type of interactions, is among the oldest notions in biology and ecology. The term can be traced back to Darwin's "struggle for existence" (Darwin 1859) and has received many different definitions over the years, some of them leading more to confusion than clarification (Grime 1977). For plants, the central part of this struggle is to find, harvest, transport and retain possession of resources (Keddy 2017). Perry et al. (2008) noted that mathematical models and—in more general terms—any attempt to quantify competition have much influenced the traditional thinking of ecologists about this concept to an extent that one might think this is a human concept imposed on nature (Keddy 1989). This relates to the fact that the physiological implications of competition processes only recently have started to be better understood including stress signal perceptions and genetic and metabolic responses (Atkinson and Urwin 2012; Pierik et al. 2013). However, what ecologists typically observe are actually the effects of competition, i.e. a *reduction in the life performance of plants due to stress, where stress is related to sharing limited resources at close proximity* (Begon et al. 2006). Burton (1993) described competition as an interference from a localised subset of other plants whilst Keddy (2017) generalised *reduction in performance* to *negative effects* that one organism has upon another. Indeed, competition and other forms of interaction are typically inferred from observed negative or positive effects of neighbouring plants without knowing in detail what resources the plants were sharing (Damgaard 2011). This lack of more direct evidence has therefore given rise to conceptual theories and much speculation.

Grime (1977) pointed out that we can always expect interaction effects, wherever plants grow in close proximity, whether they are of the same or of different species. Perry et al. (2008, p. 246) referred to this as "struggle for space". Not all of these effects, however, can be attributed to competition or even to plant interaction. It is also indicative that competition is often defined in terms of its effects rather than its mechanisms (Grime 1977), since we are still not always clear about them.

Bertness and Callaway (1994) and Keddy (2017) maintained that ecologists for a long time were preoccupied and fascinated with negative interactions between individuals whilst positive ones received little attention and were largely ignored in models. This understanding of interactions has gradually given way to a new mindset where competition is only one possible type of interaction. Cooperation is part of the struggle for survival (Keddy 2017). More specifically one could describe species and plant interactions as including negative (competition), neutral (tolerant) and positive (facilitation) relationships on a continuous scale (Díaz-Sierra et al. 2017). Plant facilitation emerges as the moderation of biotic and abiotic stress, enrichment of resources or the increased access to resources. Facilitation leads to an increase in the survivorship, growth and/or reproduction of at least one of the interacting individuals and can occur simultaneously with competition. Particularly in harsh physical envi-

Table 2.1 Types of plant interactions. The + symbol means that the respective plant benefits, the − symbol indicates inhibition and 0 stands for no effect. Modified from Perry et al. (2008)

Type of interaction	Plant 1	Plant 2
Predation	+	−
Parasitism	+	−
Competition	−	−
Amensalism	−	0
Mutualism	+	+
Commensalism	+	0
Neutralism	0	0

ronments, positive interactions during succession and recruitment as well as among established adults are very common. Perry et al. (2008, p. 220) further detailed interactions by suggesting a continuum that includes *predation, parasitism, competition, amensalism, mutualism, commensalism* and *neutralism* (tolerance), where the concept of a superorganism is an extreme form of mutualism (Oliver and Larson 1996), see Table 2.1. Facilitation in this context includes mutualism and commensalism. Symbiosis, for example, can be either mutualistic or parasitic (Perry et al. 2008).

For example shade-tolerant understorey trees are sheltered from climatic extremes by a cover of mature light-demanding trees whilst the light levels underneath the big trees are sufficient for the shade-tolerant species. In a similar way in interior Douglas fir (*Pseudotsuga menziesii* var *glauca* (Mirb.) Franco) stands in British Columbia (Canada), small regeneration trees preferably occur in the vicinity of large trees for protection from drought (LeMay et al. 2009).

The story of plant interactions is even more complex, considering that environmental changes can cause stress factors to change. The type, strength and importance of interaction depend on space and time, and as a consequence negative interactions can become positive and vice versa (as described by the stress-gradient hypothesis, SGH), i.e. plant interactions are context dependent.

2.1.1 Basic Terms and Definitions Related to Individual-Based Ecology

Very basic and traditional definitions include the terms *intra-* and *interspecific* competition, which sometimes are also referred to as *con-* and *heterospecific* competition, see, for example, Vogt et al. (2014). Intra- or conspecific competition describes a shared demand for limited resources within the same species population whereas inter- or heterospecific competition refers to this process between two different species (Kimmins 2004; Begon et al. 2006). Tilman (1982) coined the term resource-competition theory in this context. Competition typically leads to decreased performance (in terms of survivorship, growth and reproduction) and this leads to decreased fitness (i.e. number of offspring that survive to reproductive age). Because they share the same niche, others of the same species are generally the strongest potential competitors with a given individual (Perry et al. 2008). More generally speaking the *competition-trait similarity hypothesis* predicts that competitive interactions between species increase with decreasing niche distance (Kunstler et al. 2012).

The *niche theory* (Hutchinson 1957) has been referred to as the centre of gravity of community ecology (Turnbull et al. 2016) and is related to the *competition-trait similarity hypothesis*: A species' niche is essentially defined as its ecological role given a set of necessary conditions, resources and interactions. For example, a tree species' niche might be defined partly by ranges of temperature, resource availability (e.g. light, moisture), frequency and severity of disturbance, and minimal number of growing season days it can tolerate, as well as the types of interactions it can abide. The niche of a species in the absence of competition from other species is its *fundamental* niche, defined by the combination of conditions and resources that allow the species to maintain a viable population. In the presence of competitors and thus density-dependent feedback, however, the species may be restricted to a *realised* niche. This is the niche actually occupied by a species (Begon et al. 2006; Perry et al. 2008). If two competing species coexist in a stable environment, they do so as a result of *niche differentiation*, i.e. differentiation of their realised niches. If, however, the realised niche of a superior competitor completely fills the inferior competitor's fundamental niche, exclusion occurs. This principle is termed *competitive exclusion principle* or *Gause's principle* (Gause 1934; Connell 1961; Begon et al. 2006). On the other hand two or more species whose niches substantially overlap may evolve by natural selection to have more distinct niches (i.e. use different resources, occupy a different area of habitat, or grow during a different season, Pommerening and Sánchez Meador 2018) leading to *resource partitioning* (MacArthur 1965; Schoener 1974). As a consequence competing species try to diverge to achieve less niche overlap and to avoid potential extinction. In this context *niche complementarity* is defined as the tendency for coexisting species which occupy a similar position along one niche dimension to differ along another. Niche theory predicts that the loss of species is expected to reduce ecosystem functioning regardless of their specific traits (Turnbull et al. 2016) and also that the strength of interspecific interactions declines as the number of coexisting species increases. The relative strength of interspecific interactions is proportional to $1/(s-1)$ for s species (Chesson 2000; Rajala et al. 2018).

Intraspecific competition was and still often is expressed in terms of *density*, i.e. number of individuals divided by land area (as a proxy for the amount of resource). The importance of density lies in the fact that increased density reduces resource availability while increasing stress predisposes to mortality agents such as insects and disease. However, density of the population as a whole is a crude measure of competition, since the effect on an individual is rather determined by local density and particularly by the extent to which it is *crowded* or inhibited by its immediate neighbours (Begon et al. 2006).

Another important definition relates to the question of how individuals share resources. *Symmetric* competition is regarded as an equal sharing of resources amongst individuals, whilst *asymmetric* competition describes an unequal sharing, where large plants have a *disproportionate* advantage (for their relative size) in competition with smaller plants (Weiner et al. 2001) leading to pre-emption effects. As a consequence of the latter process, larger individuals have a competitive advantage over smaller ones. The word "disproportionate" plays a key role here and Weiner (1990) defined it in such a way: For competition to be asymmetric, an individual that is twice as large as another must have more than twice the competitive effect or obtain more than twice the amount of resources as its smaller neighbour. Selecting a suitable and meaningful size variable is obviously crucial in this context, as defining competitive effects in terms of different size variables of the same plant can potentially lead to different results. Asymmetric competition may arise, for example, as a consequence of variation in emergence times within a population (Freckleton and Watkinson 2001) and leads to competitive dominance or suppression of some individuals over others (Keddy 2017). The terms symmetric and asymmetric competition are collectively referred to by the "*mode of competition*". Lin et al. (2013) concluded from the literature that above-ground competition tends to be size-asymmetric, while below-ground competition is more size-symmetric, see also the discussion in Weiner (1990) and in Weiner et al. (1997). Symmetric competition is argued to produce coexistence whilst asymmetric competition leads to competitive exclusion, where the weaker species or individuals manage to disperse into gaps not yet occupied by the dominant. In the extreme case of asymmetric competition, the subordinate species or individuals are driven to evolve away from the niche of the dominant (Keddy 1989, 2017). More subtle variants of these terms including "perfect/complete/partial a/symmetry" are summarised in Fernández-Tschieder and Binkley (2018).

A related, older definition is that of *one-* and *two-sided* competition (Freckleton and Watkinson 2001; Begon et al. 2006). In a context of two species, the former implies that one species is completely dominant over another. One-sided competition can therefore be regarded as an extreme form of asymmetric competition. Competition for light is often one-sided, because light comes directionally from above so that taller plants can shade shorter ones but not *vice versa* (Kikuzawa and Umeki 1996; Falster and Westoby 2003). Weiner (1990), however, has used one-sided competition as a synonym of asymmetric competition and equates two-sided competition with symmetric competition.

Lin et al. (2012) and Keddy (2017) have argued that the concept of "mode" universally applies to plant interactions regardless of position along the continuum or point in time it is observed. Accordingly there is not only a mode of competition but also a mode of facilitation. Moreover, different modes of competition and facilitation can act simultaneously. When for example facilitation among plants is asymmetric, smaller plants receive disproportionally more benefits from larger plants. With symmetric facilitation, by contrast, all individuals receive the same benefit from one another irrespective of their sizes. The authors suggested a continuous approach to facilitative interactions ranging from completely symmetric facilitation (interacting plants receive the same amount of benefit from each other, irrespective of species and size) to completely asymmetric interaction (the beneficiary plant receives all benefits but there are no positive effects on the benefactor). As a result, mutualistic cases are expected to be at the symmetric end of the facilitation continuum and commensal cases at the asymmetric end. The authors reported model simulations involving both modes of facilitation and they have shown that both lead to increasing size inequality, however, it may be reduced as a consequence of asymmetric facilitation.

2.1.2   Theories Related to Individual-Based Ecology

A number of ecological theories have been developed that either attempt to explain or involve plant interactions.

2.1.2.1   Size-Density Relationships and Self-thinning

Size-density relationships in forest and other ecosystems are among the earliest discoveries in monospecies plantations and have played a significant role in agriculture and forestry (Keddy 2017). When individual plants grow in size, their requirements increase, they therefore compete with increasing intensity. Competition is believed to be the response to density-induced shortages (Harper 1961). This also increases the risk of dying and when some individuals eventually die, then density and intensity of competition temporarily decrease. All these processes affect growth, which in turn affects competition and survival, which again affects density etc. (Begon et al. 2006, p. 156). To summarise these effects it is possible to depict density (in terms of the number of trees per hectare) over mean plant size or weight in a graph resulting in a (negative) exponential relationship, representing the carrying capacity of a given site for a particular population with model parameters, which do not vary much for quite different plant communities. In forest science, it was Reineke (1933), who detected this relationship first, whilst in ecology the first description of this phenomenon is attributed to Yoda et al. (1963), who generalised the relationship. In ecological work, density is usually depicted on the abscissa and both variables are set in a graph with log-log scales and thus the curves are transformed to linear lines. These linear relationships, commonly represented mathematically by lines, are also referred to as self-thinning lines and the phenomenon has been called *self-thinning rule, thinning law* and *negative $^3/_2$ power law*. Another quasi-synonym and closely related term is *competition-density rule* (Sterba 1987; Shinozaki and Kira 1956; Vospernik and Sterba 2015). As populations near the thinning line, they suffer increasing amounts of competition and eventually of mortality (Begon et al. 2006). For each species independent of environmental factors a boundary line can be determined beyond which combinations of density and size or mean weight are not possible for that species. The described processes lead to size or dominance hierarchy, where some individuals for one reason or another exert dominance and others fall behind.

Fig. 2.1 The limiting relationship for Sitka spruce (yield classes 12, initial spacings from top to bottom 0.9 × 0.9 m, 1.7 × 1.7 m, 2.2 × 2.2 m, 2.6 × 2.6 m) in Britain using the Reineke (1933) approach. Derived by the authors from data of unthinned monitoring plots used to establish the British yield table system (Hamilton and Christie 1973)

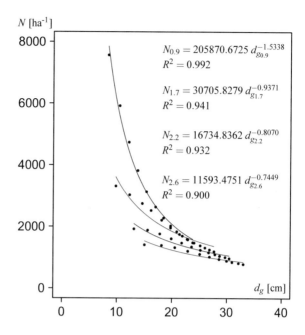

$N_{0.9} = 205870.6725 \, d_{g0.9}^{-1.5338}$
$R^2 = 0.992$

$N_{1.7} = 30705.8279 \, d_{g1.7}^{-0.9371}$
$R^2 = 0.941$

$N_{2.2} = 16734.8362 \, d_{g2.2}^{-0.8070}$
$R^2 = 0.932$

$N_{2.6} = 11593.4751 \, d_{g2.6}^{-0.7449}$
$R^2 = 0.900$

Figure 2.1 illustrates the limiting relationship using the Reineke (1933) approach for unthinned data relating to yield class 12 of Sitka spruce (*Picea sitchensis* (BONG.) CARR.) in Britain. Parameters a and b of Reineke's model can be identified by non-linear regression and the corresponding R code is given below.

```
> nls.R <- nls(N ~ a * dg^-b, data = myData, start =
+ list(a = 75568, b = -1.2689), trace = T)
> summary(nls.R)
```

Reineke (1933) defined *SDI* as the number of trees per unit area which a given forest stand with a quadratic mean diameter of 25 cm would have, i.e.

$$SDI = N \cdot \left(\frac{25}{d_g}\right)^b. \tag{2.1}$$

SDI can be implemented in R as

```
> myData$sdi <- myData$MTREE * (25 / myData$Dg)^-1.605
```

where `myData$MTREE` (N) and `myData$Dg` (d_g) can represent observed trees per hectare and quadratic mean diameter, respectively or equivalent values from forestry yield tables.

Equation (2.1) implies that the ratio of observed number of trees to maximum number of trees in relation to the observed d_g is the same as the ratio of *SDI* to maximum trees per hectare in relation to a d_g of 25 cm (originally 10 in. corresponding to

Table 2.2 Range of *SDI* values (Reineke 1933) for seven tree species calculated from Austrian yield tables (Sterba 2010). NS—Norway spruce (*Picea abies* (L.) KARST.), ESF—European silver fir (*Abies alba* MILL.), EL—European larch (*Larix decidua* MILL.), SP—Scots pine (*Pinus sylvestris* L.), DF—Douglas fir (*Pseudotsuga menziesii* (MIRB.) FRANCO), BE—European beech *Fagus sylvatica* L., OK—oak species (*Quercus spp.*)

	Species	NS	ESF	EL	SP	DF	BE	OK
SDI	min	900	800	500	600	700	650	500
	max	1100	1000	600	750	900	750	600

25.4 cm). Reineke (1933) found in unmanaged pure Douglas fir stands in Washington and Oregon as well as in other tree species and regions that $b = -1.605$ and does not vary much. Sterba (1985) could confirm this value also for European tree species including Norway spruce and beech. However, Gadow (1986), Pretzsch and Biber (2005) and Zeide (2005) have come to different conclusions. Thus if b cannot be estimated from local data, $b = -1.605$ can be assumed with the necessary caution. For a given species *SDI* varies little with age and yield class in contrast to stocking degrees, which makes *SDI* a more effective descriptor of stand density.

Sterba (2010) compiled a table of *SDI* values for seven different tree species (Table 2.2). A forest stand with $d_g = 50$ cm and 200 trees per hectare has according to Eq. (2.1) with $b = -1.605$ an *SDI* of 608. Assuming beech (*Fagus sylvatica* L.) this would qualify for a dense stand whilst considering Norway spruce (*Picea abies* (L.) KARST.) density would be low.

Nilson (1973, 2006) suggested a different approach for describing the limiting or self-thinning relationship which he termed *stand sparsity*. His concept is based on a measure, L, of distances between trees assuming regular tree dispersion as an approximation or a potential (Zeide 2010):

$$L = \sqrt{\frac{10000}{N}} = \frac{100}{\sqrt{N}} \tag{2.2}$$

Equation (2.2) can, of course, be replaced by other, more suitable estimators of mean distance between trees or by field measurements. Further assuming a linear relationship between the quadratic mean diameter, d_g, and L, Nilson (1973) expressed the actual *sparsity equation* as

$$L = a + b \cdot d_g. \tag{2.3}$$

Parameter a depends on environmental factors and b is species dependent. Both parameters can be found through simple linear regression. As a consequence of Eqs. (2.2) and (2.3), trees per hectare, N, can be calculated from

$$N = \left(\frac{100}{a + b \cdot d_g}\right)^2. \tag{2.4}$$

A possible implementation of Nilson's approach in R is provided in the following lines.

```
1  > myData$L <- 100 / sqrt(myData$N)
2  > lm.L <- lm(myData$L ~ myData$dg)
3  > summary(lm.L)
4  > par(mar = c(2, 3, 1, 1))
5  > plot(myData$dg, myData$L, las = 1, ylab = "", xlab = "",
6  + cex = .9, col = "black", pch = 16, axes = FALSE)
7  > lines(myData$dg, fitted(lm.L), col = "black")
8  > axis(1, lwd = 2, cex.axis = 1.8)
9  > axis(2, las = 1, lwd = 2, cex.axis = 1.8)
10 > box(lwd = 2)
11 > par(mar = c(2, 4.5, 1, 1))
12 > plot(myData$dg, myData$N, las = 1, ylab = "", xlab = "",
13 + cex = .9, col = "black", pch = 16, axes = FALSE)
14 > curve((100/(summary(lm.L)$coefficients[1] +
15 + summary(lm.L)$coefficients[2] * x))^2, from =
16 + min(myData$dg), to = max(myData$dg), xlab = "", lwd = 1,
17 + lty = 1, col = "black", add = TRUE)
18 > axis(1, lwd = 2, cex.axis = 1.8)
19 > axis(2, las = 1, lwd = 2, cex.axis = 1.8)
20 > box(lwd = 2)
```

In line 1, the measure L is computed as in Eq. (2.2). A linear regression following Eq. (2.3) is carried out in line 2. The results are visualised in a graph coded in lines 5–10 and shown in Fig. 2.2 (left). This is followed by the code for the right-hand graph in Fig. 2.2. In lines 14–17, the curve() command uses Eq. (2.4).

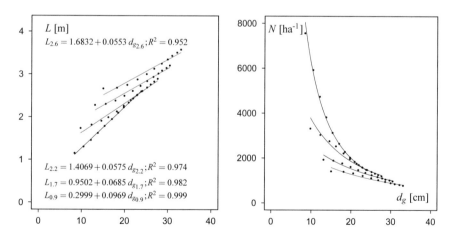

Fig. 2.2 The limiting relationship for Sitka spruce (*Picea sitchensis* (BONG.) CARR., yield classes 12 with initial spacings 0.9 × 0.9 m, 1.7 × 1.7 m, 2.2 × 2.2 m, 2.6 × 2.6 m) in Britain using the Nilson (1973, 2006) approach. Derived by the authors from data of unthinned monitoring plots used to establish the British yield table system (Hamilton and Christie 1973)

With data obtained from field experiments it is necessary to apply quantile regression (Cade and Noon 2003) to find the limiting relationships as defined by Nilson (1973) and Reineke (1933), see Sect. 5.2.5.

Zeide (2010) showed that Eq. (2.5) is Nilson's equivalent to Reineke's *SDI* Eq. (2.1):

$$SDI^* = N \left(\frac{d_g + b}{25 + b} \right)^2, \tag{2.5}$$

where b is the parameter in Eq. (2.3). Zeide (2010) concluded that Nilson's approach performs better than Reineke's.

The self-thinning rule has been widely used by forest managers as a guide to when and how much to thin forest stands by developing so-called stand-density management diagrams (Perry et al. 2008; Oliver and Larson 1996). The relationship between stand density and average tree size is also important for woodland managers who wish to optimise thinning regimes. A large basal area level is desirable for pulpwood and wood fuel stands while stands where sawtimber production is the prime objective large stem diameters are more important. Variations of this relationship have frequently been used in the past to produce silvicultural guide curves. A number of other density and stocking measures such as the *stand density index* (*SDI*) and *relative spacing* (Eq. 3.1) have been derived from this relationship (Gadow and Bredenkamp 1992; van Laar and Akça 2007).

Recent research has demonstrated that the self-thinning rule much depends on the crown geometry of trees but also on their physiology (Pretzsch and Biber 2005; Pretzsch 2006). Pretzsch and Biber (2016) also found that due to a better supply and more efficient use of resources, maximum stand density can be larger in mixed species forests compared to pure stands with similar site conditions and development stage. A related theory is the *law of constant final yield* (Shinozaki and Kira 1956; Weiner and Freckleton 2010) describing a situation at a particular point in time where in a series from low to high densities, the relationship between total stand biomass per unit area and density is initially linear, but eventually levels off at a constant biomass that does not increase further. Yield can be anything from biomass to seeds. At very low densities there is no competition leading to a linear increase in biomass. At higher densities the rate of increase in yield decreases with density. Constant final yield is a robust pattern in ecology that is key to understanding population- and community-level phenomena (Weiner and Freckleton 2010). In the context of thinning experiments and stem volume growth in forestry, Langsæter (1941) described a quite similar relationship referred to as *Langsæter's plateau* (Skovsgaard and Vanclay 2008). This was later refined by Assmann and he defined an optimum basal area concept for maximising stand volume growth (Assmann 1970), see Skovsgaard and Vanclay (2008) for a more detailed discussion.

Lastly, Shaw and Long (2007) reported evidence for a "fall-off" or asymptote in maximum stand density suggesting the assumption of linearity over the entire range of a size-density relationship is questionable. They went on to provide a more precise characterisation, stating that density-dependent mortality (self-thinning) may only influence stand conditions during a certain period of stand development, and that furthermore there may exist a transition point where other factors exert an increased influence on relative density. Shaw and Long (2007) presented this hypothesis as the *mature stand boundary* hypothesis where the resulting mortality rate of large trees is thought to be a result of the stand exceeding its capacity to capture the available growing space (Pommerening and Sánchez Meador 2018).

2.1.2.2 Stability and Resilience

A concept often referred to in forest ecology and management is that of *stability* and *resilience*. This prominence is probably also the reason for an apparent lack in the literature of agreement on what this concept includes and how it can be best defined. The nature of the terms involved is complex and has been used in contradictory ways (Kimmins 2004; Perry et al. 2008). Kimmins (2004, p. 507) suggested:

> The concept of stability and resilience usually refers to the tendency of a system to remain in its present condition or to return to that condition after a disturbance.

More specifically resilience describes the speed with which a community returns to its former state after a disturbance (Begon et al. 2006) whilst the overarching term stability is perceived as the ability of a forest to resist permanent change (Thomas and Packham 2007). A number of connotations have confused the understanding and definition of these two terms. These connotations, for example, include constancy, persistence, resistance, inertia, robustness and elasticity. Particularly important here is the term elasticity denoting the ability of a forest ecosystem to react to the consequences of disturbances in such a way that the original or another balanced system is restored (Otto 1994; Röhrig et al. 2006). Resilience and elasticity are sometimes referred to as synonyms (Kimmins 2004; Thomas and Packham 2007). Resistance mechanisms may be thought of as those properties of the system and of individuals that prevent them from succumbing to some stress so that an attack does not grow into a large disturbance. As such resistance is a process by which a community avoids displacement from a former state (Begon et al. 2006). Robustness on the other hand is the amount of perturbation that a system can tolerate before switching to another state (Perry et al. 2008).

Instability typically occurs when the system crosses some threshold from which recovery to a former state is either impossible or occurs only over relatively long time periods or with external subsidies of energy and matter (Perry et al. 2008).

Stability and resilience are associated with thresholds and exceeding them can sometimes have dramatic changes as a consequence. For example, gradual changes in temperature or other factors might have little effect until a threshold is reached at which a large shift occurs that might be difficult to reverse. Even a tiny incremental change in conditions can then trigger a large shift in some systems. Such particular thresholds are often referred to as *tipping points* (Gladwell 2000; Scheffer and Carpenter 2003; Perry et al. 2008). One such tipping point is, for example, the melting of permafrost and release of the huge stores of methane (a strong greenhouse gas) that are stored beneath the ice.

Biodiversity and tree diversity also contribute to ecosystem stability and resilience (Perry et al. 2008) and some mechanisms are explained in Sect. 2.1.2.4.

For a long time, the notion of stability was deemed essential to proper functioning of forest ecosystems. External factors that disturbed or modified this stability were often perceived negatively. For example, forest practitioners have spent tremendous efforts to eliminate disturbances such as fire and insect or pathogen outbreaks. Recent advances in ecological understanding pointed out that many disturbances such as forest fires are a crucial component of ecosystems and even may be critical for ecosystem development (Messier et al. 2013). In forest practice, stability was often understood as a resistance against biotic and abiotic influences. Forest stands were referred to as stable, if they met the production objectives without substantial losses as a result of such influences (Burschel and Huss 1997). As part of this, a distinction was made between *collective stand stability* and *individual-tree stability*. Both stability types determine the total stability of a forest stand and can be modified by thinnings and species selection. Thinning operations temporarily weaken collective stand stability, see also Sect. 2.2. However, if they occur at regular cycles, the residual trees build up individual-tree stability through gradual adaptation that helps them to withstand increased wind loads. *Adaptability* is a key attribute of ecological systems and denotes the process of an ecosystem adjusting its structure or configuration, composition, interactions or feedbacks in response to external factors (Messier et al. 2013). Good forest management practice usually attempts to balance individual-tree and collective stand stability. Individual-tree stability is particularly important in continuous cover forestry (Sect. 3.4).

2.1.2.3 Stress-Gradient Hypothesis

Naturally ecological relationships are not constant in space and time. Considering this the *stress-gradient hypothesis* (SGH; Bertness and Callaway 1994) proposes that competition and facilitation may act simultaneously and predicts that the importance of negative competitive effects is higher under benign environmental conditions, whereas positive facilitative effects increase in importance as environmental stress (either biotic or abiotic) increases (Daleo and Iribarne 2009). Later refinements of this general concept taking species differences and interactions into account were suggested by Maestre et al. (2009). The term "plant stress" is often used in a very broad sense and refers to a wide range of biological and environmental stresses that plants are subjected to including drought, weather extremes, plant competitors, herbivores and a host of diseases (Lichtenthaler 1996, 1998). SGH is valid both at intra- and interspecific level (Lin et al. 2012). Lichtenthaler (1996) harmonised stress definitions in physics and botany: According to him stress is the state of a plant under the condition of a force applied, strain is the plant's response to the stress and the resulting force applied to the plant, i.e. the expression of stress before damage occurs with damage being the result of too high a stress for which compensation can no longer be applied. Different phases of abiotic and biotic stress have been defined including a concept for adapting to stress (Lichtenthaler 1998), which shares similarities with the ecological concept of resistance and resilience (Begon et al. 2006), see the previous section. Various genetic and metabolic response patterns have recently been identified so that it is possible to measure stress not only in terms of plant performance but in terms of regulatory mechanism responses (Atkinson and Urwin 2012). Part of the difficulty of testing this concept may also be that strong competition leads to biotic stress effects whilst facilitation can be viewed as a stress relief, i.e. competition and facilitation can contribute to the overall stress balance (see also Keddy 2017). Ettinger and HilleRis-Lambers (2017) referred to SGH as *competition-environmental gradient hypothesis* (Pommerening and Sánchez Meador 2018).

2.1.2.4 Diversity Related Hypotheses

Plant competition determines the diversity and species abundance of natural communities (Pierik et al. 2013). In the ecological literature, a number of hypotheses and theories have been suggested how species diversity and coexistence is maintained naturally. Prominent examples include the *Janzen-Connell*, the *herd-immunity* and *the mingling-size hypotheses*. They describe local effects of species and size structure that usually do not extend beyond 8–10 m in temperate and boreal forests.

The *Janzen-Connell hypothesis* (Janzen 1970; Connell 1971) proposes that elevated numbers of specialist natural competitors, such as herbivores and pathogens, maintain diversity in plant communities (Fig. 2.3). They reduce the survival rates of conspecific seeds and seedlings located close to reproductive adults or in areas of high conspecific density (Comita et al. 2014) leading to elevated conspecific self-thinning (Yao et al. 2016), i.e. a progressive decline in density in a population of growing individuals of the same species (Begon et al. 2006, p. 157). An important effect of the Janzen-Connell is the negative density/distance dependence that occurs when nearby conspecific plants negatively affect performance through mechanisms such as allelopathy, intraspecific competition and pest facilitation (Wills et al. 1997; Wright 2002; Piao et al. 2013; Yao et al. 2016).

Another important ecological hypothesis in this context, the *herd immunity hypothesis*, focuses on the variation in heterospecific neighbour densities and predicts that species diversity confers protection from natural enemies by making it more difficult for specialist natural enemies to locate host plants (Wills et al. 1997). Thus the spatial spread of an infection can be slowed down or even stopped by mixtures of susceptible and resistant species (Begon et al. 2006). Therefore individual plant

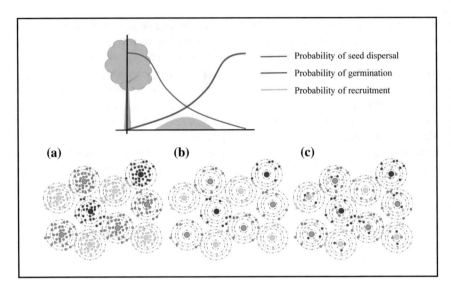

Fig. 2.3 The Janzen-Connell hypothesis suggesting that (**a**) conspecific offspring is prone to (**b**) density-dependent mortality allowing (**c**) heterospecific plants to colonise spaces near large parent trees. Different shades of green in **a–c** imply different species and the radii of the circular tree locations in these panels relate to tree size

fitness should be enhanced in stands with increased species diversity but reduced in stands with low species diversity (Wills et al. 1997; Murphy et al. 2016).

In addition, Ford (1975) and more recently Suzuki et al. (2008) demonstrated how the Janzen-Connell and the herd immunity hypotheses can affect natural populations. One observation in many natural plant populations is that self-thinning leads to *local size hierarchies* (also referred to as *size inequality*; Weiner and Solbrig 1984), where heterospecific stands include dominant plants emerging from a first colonisation cohort, which are often surrounded by patches of smaller sized plants of the same cohort. Small plants of these early colonisers are initially often of the same species as the dominant plants and according to the mechanisms of both the Janzen-Connell and herd immunity hypotheses later decrease in numbers due to self-thinning processes. Eventually the small early colonisers are partially or completely replaced by even smaller individuals of other species from subsequent colonisation cohorts. This combined effect of species and size replacement enforces both local size hierarchies and the mingling of different plant species in a given area or patch and prevents the development of monocultures. Putting the key elements of the aforementioned ecological hypotheses together, Pommerening and Uria-Diez (2017) have concluded that—as a consequence of them—there may be a tendency for plants with high species mingling (see Sect. 4.4.7.1), i.e. those with heterospecific nearest neighbours, to be larger sized plants and referred to this as the *mingling-size hypothesis*. The authors have completed an initial screening of the mingling-size hypothesis by using available forest-stand data from five climate zones. In the majority of the twelve investigated woodlands they found a confirmation of this hypothesis. However, there were also a few cases where the mingling-size hypothesis was not statistically supported. Using a different methodology Wang et al. (2018) confirmed the mingling-size hypothesis for mixed Korean pine (*Pinus koraiensis* SIEB. ET ZUCC.) broad-leaved natural forests in China.

In this context, another interesting effect is *overyielding* referring to an ecological process, in which different species in mixture through niche complementarity utilise a greater proportion of available resources than would a similar or average mono-culture, leading to larger productivity (de Wit 1960; Perry et al. 2008). The opposite is referred to as underyielding. A species mixture overyields when its production is greater than that of the average monoculture of the species contained in the mixture (Schmid et al. 2008). Finally transgressive overyielding appears when the produc-tion in mixture is larger than the single most productive species. Bulleri et al. (2016) argued that facilitation—whilst often considered a diversity-promoting interaction—under certain circumstances can reduce the forces that maintain diversity either by increasing performance differences among species or by removing opportunities for niche partitioning (decreasing the strength of complementarity). Overyielding can be interpreted as the complementarity effect of niche theory (see Sect. 2.1.1) and is positive when increases in the relative yields of some species are not exactly compen-sated by decreases in others (Chase and Leibold 2003; Turnbull et al. 2016). However, recent studies such as those by Finke and Snyder (2008) and Guderle et al. (2018) focussing on experimental manipulations of species richness, have revealed a pattern of greater resource exploitation when species diversity is increased (Pommerening and Sánchez Meador 2018). Diversity can also lead to overyielding when pests and diseases through Janzen-Connell effects have reduced incidence and severity with species grown in mixture (Turnbull et al. 2016). Bohn and Huth (2017) and Huang et al. (2018) found evidence that species diversity in some forest ecosytems can increase population productivity. Fichtner et al. (2018) demonstrated that positive effects of biodiversity on community productivity are largely driven by interactions among local neighbours, highlighting the need to promote tree species diversity at the scale of local neighbourhoods for enhancing productivity.

A more general hypothesis explaining stabilising effects of biodiversity is the *insurance hypothesis* suggesting that species that might be functionally redundant in the ecosystem increase in numbers in more favourable conditions to compensate for the reduction in performance of the dominant species thus providing "insurance" for community productivity. Biodiversity promotes greater insurance when commu-nities are made up of species that are better performers in different environments (i.e. specialists) (Yachi and Loreau 1999; Matias et al. 2013). Isbell et al. (2018) suggested methods for quantifying insurance and complementarity effects including overyielding.

2.2 Tree Mechanics and Interaction Effects on Stem Growth

Biomechanics studies functions and structures of biological systems. As part of this, tree mechanics focuses on the physical structure and functions of trees.

Metzger (1893) was the first to propose that trees develop a stem shape that is optimised to withstand vertical and horizontal mechanical loads. However, systematic studies of how plants respond to wind only started almost a century later (Berthier and Stokes, 2005).

The morphology of trees depends on environmental factors, genetics (including species and provenances) and on forest structure. Still the principles governing stem formation remain controversial despite a century of study (Dean et al. 2002).

During the cause of evolution trees have adopted the strategy of evading competition by raising their photosynthetically active biomass well above the canopy of most other vascular plants (Falster and Westoby 2003). This trait allowed them to evade competition but increasingly created problems for water conductance and environmental damage induced by wind and snow. This is a challenge to the mechanical design of trees, which is fundamental to its growth, reproductive performance and fitness (Read and Stokes 2006). Therefore trees constantly seek to adapt to changing environmental conditions and optimise their morphology to avoid windthrow and wind snap as well as similar damages from snow and ice. Particularly wind is the most constant environmental factor trees all over the world have to face. Mechanical constraints are therefore major determinants of size and shape of self-supporting plants (Spatz and Brüchert 2000). Stem taper, for example, clearly is a result of an adaptation to mechanical constraints. The more exposed a tree the larger its taper.

The commonly known effect that trees respond with increased stem diameter when their growing space is increased, e.g. as a result of removing tree neighbours, is often attributed to a decrease of competition. This is the ecological interpretation. The physical interpretation, however, is that a tree surrounded by neighbours at close proximity does not need to invest much in stem diameter as it is sheltered from the wind and supported by its neighbours. Such a tree relies on collective stand stability (see Sect. 2.1.2.2), i.e. the stability which is provided by the tree population of which it is part of. As long as no disturbance destroys some of the neighbouring trees this situation remains mechanically stable. However, if tree neighbours are removed as part of a thinning or of a disturbance, the remaining trees lose this collective support for some time to come and adapt by allocating more biomass to their stems (see also Sect. 2.1.2.2).

Several tree size ratios have been used to quantify the mechanical situation and its implication for growth performance. These ratios can be interpreted as form factors characterising geometric properties and relationships of a tree (Stoyan and Stoyan 1994). In a similar way they describe allometric relationships between different sizes of organs or parts of an organism, see Sect. 6.2.4. One example of such a ratio, the well-known *height-diameter ratio* or *slenderness* (h/d ratio, Eq. 2.6), is an important individual-tree indicator. This ratio is an allometric relationship derived from tree

Table 2.3 Interpreting height-diameter ratios (modified from Burschel and Huss 1997)

h/d value	>100	80–100	<80	<45
Individual-tree stability	Very unstable	Unstable	Stable	Open-grown tree

height and stem diameter. It is an expression of tree morphology as a result of growth conditions, namely site conditions, competition and management (Mitchell 2000). The more growing space a tree is granted, the longer its crown and the smaller its height diameter ratio. It plays an important role as a rough indicator variable of individual-tree stability in terms of wind and snow hazard particularly of trees with shallow root systems, e.g. spruce (*Picea spp.*) and birch (*Betula spp.*).

$$h/d = \frac{\text{Tree height}}{\text{dbh}} \tag{2.6}$$

The corresponding R code can be written as

```
> mydata$hd <- 100 * mydata$h / mydata$dbh
```

In this code, tree height is first converted from metre to centimetre by multiplying with 100. The height diameter ratio has no unit. Burschel and Huss (1997) suggested a simple system of interpreting individual-tree stability of coniferous trees (see Table 2.3).

The more slender trees are, the more they are prone to wind and snow damage. Open-grown trees (Hasenauer 1997; Smith et al. 1992), which have grown up in absence of interaction with other trees throughout their life, per definition have developed the highest possible degree of individual-tree stability. Forest-grown trees usually have much larger height-diameter ratios than open-grown trees. Following Pretzsch (2010) it can be useful in such a situation to combine two performance indicators, e.g. the ratio of height and stem-diameter relative growth rates (RGR, see Chap. 6), which yields the *allometric coefficient* (see Sect. 6.2.4), an indicator of resource allocation: Marked changes in allometric coefficient are usually caused by abrupt changes of environmental conditions. As a result h/d ratios for example often preserve the impact of past density patterns as a legacy effect: With increasing (local) density, h/d ratios increase and decrease with decreasing (local) density. As such slenderness is also a useful indicator of thinning urgency and hints at past management (Abetz and Klädtke 2002; Pretzsch 1996).

The h/d ratio is site dependent, i.e. on more fertile sites there tend to be larger h/d values than on less fertile sites. As an adaption to wind trees maintain a lower h/d ratio on exposed sites (Kramer 1988). Schmidt (2001) could show that branch diameters are correlated with slenderness and crown length. All other measures equal branch diameter increases with decreasing h/d ratio.

There is a natural (roughly linear) trend for the h/d ratio to decline with increasing diameter and increasing age (see Fig. 2.4, left) (Pommerening et al. 2018). Abetz

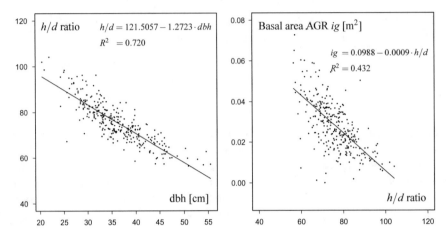

Fig. 2.4 h/d ratio over stem diameter, dbh, (left) and basal area absolute growth rate (AGR), ig, over h/d ratio in Sitka spruce (*Picea sitchensis* (BONG.) CARR.) plot 1 of the Clocaenog experiment at Cefn Du (North Wales)

(1976) found that trees with low h/d ratios respond to thinnings with larger basal area growth rates than trees with large h/d ratios. This trend is supported by Fig. 2.4 (right).

Managing light conditions is an important concern of forest management. The concept of continuous cover forestry (see Sect. 3.4) heavily relies on natural forest renewal. New cohorts of tree seedlings and saplings can only survive and eventually emerge into the main canopy, if the light conditions are adequate. For the assessment of sufficient light conditions light measurements are possible, however, there are also good correlations between more readily accessible population characteristics such as stand basal area (Hale 2003) and tree structure (Metslaid et al. 2007). A successful characteristic of the latter group is known as the *leader-to-lateral branch* or *apical dominance ratio* (*ADR*) describing an allometric relationship, see Sect. 6.2.4. There is positive correlation between this ratio and the amount of light received (Duchesneau et al. 2001; Grassi and Giannini 2005; Metslaid et al. 2007). Leader-to-lateral branch or apical dominance ratio can generally be defined as

$$ADR = \frac{\text{Length of terminal leader}}{\text{Length of lateral shoots}}. \tag{2.7}$$

Apical dominance in this context relates to the ability of the terminal shoot to have a growth advantage over lateral branches generally attributed to the plant hormone *auxin*. The length of lateral shoots in the denominator is measured at the last node before the terminal leader and can either be calculated as the maximum (Duchesneau et al. 2001) or the mean length (Grassi and Giannini 2005) of all healthy, undamaged shoots at that point. Trees with $ADR < 1$, i.e. the terminal leader is shorter than the lateral shoots, are light stressed. Trees with $ADR > 1$ have sufficient light for a

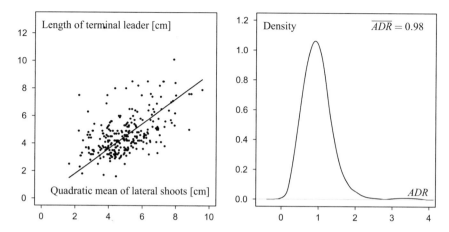

Fig. 2.5 Underplanting experiment of silver fir (*Abies alba* MILL.) under mature Sitka spruce (*Picea sitchensis* (BONG.) CARR.) at Cefn Du (compartment 5134H, block 5, Clocaenog Forest, North Wales) in autumn 2007. Left: Length of terminal leader over the quadratic mean of lateral shoots at the last node before the terminal leader. The trend line was calculated through linear regression using the model *Terminal leader* = 0.9037 · *Length of lateral shoots* (R^2 = 0.92). Right: Density distribution of the apical dominance ratio (Eq. 2.7)

successful development resulting in normal height growth and $ADR = 1$ marks the threshold or compensation point. To obtain a better idea of trends it is recommended to measure ADR several years in sequence (Grassi and Giannini 2005). Figure 2.5 gives an impression of the relationship between the length of terminal leaders and the mean of lateral shoots as well as of the distribution of ADR values in a population.

Silver fir seedlings were planted in spring 2007 at Cefn Du (compartment 5134H, block 5) of Clocaenog Forest as part of an underplanting experiment involving several species. The survey in the following autumn revealed a clear correlation between the length of the terminal leader and the mean of lateral branches at the last node. The comparatively large variation can possibly be attributed to the short time the plants had spent in situ and planting shock effects in that year. The arithmetic mean of ADR was close to 1 indicating slight light stress. Assuming only a small deviation from the normal distribution, 68% of the ADR values are between a ratio of 0.62 and 1.34. 34% of the seedlings appear to be light stressed, i.e. they had not yet adapted from the open nursery conditions to those of a closed spruce forest. Stand basal area at this stage was approximately $32 \, m^2$.

Figure 2.6 illustrates the physiological and mechanic functions of trees. Leaves are responsible for light and CO_2 assimilation and also resist wind. As part of this they also intercept precipitation and depending on various factors some of the intercepted water reaches the forest floor by stem flow. Deciduous trees shed their leaves in winter and thereby reduce the wind resistance of the crown. Branches and stems have important transport functions and on the other hand support the tree in its strategy to evade competition by other plants at forest floor level. Particularly tree

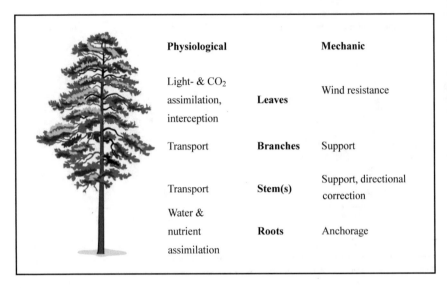

	Physiological		Mechanic
	Light- & CO_2 assimilation, interception	Leaves	Wind resistance
	Transport	Branches	Support
	Transport	Stem(s)	Support, directional correction
	Water & nutrient assimilation	Roots	Anchorage

Fig. 2.6 Physiological and mechanic tree functions (modified from Mattheck and Breloer 1994, p. 19)

stems have two primary functions, physical support and water conductance. Finally the roots fulfil the role of assimilating water and nutrients in a physiological sense. Mechanically the roots keep a tree fixed at the location of germination and provide a firm anchorage in the ground.

Mattheck and Breloer (1994) described the mechanics of a tree as a chain of equal strength and compared trees with ships: A tree crown acts like the sail of a ship collecting wind. The wind load is then passed on to the stem, which transfers all collected forces to the root plate. The root plate has a function similar to the hull of a ship, i.e. the forces are passed on to the soil except that in contrast to a ship a tree is not supposed to move. Therefore crown, stem and root plate have to be able to sustain wind loads more or less unharmed. A tree with a large crown thus also requires a sizable stem to cope with moderate to strong winds. Adaptation mechanisms include the shedding of leaves in winter (usually a time of increased wind and snow occurrence) and the reduction of the crown on exposed sites.

In individual-based tree models (see Sect. 5.2), a crucial element is to describe how the growth of tree stems depends on tree interactions. Based on the aforementioned concepts of plant interactions, competition has often been used to motivate reductions or increases in stem diameter growth. This is supported by empirical comparisons between open- and forest-grown trees. The former usually tend to have larger stem diameters and tapers compared to forest-grown trees on comparable sites and at the same development stage. In fact, open-grown trees represent the empirical maximum stem diameters (Hasenauer 1997). This is often motivated by the argument that forest-grown trees typically face competition from (or at least have interaction with) surrounding trees compared to open-grown trees. This rationale has given rise to a larger number of methods for quantifying tree competition, i.e. the so-called competition indices.

An alternative explanation is offered by the field of biomechanics: Wind, not direct tree interaction, is a major factor influencing the growth of tree stems, because they have to withstand vertical and horizontal mechanical loads and wind is the most persistent environmental factor causing such loads around the world (Metzger 1893; Brüchert and Gardiner 2006). Stem growth is therefore increasingly triggered whenever wind load increases, i.e. what often is interpreted as a relief or release effect (by a thinning operation) from biotic stress caused by competition, may in fact be interpreted as an effect of adding abiotic stress.

Wind load typically increases when local density around a given tree decreases, e.g. as a consequence of thinnings or disturbances. By contrast, when local tree density increases, wind load deceases as a given tree is increasingly sheltered by others. As a result stem growth is inhibited or altered. These processes of adaptive growth lead to an optimisation capable of withstanding mechanical loads. Despite the fact that neither the mechanoreceptor or -sensor nor the signal transduction chain has yet been identified in trees, mechanical constraints are major determinants of size and shape of self-supporting plants (Spatz and Brüchert 2000).

In this context it may be helpful to revise important allometric crown relationships and crown form factors in trees. Figure 2.7 illustrates the most important crown variables measured in field work. The *crown radius* is the distance between the stem centre and the outer edge of the crown. Tree crowns can be excentric, for this reason the crown radius is usually determined as quadratic mean of 4–8 radius measurements

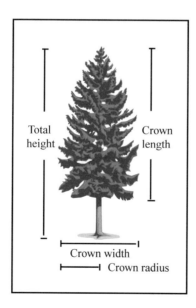

Fig. 2.7 Crown measures

Table 2.4 Crown indices and ratios (van Laar and Akça 2007; Philip 1994)

Eq. #	Name	Ratio	Other name	R code
(2.8)	Crown ratio	$\frac{\text{Crown length}}{\text{Tree height}}$	c/h ratio	> myData$cl / myData$h
(2.9)	Crown form index	$\frac{\text{Crown length}}{\text{Crown width}}$	–	> myData$cl / myData$cd
(2.10)	Linear crown index	$\frac{\text{Crown width}}{\text{dbh}}$	k/d ratio	> myData$cd / (myData$dbh / 100)
(2.11)	Crown spread ratio	$\frac{\text{Crown width}}{\text{Tree height}}$	–	> myData$cd / myData$h

in different directions. *Crown width* is crown radius multiplied by two. For *height to base of crown* there are various definitions in the literature (van Laar and Akça 2007; Pretzsch 2009). A sensible definition is "the first living branch (broadleaves), the first whorl with at least three living branches (conifers) from the base of the tree that is contiguous with the rest of the crown". *Crown length* or *crown depth* is the difference between total tree height and height to base of crown. Based on these crown measures a number of indices or ratios have been developed which play a certain role in individual-tree analysis and modelling (see Table 2.4, cl—crown length, cd—crown diameter = crown width).

The *crown ratio* is often used to assess individual-tree stability particularly of coniferous trees in a similar way as the h/d ratio, although the first more likely is an indicator for resistance to stem breakage while the latter indicates resistance to windthrow. An interpretation guide for the c/h ratio is given in Table 2.5.

Both c/h and h/d ratios are often used to assess thinning requirements in managed forests (Pretzsch 1996). The crown ratio is also related to photosynthesis and assimilation to answer the question how much of a tree's crown can be reduced in prunings or is naturally reduced in dense forests without major assimilation losses. This is why the crown ratio is often used as an indicator of vigour and vitality. A common silvicultural requirement is that frame trees (see Sect. 3.6.1) have a crown ratio of 50–66% (Röhrig et al. 2006). The *crown form index* is the ratio of the assimilating part of a crown to its demand on growing space. With a given growing space defined by the crown projection area a large crown form index is associated with a large assimilating crown surface and an efficient use of growing space. The *linear crown index* is a traditional and important crown measure. In Germany, it is also known as Seebach's growing space

Table 2.5 Interpreting crown ratios (modified from Schütz 2001)

c/h value	<0.30	0.30 < c/h < 0.50	>50	>0.62
Individual-tree stability	Very unstable	Unstable	Stable	Open-grown tree

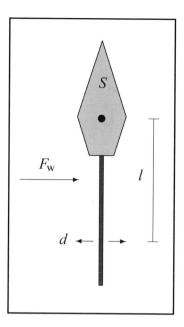

Fig. 2.8 Variables relating to the calculation of the potential bending moment (modified from Lundqvist and Elfving 2010)

measure. The squared reciprocal of this measure can be expressed and interpreted as a tree measure of basal area density, i.e. basal area/crown projection area with crown projection area = (crown width $/2)^2 \times \pi$. It is also common to use the square of the linear crown index. Spiecker (1994) found a linear relationship between linear crown index and absolute diameter growth rate (AGR) of individual wild cherry trees (*Prunus avium* (L.) L.). The *crown spread ratio* has often been used to describe growing space requirements of trees depending on stand height, because it does not change much in dominant trees of a given species with time. Based on these studies tree-number guide curves have been developed for practical use in forest management (see Fig. 3.12). With square spacing, $N = 10000/(\text{crown spread ratio}^2 \times \text{stand height}^2)$ and for other tree dispersion patterns this relationship can be adapted (Pretzsch 2009; Kramer 1988).

Dean et al. (2012) applied the *uniform-stress model* of stem formation to predict stem diameter at any height of the stem. The usefulness of the uniform-stress model for explaining interaction and growth processes was also confirmed by Lundqvist and Elfving (2010) among others. Based on the uniform-stress model and work by Dean and Long (1986) these authors derived a model that predicts stem diameter d at a given height on the stem as a simple power function of the bending moment M acting at that height (Eq. 2.8; Dean et al. 2002). Here ϕ and δ are model parameters and δ is theoretically known to be $1/3$. The bending moment M can be approximated by the product of crown size S, length l of the lever arm and wind load F_w. The lever arm is the distance between crown centre of gravity (marked by the black filled circle in Fig. 2.8) or centre of leaf area and the height where d is measured, e.g. 1.3 m (Fig. 2.8). The approximations turned out to be surprisingly accurate (Dean et al. 2002; Lundqvist and Elfving 2010). The relationship of Eq. 2.8 can be used for developing a growth model (Dean 2004).

Niklas and Spatz (2004), however, suggested that the proportional relationships of tree size are governed by hydraulic constraints rather than by mechanical stability.

$$d = \phi \cdot M^{\delta} \approx (S \cdot l \cdot F_w)^{\frac{1}{3}} \tag{2.8}$$

The biomechanical theory sheds a different light on the ecological interpretation of tree interactions and complements it. Stating that tree stem growth is completely driven by wind and other mechanical forces would certainly be an immense over-simplification, but biomechanics does indeed contribute to the complex story of tree interactions. Keddy (1989) based on Morowitz (1968) offers a thermodynamic interpretation of competition.

References

Abetz P (1976) Beiträge zum Baumwachstum: Der h/d-Wert – mehr als ein Schlankheitsgrad! [On tree growth – h/d ratio – more than a measure of slenderness]. Forst- und Holzwirt 31:389–393

Abetz P, Klädtke J (2002) The target tree management system. Forstwissenschaftliches Centralblatt 121:73–82

Armas C, Ordiales R, Pugnaire FI (2004) Measuring plant interactions: a new comparative index. Ecology 85:2682–2686

Assmann E (1970) The principles of forest yield study. Studies in the organic production, structure, increment and yield of forest stands. Pergamon Press, Oxford, 506 p

Atkinson NJ, Urwin PE (2012) The interaction of plant biotic an abiotic stresses: from genes to the field. J Exp Bot 63:3523–3544

Begon M, Harper JL, Townsend CR (2006) Ecology: individuals, populations and communities, 3rd edn. Blackwell Science, Oxford, 1092 p

Bertness MD, Callaway R (1994) Positive interactions in communities. Trends Ecol Evol 9:191–193

Bohn FJ, Huth A (2017) The importance of forest structure to biodiversity-productivity relationships. R Soc Open Sci 4:160521

Brüchert F, Gardiner B (2006) The effect of wind exposure on the tree aerial architecture and biomechanics of Sitka spruce (Picea sitchensis, Pinaceae). Am J Bot 93:1512–1521

Bulleri F, Bruno JF, Silliman BR, Stachowicz JJ (2016) Facilitation and the niche: implications for coexistence, range shifts and ecosystem functioning. Funct Ecol 30:70–78

Burschel P, Huss J (1997) Grundriss des Waldbaus [Outline of silviculture]. Parey Buchverlag, Berlin, 488 p

Burton PJ (1993) Some limitations inherent to static indices of plant competition. Can J For Res 23:2141–2152

Cade BS, Noon BR (2003) A gentle introduction to quantile regression for ecologists. Front Ecol Environ 8:412–420

Chase JM, Leibold MA (2003) Ecological niches: linking classical and contemporary approaches. University of Chicago Press, Chicago, 216 p

Chesson P (2000) Mechanisms of maintenance of species diversity. Annu Rev Ecol Evol Syst 31:343–366

Comita LS, Queenborough SA, Murphy SJ, Eck JL, Xu K, Krishnadas M, Beckman N, Zhu Y (2014) Testing predictions of the Janzen-Connell hypothesis: a meta-analysis of experimental evidence for distance- and density-dependent seed and seedling survival. J Ecol 102:845–856

Connell JH (1961) The influence of interspecific competition and other factors on the distribution of the barnacle Chthamalus stellat. Ecology 42:710–723

Connell JH (1971) On the role of natural enemies in preventing competitive exclusion in some marine animals and in rain forests. In: den Boer PJ, Gradwell GR (eds) Dynamics of populations. Centre for Agricultural Publishing and Documentation, Wageningen, the Netherlands, pp 298–312

Daleo P, Iribarne O (2009) Beyond competition: the stress-gradient hypothesis tested in plant-herbivore interactions. Ecology 90:2368–2374

Damgaard C (2011) Measuring competition in plant communities where it is difficult to distinguish individual plants. Comput Ecol Softw 1:125–137

Darwin C (1859) The origin of species by means of natural selection or the preservation of favoured races in the struggle for life. Murray, London, 576 p

de Wit CT (1960) On competition, vol 66. Verslagen van Landbouwkundige Onderzoekingen (Agricultural Research Reports), pp 1–82

Dean TJ (2004) Basal area increment and growth efficiency as functions of canopy dynamics and stem mechanics. For Sci 50:106–116

Dean TJ, Long JN (1986) Validity of constant-stress and elastic instability principles of stem formation in Pinus contorta and Trifolium pratense. Ann Bot 54:833–840

Dean TJ, Roberts SD, Gilmore DW, Maguire DA, Long JN, O'Hara KL, Seymore RS (2002) An evaluation of the uniform stress hypothesis based on stem geometry in selected North American conifers. Trees 16:559–568

Dean TJ, Jerez M, Cao QV (2012) A simple stand growth model based on canopy dynamics and biomechanics. For Sci 59:335–344

Díaz-Sierra R, Verwijmeren M, Rietkerk M, Resco de Dios V, Baudena M (2017) A new family of standardized and symmetric indices for measuring the intensity and importance of plant neighbour effects. Methods Ecol Evol 8:580–591

Duchesneau R, Lesage I, Messier C, Morin H (2001) Effects of light and intraspecific competition on growth and crown morphology of two size classes of understory balsam fir saplings. For Ecol Manag 140:215–225

Ettinger A, HilleRisLambers J (2017) Competition and facilitation may lead to asymmetric range shift dynamics with climate change. Glob Chang Biol 23:3921–3933

Falster DF, Westoby M (2003) Plant height and evolutionary games. Trends Ecol Evol 18:337–343

Fernández-Tschieder E, Binkley D (2018) Linking competition with growth dominance and production ecology. For Ecol Manag 414:99–107

Fichtner F, Härdle W, Bruelheide H, Kunz M, Li Y, von Oheimb G (2018) Neighbourhood interactions drive overyielding in mixed-species tree communities. Nat Commun 9:1144

Finke DL, Snyder WE (2008) Niche partitioning increases resource exploitation by diverse communities. Science 321:1488–1490

Ford ED (1975) Competition and stand structure in some even-aged plant monocultures. J Ecol 63:311–333

Freckleton RP, Watkinson AR (2001) Asymmetric competition between plant species. Funct Ecol 15:615–623

Gause GF (1934) The struggle for existence. Williams and Wilkins, Baltimore, 184 p

Gladwell M (2000) The tipping point: how little things can make a big difference. Abacus, New York, 288 p

Grassi G, Giannini R (2005) Influence of light and competition on crown and shoot morphological parameters of Norway spruce and silver fir saplings. Ann For Sci 62:269–274

Grime JP (1977) Evidence for the existence of three primary strategies in plants and its relevance to ecological and evolutionary theory. Am Nat 111:1169–1194

Guderle M, Bachmann D, Milcu A, Gockele A, Bechmann M, Fischer C, Roscher C, Landais D, Ravel O, Devidal S, Roy J, Gessler A, Buchmann N, Weigelt A, Hildebrandt A (2018) Dynamic niche partitioning in root water uptake facilitates efficient water use in more diverse grassland plant communities. Funct Ecol 32:214–227

Hale SE (2003) The effect of thinning intensity on the below-canopy light environment in a Sitka spruce plantation. For Ecol Manag 179:341–349

Hamilton GJ, Christie JM (1973) Construction and application of stand yield models. Forestry commission research and development paper, vol 96. Edinburgh, 120 p

Harper JL (1961) Approaches to the study of plant competition. Symp Soc Exp Biol 15:1–39

Hasenauer H (1997) Dimensional relationships of open-grown trees in Austria. For Ecol Manag 96:197–206

Huang Y, Chen Y, Castro-Izaguirre N, Baruffol M, Brezzi M, Lang A, Li Y, Härdtle W, von Oheimb G, Yang X, Liu X, Pei K, Both S, Yang B, Eichenberg D, Assmann T, Bauhus J, Behrens T, Buscot F, Chen X-Y, Chesters D, Ding B-Y, Durka W, Erfmeier A, Fang J, Fischer M, Guo L-D, Guo D, Gutknecht JLM, He J-S, He C-L, Hector A, Hönig L, Hu R-Y, Klein A-M, Kühn P, Liang Y, Li S, Michalski S, Scherer-Lorenzen M, Schmidt K, Scholten T, Schuldt A, Shi X, Tan M-Z, Tang Z, Trogisch S, Wang Z, Welk E, Wirth C, Wubet T, Xiang W, Yu M, Yu X-D, Zhang J, Zhang S, Zhang N, Zhou H-Z, Zhu C-D, Zhu L, Bruelheide H, Ma K, Niklaus PA, Schmid B (2018) Impacts of species richness on productivity in a large-scale subtropical forest experiment. Science 362:80–83

Hutchinson GE (1957) Concluding Remarks. Cold Spring Harb Symp Quant Biol 22:415–427

Isbell F, Cowles J, Dee LE, Loreau M, Reich PB, Gonzalez A, Hector A, Schmid B (2018) Quantifying effects of biodiversity on ecosystem functioning across times and places. Ecol Lett 21:763–778

Janzen DH (1970) Herbivores and the number of tree species in tropical forests. Am Nat 104:501–528

Judson O (1994) The rise of the individual-based model in ecology. Trends Ecol Evol 9:9–14

Keddy PA (1989) Competition. Chapman and Hall, London, 552 p

Keddy PA (2017) Plant ecology: Origins, processes, consequences, 2nd edn. Cambridge University Press, Cambridge, 624 p

Kikuzawa K, Umeki K (1996) Effect of canopy structure on degree of asymmetry of competition in two forest stands in Northern Japan. Ann Bot 77:565–571

Kimmins JP (2004) Forest ecology - a foundation for sustainable management, 3rd edn. Pearson Education Prentice Hall, Upper Saddle River, 700 p

Kramer H (1988) Waldwachstumslehre [Forest growth and yield science]. Verlag Paul Parey, Hamburg and Berlin, 374 p

Kunstler G, Lavergne S, Courbaud B, Thuiller W, Vieilledent G, Zimmermann NE, Kattge J, Coomes DA (2012) Competitive interactions between forest trees are driven by species' trait hierarchy, not phylogenetic or functional similarity: implications for forest community assembly. Ecol Lett 15:831–840

Langsæter A (1941) Om tynning i enaldret gran- og furuskog [About thinnings in even-aged spruce and pine forests]. Medd Nor Skogforsoksves 8:131–216

LeMay V, Pommerening A, Marshall P (2009) Spatio-temporal structure of multi-storied, multi-aged interior Douglas fir (Pseudotsuga menziesii var. glauca) stands. J Ecol 97:1062–1074

Lichtenthaler HK (1996) Vegetation stress: an introduction to the stress concept in plants. J Plant Physiol 148:4–14

Lichtenthaler HK (1998) The stress concept in plants: an introduction. Ann N Y Acad Sci 851:187–198

Lin Y, Berger U, Grimm V, Quian-Ru J (2012) Differences between symmetric and asymmetric facilitation matter: exploring the interplay between the modes of positive and negative plant interactions. J Ecol 100:1482–1491

Lin Y, Berger U, Grimm V, Huth F, Weiner J (2013) Plant interactions alter the predictions of metabolic scaling theory. PLOS ONE 8:e57612

Lundqvist L, Elfving B (2010) Influence of biomechanics and growing space on tree growth in young Pinus sylvestris stands. For Ecol Manag 260:2143–2147

MacArthur RH (1965) Patterns of species diversity. Biol Rev Camb Philos Soc 40:510–533

Maestre FT, Callaway RM, Valladares F, Lortie CJ (2009) Refining the stress-gradient hypothesis for competition and facilitation in plant communities. J Ecol 97:199–205

Matias MG, Combe M, Barbera C, Mouquet N (2013) Ecological strategies shape the insurance potential of biodiversity. Front Microbiol 3:432

Mattheck C, Breloer H (1994) The body language of trees – a handbook for failure analysis. HMSO, London

Messier C, Puettmann KJ, Coates KD (2013) Managing forests as complex adaptive systems. Building resilience to the challenge of global change. Routledge, Oxon, 353 p

Metslaid M, Jõgiste K, Nikinmaa E, Moser WK, Porcar-Castell A (2007) Tree variables related to growth response and acclimation of advance regeneration of Norway spruce and other coniferous species after release. For Ecol Manag 250:56–63

Metzger K (1893) Der Wind als maßgebender Faktor für das Wachstum der Waldbäume [Wind as a crucial factor for the growth of forest trees]. Mündener Forstliche Hefte 3:35–86

Mitchell SJ (2000) Stem growth responses in Douglas fir and Sitka spruce following thinning: implications for assessing windfirmness. For Ecol Manag 135:105–114

Morowitz HJ (1968) Energy flow in biology. Academic Press, New York, 234 p

Murphy SJ, Xu K, Comita LS (2016) Tree seedling richness, but not neighbourhood composition, influences insect herbivory in a temperate deciduous forest community. Ecol Evol 6:6310–6319

Niklas KJ, Spatz H-Ch (2004) Growth and hydraulic (not mechanical) constraints govern the scaling of tree height and mass. Proc Natl Acad Sci USA 104:15661–15663

Nilson A (1973) Hooldusraiete arvutusliku projekteerimise teooriast [On the theory of programming thinnings]. EPA teaduslike tööde kogumik 89:136–142

Nilson A (2006) Modeling dependence between the number of trees and mean tree diameter of stands, stand density and stand sparsity. In: Cieszewski CC, Straub M (eds) Proceedings of the second international conference on forest measurements and quantitative methods and management & The 2004 southern mensurationists meeting. Athens GA, pp 74–94

Oliver CD, Larson BC (1996) Forest stand dynamics, Update edn. Wiley, New York, 520 p

Otto H-J (1994) Waldökologie [Forest ecology]. Ulmer, Stuttgart, 391 p

Perry DA, Oren R, Hart SC (2008) Forest ecosystems, 2nd edn. The Johns Hopkins University Press, Baltimore, 632 p

Philip MS (1994) Measuring trees and forests, 2nd edn. CABI Publishing, Wallingford, 310 p

Piao T, Comita LS, Jin G, Kim JH (2013) Density dependence across multiple life stages in a temperate old-growth forest of northeast China. Oecologia 172:207–217

Pierik R, Mommer L, Voesenek LACJ (2013) Molecular mechanisms of plant competition: neighbour detection and response strategies. Funct Ecol 27:841–853

Pommerening A, Sánchez Meador AJ (2018) Tamm review: tree interactions between myth and reality. For Ecol Manag 428:164–176

Pommerening A, Uria-Diez J (2017) Do large trees tend towards high species mingling? Ecol Inform 42:139–147

Pommerening A, Pallarés Ramos C, Kędziora W, Haufe J (2018) Rating experiments in forestry: how much agreement is there in tree marking? PLOS ONE 13:e0194747

Pretzsch H (1996) Erfassung des Pflegezustandes von Waldbeständen bei der zweiten Bundeswaldinventur [Monitoring forest management in the second national forest inventory of Germany]. AFZ/DerWald 15:820–823

Pretzsch H (2006) Species-specific allometric scaling under self-thinning: Evidence from long-term plots in forest stands. Oecologia 146:572–583

Pretzsch H (2009) Forest dynamics, growth and yield: From measurement to model. Springer, Heidelberg, 664 p

Pretzsch H (2010) Re-evaluation of allometry: state-of-the-art and perspective regarding individuals and stands of woody plants. In: Lüttge U, Beyschlag W, Nüdel B, Francis D (eds) Progress in Botany, vol 71. Springer, Heidelberg, pp 339–369

Pretzsch H, Biber P (2005) A re-evaluation of Reineke's rule and stand density index. For Sci 51:304–320

Pretzsch H, Biber P (2016) Tree species mixing can increase maximum stand density. Can J For Res 46:1179–1193

Rajala T, Olhede SC, Murrell DJ (2018) When do we have the power to detect biological interactions in spatial point patterns? J Ecol 107:711–721

Read J, Stokes A (2006) Plant biomechanics in an ecological context. Am J Bot 93:1546–1565

Reineke LH (1933) Perfecting a stand-density index for even-aged forests. J Agric Res 46:627–638

Röhrig E, Bartsch N, von Lüpke B (2006) Waldbau auf ökologischer Grundlage [Silviculture on an ecological basis]. Verlag Eugen Ulmer Stuttgart, Stuttgart, 479 p

Scheffer M, Carpenter SR (2003) Catastrophic regime shifts in ecosystems: linking theory to observation. Trends Ecol Evol 18:648–656

Schmid B, Hector A, Saha P, Loreau M (2008) Biodiversity effects and transgressive overyielding. J Plant Ecol 1:95–102

Schmidt M (2001) Prognosemodelle für ausgewählte Holzqualitätsmerkmale wichtiger Baumarten [Modelling timber quality of important tree species]. PhD thesis, Göttingen University, Göttingen, 302 p

Schoener TW (1974) Resource partitioning in ecological communities. Science 185:27–39

Schütz JP (2001) Der Plenterwald und weitere Formen strukturierter und gemischter Wälder [The selection forest and other types os structured and mixed species forests]. Parey Buchverlag, Berlin, 207 p

Seifan T, Seifan M (2015) Symmetry and range limits in importance indices. Ecol Evol 5:4517–4522

Shaw JD, Long JN (2007) A density management diagram for longleaf pine stands. South J Appl For 31:28–38

Shinozaki K, Kira T (1956) Intraspecific competition among higher plants VII. Logistic theory of the C-D effect. J Inst Polytech Osaka City Univ D7:35–72

Skovsgaard JP, Vanclay JK (2008) Forest site productivity: a review of the evolution of dendrometric concepts for even-aged stands. Forestry 81:13–31

Smith WR, Farrar RM Jr, Murphy RA, Yeiser JL, Meldahl RS, Kush JS (1992) Crown and basal area relationships of open-grown southern pines for modelling competition and growth. Can J For Res 22:341–347

Spatz H-C, Brüchert F (2000) Basic biomechanics of self-supporting plants: Wind loads and gravitational loads on a Norway spruce tree. For Ecol Manag 135:33–44

Spiecker H (1994) Wachstum und Erziehung wertvoller Kirschen. [Growth and management of valuable cherry trees] Mitteilungen der Forstlichen Versuchs- und Forschungsanstalt Baden-Württemberg, vol 181. Freiburg, 92 p

Sterba H (1985) Das Ertragsniveau und der maximale Stand-Density-Index nach Reineke [Yield level and maximum stand density index according to Reineke]. Centralblatt für das gesamte Forstwesen 102:78–86

Sterba H (1987) Estimating potential density from thinning experiments and inventory data. For Sci 33:1022–1034

Sterba H (2010) Forstliche Ertragslehre [Forest growth and yield science]. Lecture notes. BOKU University Vienna, Vienna, 120 p

Stoyan D, Stoyan H (1994) Fractals, random shapes and points fields. Wiley, Chichester, 406 p

Suzuki SN, Kachi N, Suzuki J-I (2008) Development of local size hierarchy causes regular spacing of trees in an aven-aged Abies forest: analyses using spatial autocorrelation and the mark correlation function. Ann Bot 102:435–441

Thomas PA, Packham JR (2007) Ecology of woodlands and forests: description, dynamics and diversity. Cambridge University Press, Cambridge, 528 p

Tilman D (1982) Resource competition and community structure. Princeton University Press, Princeton, 310 p

Turnbull LA, Isbell F, Purves DW, Loreau M, Hector A (2016) Understanding the value of plant diversity for ecosystem functioning through niche theory. Proc R Soc B 283:20160536

van Laar A, Akça A (2007) Forest mensuration. Managing forest ecosystems, vol 13. Springer. Dordrecht, 383 p

Vogt J, Lin Y, Pranchai A, Frohberg P, Mehlig U, Berger U (2014) The importance of conspecific facilitation during recruitment and regeneration: a case study in degraded mangroves. Basic Appl Ecol 15:651–660

von Gadow K (1986) Observation on self-thinning in pine plantations. S Afr J Sci 82:364–368

von Gadow K, Bredenkamp B (1992) Forest management. Academia, Pretoria, 151 p

Vospernik S, Sterba H (2015) Do competition-density rule and self-thinning rule agree? Ann For Sci 72:379–390

Wang H, Peng H, Hui G, Hu Y, Zhao Z (2018) Large trees are surrounded by more heterospecific neighboring trees in Korean pine broad-leaved natural forests. Sci Rep 8:9149

Weiner J (1990) Asymmetric competition in plant populations. Trends Ecol Evol 5:360–364

Weiner J, Freckleton RP (2010) Constant final yield. Annu Rev Ecol Evol Syst 41:173–192

Weiner J, Solbrig OT (1984) The meaning and measurement of size hierarchies in plant populations. Oecologia 61:334–336

Weiner J, Wright DB, Castro S (1997) Symmetry of below-ground competition between Kochia scoparia individuals. Oikos 79:85–91

Weiner J, Stoll P, Muller-Landau H, Jasentuliyana A (2001) The effects of density, spatial pattern, and competitive symmetry on size variation in simulated plant populations. Am Nat 158:438–450

Wills C, Condit R, Foster RB, Hubbell SP (1997) Strong density- and diversity-related effects help to maintain tree species diversity in a neotropical forest. Proc Natl Acad Sci USA 94:1252–1257

Wright SJ (2002) Plant diversity in tropical forests: a review of mechanisms of species coexistence. Oecologia 130:1–14

Yachi S, Loreau M (1999) Biodiversity and ecosystem productivity in a fluctuating environment: the insurance hypothesis. Proc Natl Acad Sci USA 96:1463–1468

Yao J, Zhang X, Zhang C, Zhao X, von Gadow K (2016) Effects of density dependence in a temperate forest in northeastern China. Sci Rep 6:32844

Yoda K, Kira T, Ogawa H, Hozumi K (1963) Self-thinning in overcrowded pure stands under cultivated and natural conditions. (Intraspecific competition among higher plants XI). J Inst Polytech Osaka City Univ Ser D 14:107–129

Zeide B (2005) How to measure density. Trees Struct Funct 19:1–4

Zeide B (2010) Comparison of self-thinning models: an exercise in reasoning. Trees Struct Funct 24:1117–1126

Chapter 3
Theories and Concepts in Individual-Based Forest Management

Abstract The academic field of forest management and silviculture has a very rich and long tradition, since this subject area once was the cradle of forestry. The methods used were originally based on experience in agriculture which later gave way to ecological principles and can be described as resource management for the purpose of providing goods and services to human societies. With increasing ecological and physiological knowledge forest management methods have become individual-based and many of them are useful in a wide range of contexts including timber production, production of non-timber forest products, conservation and recreation to name but a few. Generic methods have been developed partly based on research results and partly based on practical experience. This chapter outlines the basic principles of individual-based forest management providing the basis for the subsequent chapters of this book. Innovative methods of individual-based forest management focussing on local neighbourhood relationships have recently been introduced in many countries and are likely to form an important part of future, sustainable forest management.

3.1 Introduction to Forest Management

Many authors agree that the prime objective of forestry is to satisfy the forest related demands of society in a sustainable way with minimum input of scarce resources, e.g. energy and money (Köstler 1956; Röhrig et al. 2006). These demands include the provision of various goods and services, namely of raw materials, environmental conservation and the conservation of aesthetical and spiritual properties. For a long time the production of timber has been the only or at least the dominant objective of forestry. This has changed significantly in the last few decades in many parts of the world.

To achieve these general objectives of forestry, there are a number of academic and practical fields within forest science and forestry that help to deliver them. The most central one is forest management or *silviculture*. In analogy to ecosystem management and conservation management, *forest management* is often used as a synonym of silviculture and vice versa (Helms 1998). Köstler (1956) wrote that silviculture is the kernel of forestry and forest science, for it includes direct human

© Springer Nature Switzerland AG 2019
A. Pommerening and P. Grabarnik, *Individual-based Methods
in Forest Ecology and Management*, https://doi.org/10.1007/978-3-030-24528-3_3

action in the forest, and in it, all objectives and all technical considerations ultimately converge. Silviculture has a long history and is the oldest and possibly most traditional subject of forest science and education.

Successful long-term forest management techniques have to be based on biological-ecological requirements because there is much less scope for technical manipulation, which is also increasingly being restricted by law in many countries. Therefore forest managers are bound to understand and to employ natural processes to meet economic objectives. Economic objectives have to be based on eco-physiological and environmental site limitations rather than keeping highly artificial, industrial and risky forest stands alive by tending symptoms through chemical forest protection, fertilisation and weeding (Mayer 1984).

Dengler (1944) noted that silviculture is concerned with the building or design of forests by arranging their individual components, the trees and forest stands, which significantly influence production, health and utilisation of the forest.

Silviculture or forest management as we know this academic field today is a process of forest engineering aimed at creating structures or developmental sequences that will serve the intended purposes, whilst being in harmony with the environment, and withstanding the loads imposed by environmental influences. Because forests grow and change with time, their design is more sophisticated and difficult to envision than that of static buildings. This has made foresters uneasy in the past and, as an expression of this, natural disturbances have often been labelled as "catastrophes" and "risks" (Putz et al. 2012; Puettmann et al. 2009, p. 117ff.). Furthermore, forest stands alter their own environment sufficiently that the forest manager is partly creating a new ecosystem and partly adapting to the one that already exists (Smith et al. 1997). To summarise these aspects we can put forward the following definition:

> The term "forest management" or "silviculture" describes the main activities of forestry, which are the establishment of new forests and the management and regeneration of existing ones. Forest management activities should aim to maintain and improve site quality and growth, stability, quality and diversity of forest vegetation to meet the targeted diverse needs and values of landowners and society on a sustainable basis.

Thus forest management is concerned with the technology of growing tree vegetation. It contributes a major part of the biological technology that carries ecosystem management into action (Smith et al. 1997) and silvicultural activities reflect the forest manager's efforts to imitate natural succession and disturbance.

Forest management heavily draws on a wide range of basic sciences as does practical silviculture carried out by forest managers in the field. These basic sciences include soil science, plant physiology, climatology, geology, dendrology and many more. Silvicultural and forest management methods, however, are essential for forest planning, nature and landscape conservation.

3.2 Sustainability

Concern over the sustainability of timber resources gave birth to state organised forestry. On the European continent, the idea of sustainability of timber resources can be traced back as far as the 14th century (L'ordonnance de Brunoy by Philippe VI de Valois, see (Hasel 1985). The essence of this idea was to achieve a balance between growth and harvesting, i.e. not to harvest more timber than would regrow at any one time. This concept was finally put into action in Germany at the beginning of the 18th century when timber shortages became a serious constraint and the eminent silviculturists Hartig, Cotta and Gayer emphasised the sustainability principle in the 18 and 19th centuries.

Simple conceptual models such as the normal forest were developed to ensure sustainable cutting (Gadow and Bredenkamp 1992; Bettinger et al. 2009). Sustained yield was achieved by what has come to be called the *area method of regulation of the cut*. This consists basically of dividing the total forest area into as many equally productive units as there are years in the planned rotation and harvesting one unit each year. The method was applied to growing conifers by clearcutting and planting, a system that imitated agriculture (Smith et al. 1997).

Such tools, ensuring the sustainability of timber resources, were constantly improved by forest planning methods. In many countries where plantation silviculture is the dominant forest management type, the normal forest concept with its area-control method still has a considerable influence on the landscape. In some countries such as Britain, attempts have even been made to apply the method of area control to continuous cover forest (CCF) management (see Sect. 3.4). For example the so-called Bradford-Hutt plan and even the British interpretation of the group selection system are in fact small-scale applications of the area-control method (see Garfitt 1994, Hart 1991, for details).

The concept of sustainability has been through a considerable process of evolution (Aplet et al. 1993; Toman and Ashton 1996) and in many countries the *area-control method* of sustainable management has given way to individual-tree management and the *size-control method*, particularly in those countries where CCF was favoured. Area-control basically implies that trees to be managed are identified by their location in certain areas, e.g. a certain compartment comprises the oldest trees in a forest district and can be clearfelled. By contrast, in CCF management requirements are determined by the size of individual trees, e.g. by stem diameter or total height.

Traditionally the most common size variable used at forest estate/district and stand levels was standing volume (Bettinger et al. 2009, p. 213f.), which is now increasingly replaced by basal area. At individual tree level, stem diameter at breast height is very common and thinning/harvesting criteria are defined as target diameters, see Sect. 3.6.1. Stand height is also sometimes used as thinning criterion (see for example Pretzsch 2009, p. 175f.).

Speidel (1972) put forward a constructive definition of sustainability as "a forest enterprise's ability to continuously and optimally provide timber and non-timber products and infrastructure, e.g. increment, timber, volume, timber quality, revenue, employment, mushrooms, berries, infrastructure (water, conservation, recreation), for the purpose of present and future generations."

Bettinger et al. (2009, p. 186) emphasised that the term sustainability often refers to the general ability to maintain a resource indefinitely into the future, with no decline in quality or quantity, regardless of outside influences.

A milestone in defining sustainability was agreed by the United Nations (2001) as part of the Agenda 21. This document draws on the principles put forward at the UN Conference on Environment and Development held at Rio de Janeiro in 1992. The Agenda 21 is a comprehensive environmental strategy and Chap. 11 of this agenda explicitly deals with forests. This was the first international agreement on the management, conservation and sustainable development of all forest types.

"Forest resources and forest lands should be sustainably managed to meet the social, economic, ecological, cultural and spiritual needs of present and future generations."

According to this definition sustainable forest management involves practising a land stewardship ethic that integrates reforestation, management, growing, nurturing and harvesting of trees for useful products with the conservation of soil, air and water quality, wildlife and fish habitat, and aesthetics. This also includes balancing long-term carbon storage levels, minimising erosion, avoiding the depletion of soil nutrient stores among other things (Bettinger et al. 2009). Usually sustainability of timber resources was defined at forest estate/enterprise or forest district level.

The traditional concept of forest ecosystem functions is closely connected with the idea of sustainability. de Groot et al. (2002) defined ecosystem functions as *the capacity of natural processes and components to provide goods and services that satisfy human needs, directly or indirectly.* During the evolution of forestry and forest science the traditional function of timber production has increasingly given way a great deal of its former importance to other functions or purposes. Woodlands—especially in the densely populated European countries—are often considered as a multi-purpose resource. All forest functions can be allocated to three major themes—production, social, conservation/protection functions.

Forest functions are a good way of highlighting the various interests the society may have in the same parcel of land and need to be considered and weighted in forest planning. Their significance varies locally although very often many functions must be optimised simultaneously on the same site. This is particularly crucial in the comparatively small-scale European forests. There are different views as to the degree of spatially *integrating* or *separating* forest functions. These can range from *large-scale segregation* to *small-scale segregation, integration with elements of segregation and integration* (Bončina 2011). In upland or coastal protection forests, the conservation/protection function largely overrules the other two functions whilst the social and spiritual functions are paramount in forest cemeteries or at recreation hotspots. Forest functions, in turn, provide the ecosystem goods and services that are valued by humans (de Groot et al. 2002). They are a consequence of the complex interplay between ecosystem structure and processes.

Undoubtedly sustainability has become a major buzz word of this day and age. However, the various definitions offered, are in most cases, not clear enough for direct implementation in field operations (Kimmins 2004). As a result of the Ministerial Conference on the Protection of Forests in Europe (Helsinki 1993) the following definition was put forward: *"Sustainable forest management (SFM) is the stewardship and use of forests and forest lands in a way, and at a rate, that maintains their biodiversity, productivity, regeneration, capacity, vitality, and potential to fulfil, now and in the future, relevant ecological, economic and social functions at local, national and global levels and does not cause damage to other ecosystems."* This formulation remains very general and does not suggest any detailed ways of conducting forest management. It is, for example, unclear whether "stewardship" and "use" are in opposition and whether the stated criteria are in a particular ranked sequence (Röhrig et al. 2006; Helms 1998).

General political objectives need a detailed breakdown at national and regional level. Long-term forest management programmes and certification schemes are expected to build on the framework provided by the international conferences on sustainability.

Monitoring sustainability requires a set of operational criteria and indicators of sustainable forest management. As a result of the Ministerial Conference on the Protection of Forests in Europe (Lisbon 1998) a catalogue with 6 criteria, 27 indicators and 45 guidelines was agreed. The certification of sustainable forest management is based on such criteria and indicators. Woodland certification provides an independent assurance that a woodland under study meets a recognised standard of management. Different international certification schemes such as the Programme for the Endorsement of Forest Certification schemes (PEFC) and the Forest Stewardship Council (FSC) are concerned with the standardization and promotion of sustainable forest management. The national interpretations and variants of these schemes, however, can differ substantially.

3.3 Silvicultural Regimes and Types of Forest Management

Naturally there are many possible ways of classifying silvicultural methods. The system we devised in this book may aid the understanding of all these terms in a challenging way.

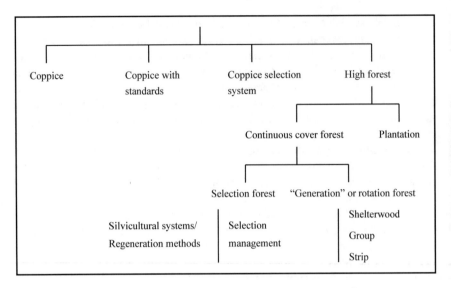

Fig. 3.1   The relationship between silvicultural regimes and basic silvicultural systems

Silvicultural regimes are technically different methods which give whole forest units their specific character, the basis of differentiation lies mainly in the regeneration method (Köstler 1956, p. 361). In the Anglo-American literature both silvicultural regimes and forest management types are usually lumped together by the term "silvicultural systems" (see for example Matthews 1991, Nyland 2002). In this tradition, silvicultural systems are perceived as "plans for management" (Nyland 2002, p. 17) or "planned programmes of silvicultural treatment" (Smith et al. 1997, p. 301) including and fully integrating the three domains of silviculture, i.e. establishment, tending and harvesting, extending throughout the life of a forest stand. This concept differs from the European view where most silvicultural systems are purely seen as regeneration methods whilst coppice, coppice with standards and high forest are silvicultural regimes (see, for example, Burschel and Huss 1997, Röhrig et al. 2006). In Europe, silvicultural programmes for a whole woodland community are better described by the format of Table 3.1. In the central parts of Europe, it was felt that silvicultural regimes are so different from silvicultural systems with respect to resulting structure and in their technical handling that they were separated from them as a matter of principle (Köstler 1956) (Fig. 3.1).

One of the oldest silvicultural regimes is *coppice* or *low forest* (in some of the European terminologies like for example in German and Spanish). It is believed that this silvicultural regime was first introduced in the Bronze Age as a natural consequence of clearing forest vegetation for settlements. Some of the trees resprouted from dormant buds at the remaining tree stumps or at the roots (root suckers) and this gave rise to a secondary forest that eventually developed into a coppice forest. Coppice forests typically have a short rotation length, i.e. all trees are cut every

3.3 Silvicultural Regimes and Types of Forest Management

20–30 years because the sprouting ability of trees decreases with age and because traditionally the focus was on small-sized timber assortments (Rittershofer 1999; Röhrig et al. 2006). In England, hazel (*Corylus avellana* L.) grown in coppice forests for thatching spars are cut every 5–7 years. After coppicing, which essentially is a clearfelling operation, the forest then regenerates from stool shoots and root suckers. Due to their fairly short lifetime these forests are normally comparatively short in height (hence the ancient Germanic term "low forest") and tree diameters remain small. In coppice forests, broadleaved species are predominantly used not least for their resprouting ability. Coppiced trees typically comprise clusters of stems and share similarities with the basitonic growth pattern of shrubs.

The main products of coppice forests included firewood, fencing material, posts, roofing materials, charcoal, bark and other small-sized items. A special form of coppice management is *pollarding*, in which the tops of trees are removed, thus inducing them to sprout at points above the reach of browsing animals (Smith et al. 1997), i.e. coppicing can be carried out at different stem heights. Whilst being a simple and ancient regime it is currently re-visited as a source for animal fodder and fuelwood contributing to renewable energy.

By ways of gradual evolution *coppice with standards* or *middle forest* (in some of the central European terminologies) developed when the need for larger-sized products arose along with the traditional coppice products. Essentially coppice with standards is a combination of trees grown from coppice shoots and from seedlings. Coppice forests have received a lot of attention in recent years because they usually have a considerably high biodiversity and conservation value and simultaneously provide fuelwood and other timber and non-timber products.

High forest regimes can be characterised as forests regenerated from seeds or planted seedlings (sometimes referred to as virgin trees). This contrasts with *coppice* or *low forest* systems that originate vegetatively as natural sprouts from the stools of felled trees. The name of this regime comes from the fact that trees grown from seeds usually develop larger total heights than those that have regenerated vegetatively. Also the production period (= rotation) is usually longer. In many parts of Europe, coppice and coppice-with-standards forests were converted to high forests towards the end of the 19th century, a process which is currently being reversed in some regions. Many high forests are traditionally dominated by conifers. High forests came into fashion when increasingly a need arose for construction and sawn timber. At the same time the demand for fuel wood declined due to an increasing availability of fossil fuels. The structure of high forests most closely resembles that of natural forests, since trees are usually allowed to have longer lifespans and larger total heights than in the other two regimes. High forest trees typically have single stems that show more or less acrotonic growth in contrast to shrubs and coppiced trees.

High forest regimes can be further subdivided into plantation forest management and continuous cover forestry (CCF) or near-natural forest management, based on the development and continuity of tree biomass over time (Pukkala and Gadow 2012, p. v), see Sect. 3.4. Other common synonyms include *all-aged, uneven-aged, multi-aged* as opposed to *even-aged* forest management (for more synonyms see

Fig. 3.2 Biomass
development in different
management approaches.
Plantation (top), CCF
(centre) and transformation
management (bottom). R is
rotation age

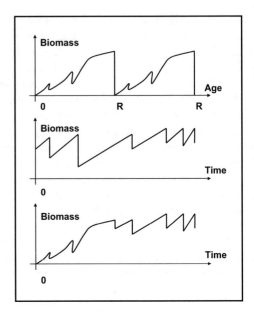

Pommerening and Murphy 2004, O'Hara 2014), although terms involving structure
rather than age are more meaningful. Associated with the first type of management is
a rather abrupt or sudden transition from one forest generation or rotation to another
one, usually by clearfelling all trees of a stand (see Fig. 3.2). Mason and Kerr (2001)
used the terms *complex* and *simple* forest structures. They defined complex forest
structures to have more than two distinct storeys.

   Rotation is the period during which a generation of a single forest stand is allowed
to grow or in other words the period between establishment and final cutting. It is
also known as either economic or natural maturity (Smith et al. 1997). The length
of a rotation may be based on many criteria including species, mean size, age, increment culmination, growth rates, wind hazard and biological condition among others.
Typical properties of plantation forest management include

- A very short period of stand establishment with instant artificial regenera-
  tion,
- The origin of seedlings is often not local and in many cases includes genet-
  ically improved material,
- Low genetic diversity,
- Hardly any age difference between trees of the same stand,
- Clearfelling is the predominant harvesting method,
- Highly industrial use of timber products (e.g. pulp and paper, fibreboards).

Plantation forest management is the most widespread type of forest management on the planet but compared with natural forests, largely unaffected by human management at least for some time, it is also the most extreme one in terms of species composition and structure. The share of the global timber production coming from plantations is high and increasing. However, this forest type remains a small portion of the earth's total forest cover. Also plantations do not necessarily need to involve nonnative species: In the US, which has a sizeable portion of the world's planted forests, practically all plantations are of native species.

In contrast continuous cover forestry is usually characterised by selective thinnings and natural regeneration, resulting in uneven-aged structures and frequently, multi-species forests (see also next section). Stand age is typically undefined in such forests and the growing stock usually oscillates about a specified level (Pukkala and Gadow 2012). Interestingly CCF shares similarities with the horticultural concept of *permaculture* (Whitefield 2004). Both approaches have in common that the soil is never completely exposed at large scale and covered by some level of vegetation. In every country, certain thresholds for allowable gap size have entered legislation. For example in Britain the maximum size of an area cleared from tree vegetation is 0.25 ha (Hart 1991). In this context it is remarkable that already Anderson (1953) referred to the *permanent forest* when writing about what is known as continuous cover forestry and near-natural forestry today.

Depending on how abruptly the transition from one forest generation to the next is carried out there are grey zones and overlaps between the *age-class* or "*generation*"/rotation forest system and the selection forest system (see Sect. 3.7.7), where no distinct tree generations and rotations exist. In the former, processes of natural regeneration are also used but forest development still progresses in distinctive generations or rotations usually allocated to two distinctive storeys. The basic variants of shelterwood, group and strip systems are silvicultural systems that more or less propagate age-class or generation forests. As a result the tree biomass development over time is fairly similar to the top graph in Fig. 3.2 with the difference that the transition from one generation or rotation to another is less abrupt than in plantation management. Still there can be a considerable amount of age and size differences in such forests. This is contrasted by plantation forestry that can be considered as an extreme form of rotation forest management with no temporal overlap whatsoever between two successive forest generations. Also, regeneration in plantation forestry is usually established by replanting. The overstorey removals in silvicultural systems often reflect geometric shapes, i.e. in group systems overstorey trees in circular areas are removed whilst in strip systems overstorey trees in elongated rectangles are cut.

Selection or "*plenter*" forests (see Sect. 3.7.7) are a very specific type of CCF management with a wide range of age and size classes, and tree canopies present throughout the vertical growing space (Schütz 2001b, p. 27). There is evidence that any attempt to remove the age-class or generation structure of forests, for example by maintaining a high forest with two permanent storeys, ultimately results in a selection system (Sterba and Zingg 2001). Also conifer species appear to play a decisive role in achieving a diverse vertical stand structure, which is much more difficult in pure broadleaved forests (Schütz 2001b). Selection systems are the only silvicultural systems where sustainability of timber resources applies at stand and not at estate or district level. Also, the selection system is the only silvicultural system that comes close to the Anglo-American view of "planned programmes of silvicultural treatment" (Smith et al. 1997, p. 301) because the overall structure of the resulting forest more or less stays the same at all times. It should also be mentioned, that the *coppice selection system* (Matthews 1991) as a rare exception is an interesting combination of coppicing and selection system. In contrast to conventional coppicing not all trees are cut at the same time like in a clearfelling operation, but rather individual trees and small groups of trees are coppiced at any one time. This type of short-rotation (12–15 years) selection system was, for example, traditionally practised in the Swiss canton Ticino to produce larger stems and to avoid soil erosion (Schweizerischer Forstverein 1925).

Often silviculturists are concerned with the *transformation* of one silvicultural regime or system to another (see Sect. 3.4; Matthews 1991, p. 225). As mentioned before, a widespread transformation task of the 19th and early 20th century in many European countries was that of coppice forests to high forests, whereas for environmental and conservation reasons this process is now being reversed in some countries. The transformation of plantation forests to continuous cover woodlands is currently a very frequent activity of silviculturists in many countries. Some authors give transformation forest management the same attention as plantation and CCF management (Pukkala and Gadow 2012). This group of activities concerns the active gradual change of woodland structure and or species composition. The biomass curve of transformation management consequently has elements of both, plantation management in the beginning and continuous cover management later on.

Altogether there is a wide range of silvicultural possibilities within CCF including many combinations of silvicultural systems and treatments (Pommerening and Murphy 2004).

3.4 Continuous Cover Forestry and Individual-Based Forest Management

Near-natural forestry or continuous cover forestry (CCF) is not a new phenomenon but over the last decades there has been a renewed worldwide debate regarding its position in forest management (Pommerening and Murphy 2004). Recently CCF has increasingly been perceived as a robust strategy for mitigating climate change and loss of biodiversity (Pukkala and Gadow 2012).

Continuous cover forestry stretches from even-aged monospecific coniferous woodlands managed on a non-clearfelling basis to complex selection forests involving several tree species. As Pommerening and Murphy (2004) pointed out, the definition of CCF often includes a range of criteria:

- Continuity of woodland conditions,
- Emphasis on vertical and horizontal structure,
- Mixed age classes and tree species,
- Attention to site limitations,
- Selective individual tree silviculture,
- Conservation of old trees, deadwood and protection of endangered plant and animal species,
- Promotion of native tree species/provenance and broadleaves,
- Ecologically sensitive forest protection, thinning and harvesting operations,
- Ecologically sensitive wildlife management,
- Establishment of forest margins and a network of protected woodlands.

The general idea of near-natural forestry or continuous cover forestry is to promote managed forests with structures, management practices and/or species compositions that are more akin to the potentially natural stages of development and to the potentially natural processes of tree vegetation on any particular site than those that are commonly observed in rigid plantation management (O'Hara 2014). This concept can be regarded as a naïve understanding of and a step towards forestry or silviculture on an ecological or environmental basis.

The definitions and criteria mostly stress the idea of the continuity of woodland conditions over time hence the name "continuous cover forestry", a term which has given rise to many misunderstandings. Often it has been misunderstood as an intention to create and maintain dense forests with closed canopies where only shade tolerant species can survive. The term, however, does not imply any degree of canopy closure and is fully compatible with the creation of smaller or larger gaps for promoting natural regeneration, the conservation of wildlife or for the establishment of viewpoints should the necessity arise. CCF does not necessarily imply a lack of management (as the quasi-synonym low-impact silviculture may suggest) but emphasises the need to avoid clearfelling over very large areas and within this broad concept a range of silvicultural systems are possible.

However, CCF is more than the mere avoidance of large-scale clearcutting. Some of the definitions above highlight other important components such as the selective removal of trees, allowable gap size, suitable silvicultural systems and vertical structure. In particular CCF is being seen as compatible with a holistic approach to forestry with multi-purpose management objectives (O'Hara 2014).

According to Gadow (pers. comm.) there are three basic CCF situations: establishment on bare land, transformation of even-aged plantations and maintenance of existing CCF woodlands. In the traditional British literature (Troup 1928), the terms *transformation* and *conversion* are treated as synonyms. They are regarded as very general terms implying the active change from one silvicultural system to another, e.g. from coppice to high forest, from high forest to coppice, from systems involving clearfelling to CCF, from coniferous plantations to semi-natural broadleaved woodlands and the other way round. Later suggestions have been made to distinguish between the two terms (Spiecker et al. 2004):

Transformation
Active gradual change of woodland structure and/or species composition (in the German terminology referred to as *Überführung*), e.g. the transformation of even-aged Sitka spruce plantations to uneven-aged Sitka spruce woodlands (with possibly some broadleaved enrichment).

Conversion
Active abrupt change of species composition (thus coinciding with the German term *Umwandlung*) used in the context of ecosystem restoration, e.g. the conversion of coniferous plantations to restored broadleaved woodlands on ancient woodland sites.

At present most interest focuses on the transformation or conversion of existing forests, such as monospecies even-aged coniferous plantations to diverse uneven-aged continuous woodlands or the restoration of native woodlands on ancient woodland sites (O'Hara 2014). For stands where direct transformation is considered too risky, it is generally proposed that a pure stand should be re-established after clear-felling. The new stand could then be managed in such a way to establish continuous forest conditions (Schütz 2001a). Having succeeded in transformation the uneven-aged forest needs to be maintained, i.e. managed in a way that sustainable and uninterrupted harvesting, regeneration and recruitment is possible. However, there is another silvicultural option, that of establishing mixed forests under CCF prescription directly from scratch on bare land, irrespective of whether it has not been recently under forest or it is a restock site. Direct establishment of mixed forests based on the nurse-crop technique has been very successful especially where severe climatic conditions, such as strong winds and high precipitation, along the North Sea coast of Denmark and Germany made other methods impossible (Pommerening and Murphy 2004).

Individual-based forest management is crucial to CCF. Here individual-based forest management is in fact needed most and also most frequently applied. Important criteria in selective, individual-based thinning and harvesting are size and distance between trees. Target diameter harvesting (see Sect. 3.6.1) ensures harvesting of individual trees when the value growth rate culminates and with respect to ecological and genetic requirements (Messier et al. 2013). Such management requires a range of skills and in-depth ecosystem knowledge that exceed the skill set required in plantation forestry by far, therefore the introduction of CCF is always also an educational challenge. The emphasis on woodland structure and conservation of old trees also implies individual-based approaches. In forests managed for commercial reasons, another consequence of continuous cover forestry for managed forests is moving away from maximum timber production to maximum timber quality in individual trees. This implication may also lead to a species change on many sites. As the retention of woodland conditions in space and time is the most important criterion of CCF, large-scale harvesting is replaced by continuous selective thinnings that include the selective harvesting of individual mature trees. In near-natural or continuous cover forestry, there is a trend towards longer production cycles in managed forests. This implies that at least some of the trees in such forests are increasingly allowed to approach natural life expectancies. Naturally trees managed under such conditions also reach larger sizes than those grown in standard plantation regimes and there is greater variability of tree sizes and timber quality (Röhrig et al. 2006). This in turn has consequences in terms of carbon sequestration, sampling, modelling, timber extraction and processing.

3.5 Silvicultural Planning

Many methods of individual-based forest management support silvicultural planning and the subsequent process of controlling the implementation. The silvicultural planning process at stand level is also a good reflection of the philosophy of general silvicultural analysis.

To begin with, the current state of the respective planning unit needs to be sampled and analysed (Fig. 3.3). In the same step the processes that have led to the current state have to be taken into consideration. Any information on the history of stand development may prove useful in order to get a feeling for the velocity of the dynamics involved. Particularly the questions of how the given forest ecosystem will develop with and without forest management, in what directions and how fast, are important in this context (see also Appendix A for more details).

Based on the analysis, projections of potential forest development paths are undertaken which can be model aided (Coates et al. 2003; Wikström et al. 2011). Usually a number of different forest management possibilities or scenarios are explored in a scenario analysis and the best option under the given (legal) constraints and management objectives is identified. This process can be formalised by methods of optimisation and operations research that are usually presented in forest planning textbooks (see Bettinger et al. 2009). The silvicultural scenarios include key processes and methods of forest management such as species choice, silvicultural regime, silvicultural system and forest management types.

Both the results of the sampling analysis and scenario analysis then feed into the silvicultural management plan. The core part of this plan is a set of silvicultural prescriptions usually for the next 5–15 years. A silvicultural prescription is a planned series of treatments designed to change current stand structure to one that

Fig. 3.3 The general process of silvicultural planning (modified from Gadow 2005, p. 24)

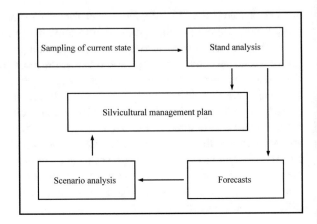

meets management objectives (Helms 1998) and can be part of a larger silvicultural programme for a woodland community, see Table 3.1 for an example.

After reaching a conclusion the forest management plan needs to be translated into a clear, transparent and reproducible work description for practical implementation.

The practical implementation should ideally be followed by a control element. Control should not be thought of as having negative connotations and can already be taking place while the actual work is under way. In plantings and thinnings for example, major mistakes can be identified and mitigated during on-site visits. On the other hand some results will only become evident several years after the actual work has finished, such as the survival rate of plants on a restocking or underplanting site. Long-term monitoring is therefore important and it is crucial to record even seemingly minor details, which also help to understand cause and effect relationships.

Also, in practical or applied forest management, the benefit of monitoring or control can be enhanced by record keeping that allows further statistical analysis. Statistical analysis can provide a better and deeper understanding of advantages and disadvantages of individual components used. In the long run this can lead to a forest enterprise specific optimisation of silvicultural planning through adaptive management (Thomasius 1990). Other aspects of silvicultural controlling include recording the density and height of natural regeneration, the impact of felling and extraction on remaining trees, the impact of browsing and bark stripping by animals, the growth performance, the impact of natural disturbances, the natural mortality of and the interaction among trees.

The methodology employed for monitoring the implementation of silvicultural plans (see for example Gadow and Stüber 1994, Pretzsch 1996) can also be used for quantifying the impact of disturbances and vice versa (see Chap. 7). Recently some of this methodology has also been adopted for use in forest management training which has received a lot of attention in forest practice in France, Switzerland, Britain and Ireland. For this purpose all trees of a rectangular or circular sample plot are marked with tree numbers and are callipered. These training sites are frequently referred to as *marteloscopes* (Bruciamacchie et al. 2005; Poore 2011; Susse et al. 2011, p. 129) (from French *martelage*—marking). Participants of such training seminars are then provided with a list of all trees and are asked to mark trees for thinnings. Methods, that are discussed in Chap. 7 in detail, are used after the exercise to assess how each participant has carried out the silvicultural objectives compared to others in their group by quantifying how the marking will modify the current state of the forest after implementation (Messier et al. 2013).

Finally, it should be emphasised that this traditional procedure of preparing silvicultural plans, implementing, checking up on the implementation and revising the plan after 10–15 years is a good example of what is described as adaptive management.

3.6 Thinning Interventions

There are many different activities or interventions in silviculture and forest management such as the planting of trees, pruning and soil preparation among others. They have in common that they disturb natural vegetation development by goal-oriented human activities following textbook advice such as that in Nyland (2002), Röhrig et al. (2006) and Smith et al. (1997) or other guidelines. Such human interventions in ecosystem processes are necessary where the provision of ecosystem goods and services need optimisation to produce these outputs more quickly and/or in greater quantities than is possible under purely natural conditions (Smith et al. 1997).

Among those that have the strongest effects on forest developments are thinnings. Originally designed to reduce tree density by mimicking self-thinning (see Sect. 2.1.2.1) in a controlled, goal-oriented way, they are closely related to individual-based forest management and also play an important role in silvicultural planning. The general rationale of thinning interventions is to steer interactions among trees and between trees and the environment to meet the objectives assigned to a particular forest stand. As such thinnings can accelerate the growth of residual trees, i.e. of the trees remaining in the forest stand after the thinning operation has been carried out. The increasing demand of trees for growing space leads to natural size differentiation and self-thinning. Interventions in forest management aim to steer this process, in particular to

- Maximise the total volume production of a forest stand,
- Maximise the production of certain, individual trees or groups of trees,
- Adjust the available growing space to the actual requirements of the trees,
- Remove diseased and damaged trees and trees that cause damage to others,
- Steer the species composition,

- Increase tree diversity,
- Promote the individual stability of trees,
- Retain particular structures and processes on a long-term basis (process conservation).

The particular strategy of a thinning intervention depends on the overall objectives associated with a particular forest stand. Maximising overall volume production has been an important traditional strategy of forest management, whilst maximising the production of individual trees has in recent decades replaced this maxim in many countries. Such individual trees or groups of trees can include rare species, particular habitat trees and scenic trees. Process conservation is, for example, used in maintaining forest margins, i.e. strips of 20–30 m width along forest boundaries where shrubs and secondary tree species form transition zones between open landscapes and forests and provide valuable habitats. Also, the single-tree selection or plenter system is a kind of process conservation, where the regeneration phase is artificially preserved on a long-term basis (Schütz 2001b; O'Hara 2014). Considering these generic strategies many different objectives ranging from commercial timber production to conservation and forest management for carbon sequestration can be accommodated.

Thinning interventions can be interpreted as temporary disturbances to current stand structure and growth processes. The removal of elements of the main canopy leads to a temporary destabilisation of the stand in terms of wind and snow. The time required to re-establish the original level of stability depends on how quickly the gaps in the canopy close again. This, in turn, depends on species-specific growth patterns, stand age and local environmental factors. Similarly, removing productive organic matter may mean a temporary decrease in stand growth rates (so-called release shock). Only dense young stands are capable of responding to interventions by an immediate acceleration of growth. The felling and extraction of trees can also cause physical damage to the remaining stand. Finally, the creation of gaps in the canopy leads to reduced rainfall interception and increased solar radiation reaching the forest floor, which in consequence accelerates humus decomposition and creates better conditions for the establishment of ground vegetation. At the same time habitat properties for wildlife are modified. All these effects are rather localised, however, and disappear as the canopy gaps close (Davies et al. 2008).

In traditional forest management and silviculture, there are different terms for the goal-oriented removal of trees and they depend on the development stage of the forest and/or the purpose of removal. "Respacings" or "pre-commercial thinnings" are applied to small and young trees up to a stand height of approximately 12–15 m. "Harvesting" on the other hand is referred to the removal of large, mature trees with a certain economic value. Interventions in between are termed "thinnings". From a generic, ecological as well as statistical point of view, there is no reason to distinguish much between these different terms. Technically they are all thinnings and involve the removal of trees, either selectively or as a whole.

In a way similar to natural disturbances, thinnings are generally characterised by their *type*, *intensity* and *cycle* (Röhrig et al. 2006; Kimmins 2004). The thinning type describes the general properties of trees that are removed in the intervention. Thinning intensity defines the severity of thinning, i.e. how many trees are removed in terms of number, basal area or volume per area. Finally the thinning cycle provides information on when the first thinning is scheduled and how often after the first intervention new thinning interventions are planned.

3.6.1 *Thinning Types*

Generally we can distinguish 1. *global* and 2. *local* or *individual-based* thinning types. Global thinning types address the whole forest stand as a population and only marginally consider tree interactions at local scale. A classic representative of global thinning types is the *systematic* or *mechanical thinning*. Here trees are removed from across the whole stand area without considering their individual characteristics. One application of this approach is the removal of complete rows of (planted) trees to open extraction lines during the first intervention (Davies et al. 2008). Systematic thinnings are useful in young stands growing at high densities where differences in individual tree properties are not apparent to the naked eye. Global thinnings, however, can also be selective, i.e. individual trees are selected according to certain criteria but without taking neighbourhood relationships much into account. Global systematic and selective thinnings can also be carried out in combination, e.g. the complete removal of every seventh row of trees in a plantation combined with a selective removal of individual trees in the stand matrix between these rows (Wenk et al. 1990).

Global Thinning Types

The next step in the evolution of thinning methods was to distinguish between certain tree properties. Any thinning operation that removes individual trees on the basis of their specific characteristics is termed *selective thinning*, regardless of its type or intensity. To make selective thinnings possible silviculturists devised tree classification systems. These classifications were intended to guide forestry staff which trees to select for a given objective. Classifying trees according to "social" or "crown" classes goes as far back as 1844 (Rozsnyay 1979). *Crown* or *canopy classes* (Hart 1991, p. 292f.) were originally devised for homogeneous even-aged forests and have traditionally been the basis for defining thinning types and intensities (Pretzsch 2009). According to the crown-class system trees are classified according to their total heights, i.e. their relative position in the forest stand, and their crown morphology. This visual assessment uses correlations between crown size and shape and competitive status of trees in a forest stand based on the assumption that light is the limiting environmental factor. For practical and scientific use it is also important to

Fig. 3.4 Crown classes
according to Kraft (1884)

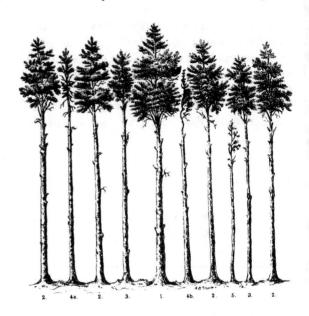

distinguish in this context between light demanding and shade tolerant tree species. For example a mixed broadleaved forest stand with light demanding tree species in the overstorey can have overtopped beech (*Fagus sylvatica* L.), hornbeam (*Carpinus betulus* L.) and lime (*Tilia spp.* L.) trees with well developed crowns (crown class 5a) (Fig. 3.4).

There are different numbers of classes, names and coding systems in the literature (Burschel and Huss 1997; Köstler 1956; Assmann 1970; Burschel and Huss 1997; Röhrig et al. 2006; Smith et al. 1997). Anglo-American sources often use letters (D, CD, SD, S) while numbers are common on the European continent (1–5). Also, continental European systems tend to assess both competitive status and crown shape whilst Anglo-American consider the perceived competitive status only. Assmann (1970) associated classes 1–3 with the overstorey, class 4 with the middle and class 5 with the understorey. Often a more simplified version of Kraft's original system is used (Röhrig et al. 2006). This has, of course, limitations in more complex woodlands involving tree species with very different light demands. Based on these classifications, other global thinning types include *thinnings from below* and *thinnings from above* (also termed *crown thinnings*). In thinnings from below, dominated trees (crown classes 4–5, SD–S) are removed first. The selection process is a negative one, i.e. trees with seemingly undesirable characteristics are marked for removal. Colloquially this is also referred to in forest practice as "tidying up a forest stand". The method typically targets trees of smaller sizes from the left hand side of the diameter distribution.

1. Predominant trees	Most dominant trees of a forest stand with exceptionally strongly developed crowns often above the level of the main canopy.
2. Dominant trees	Dominant trees forming the main canopy and having comparatively well developed crowns.
3. Co-dominant trees	Crowns extend into main canopy, but comparatively weakly developed and narrow. Crowns start to degenerate. Lower limit of dominant trees.
4. Dominated trees	Dominated trees with heavily squeezed or one-sided crowns (flag-shaped).
	a. Free crowns tops in the middle storey.
	b. Partly overtopped crowns in the understorey with beginning crown dieback.
5. Suppressed trees	Crowns completely overtopped
	a. but surviving (shade tolerant species only).
	b. dying or dead.

Thinnings from below aim to maximise the area-related volume production, generally lead to the development of a uniform, single-storey stand structure and promote the collective stability of the entire stand. Assmann (1970) termed this the "thinning method of nature", since in natural self-thinnings the same crown classes contribute to the majority of mortality cases.

1. Dominant trees (D)	Most dominant trees of a forest stand with crowns above the level of the main canopy facing hardly any lateral competition.
2. Co-dominant trees (CD)	Dominant trees forming the main canopy with little lateral competition.
3. Sub-domin. trees (SD)	Crowns extend into main canopy, but face strong lateral competition. Crowns are therefore smaller and irregular in shape.
4. Suppressed trees (S)	Trees with overtopped crowns under the canopy of the main canopy.

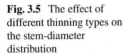

Fig. 3.5 The effect of different thinning types on the stem-diameter distribution

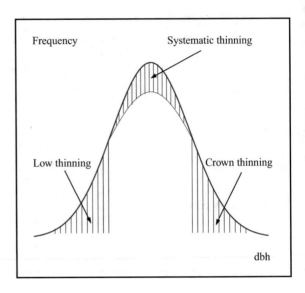

In crown thinnings, interventions mainly affect dominant trees. This involves a positive selection process of dominant and co-dominant trees (crown classes 1–3, D-SD), i.e. trees from the right-hand side of the diameter distribution (Fig. 3.5).

This sometimes is colloquially referred to as "creaming" in the forestry profession (Price and Price 2006). Unlike thinnings from below, crown thinnings result in measurable growth acceleration of the promoted trees and provide early revenues in commercial forestry. Crown thinnings aim to achieve maximum volume and value of individual trees rather than high overall yields. They usually lead to more diverse, often multi-storeyed stand structures and promote the individual stability of the most valuable or important trees (Röhrig et al. 2006; Davies et al. 2008). For these reasons crown thinnings are typically preferred in continuous cover forestry.

In the western United States and Canada, new silvicultural concepts such as *variable-density thinning* (VDT; Roberts and Harrington 2008; Dodson et al. 2012) and the *individual, clumps and openings* (ICO) method (Churchill et al. 2013) have to some degree replaced previous systematic thinnings. They distribute resources unevenly within a stand by subdividing the stand area into patches between 0.1 and 0.5 ha where canopy gaps are created, patches where selective thinnings are carried out and other patches with no thinnings (see Fig. 2 in Willis et al. 2018). Thus a stand density gradient is achieved with the intention to accelerate the development of late-successional habitat (Willis et al. 2018). In the UK and Ireland, *graduated-density thinning* (GDT) has been proposed and applied to transforming young conifer stands to CCF (Vítková and Ní Dhubháin 2013). During the first thinning extraction racks are cut in every eighth row and 40% of trees are selectively or randomly removed from the rows immediately adjacent to an extraction rack. In the second row from the rack, 20% of the trees are selectively or randomly removed followed by 10% in the third row. The fourth row is situated half way between the extraction racks and is left unthinned. In a subsequent thinning, the unthinned rows of trees are completely removed to make new or additional extraction racks with further selective thinnings on either side of the new racks with the same or modified graduated thinning intensities (Vítková and Ní Dhubháin 2013).

Although partly selective these methods are not local or individual-based thinnings as per the definition in the following section but global, selective thinnings. Both aforementioned thinning methods are largely based on the tradition of the area-control method as described in Sect. 3.2. VDT even appears to accommodate elements of sylvicultural systems, namely the group (shelterwood) system, see Sect. 3.7.

Local Thinning Types

Since they follow the concept of a strict individual-based bottom-up approach, local thinning types are fundamentally different from global thinning types (Li et al. 2014). Schütz (2003) referred to local thinnings as *situative thinnings*. Here individual trees are considered in the context of their local tree neighbourhood based on the size-control method explained in Sect. 3.2.

A truly local or individual-based thinning type is the frame-tree method, see also Sect. 1.2. *Frame trees* are those trees intended to remain until the end of the current forest generation or long-term planning period. They are selected at a very early stage of stand development, e.g. when a top height of 12 m is reached. Wilhelm and Rieger (2018) proposed to select frame trees when their height to base of crown has reached 25% of expected final total height.

Frame trees are temporarily or permanently marked and promoted in every subsequent intervention by removing some of the nearest, competitive neighbours. Forest managers identify competitors as an interpretation of the individual frame tree's "eye view". Competitiveness is usually defined by a combination of size (crown and total height) and intertree distance (see Figs. 3.6 and 3.8 for visual impressions). Note that in some parts of the world, particularly in arid zones and in areas with nutrient deficiencies, competition is strongest below ground and therefore not necessarily so easy to identify by naked eye. The number of frame trees per hectare normally varies from

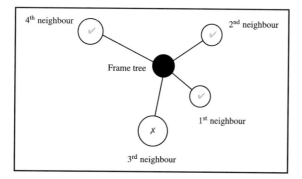

Fig. 3.6 Hypothetical example of a frame tree and four potential, most competitive neighbours. The frame-tree concept is clearly based on the nearest-neighbour principle (see Sect. 4.4.7.1), where the perceived interaction between crowns (judged by whether they touch or even intersect) in most cases drives the decision, whether neighbouring trees are marked for thinning. In this case, the forest manager has decided to remove the 3rd neighbour only. The circle diameters indicate stem size

site to site and in accordance with silvicultural objectives, e.g. so-called *target diameters* specifying the diameter when frame trees have sufficiently matured so that they can be removed for commercial use. Thus for practical purposes the trees of a forest stand can be divided into frame trees and matrix (=non-frame) trees. Normally frame trees would not be removed in thinnings and in commercial scenarios the majority are finally felled through *target-diameter harvesting*, i.e. not at the same time but staggered in time depending on individual size maturity. Some frame trees are kept on a long-term basis as habitat and/or seed trees, hence this type of "relaxed" target-diameter harvesting is sometimes referred to as *variable target-diameter harvesting*. Matrix trees are meant to serve frame trees through "mild, healthy competition" and provide by-products such as energy wood or pulp. In commercial scenarios, frame trees[1] usually have the following properties:

- Vigorous (no diseases, no physical damage, high growth rate, large stem diameter and total height, crown class 1–3, D and CD).
- Good timber quality (straight stems, low branchiness, little taper).
- Non-deciduous trees particularly with shallow root systems (e.g. spruce (*Picea spp.*)) should have a total height to stem diameter ratio (h/d ratio) which does not exceed a value of 80.
- Dispersion (as uniform as possible or clustered).

Frame trees are the cell nuclei of small local management units (Schädelin 1934) within a forest stand that include frame trees and their nearest tree neighbours (Fig. 3.7). Following the idea of a bottom-up approach, all local management units aggregate to a forest stand or tree population. This implies that all local management units are connected with neighbouring units that surround them and interact with them. In the process of tree marking, this needs to be considered. For example in Fig. 3.7, for four frame trees (no. 17, 23, 35 and 54) the forest manager has only selected one nearest neighbour or competitor for removal. For trees no. 12, 36 and 42 two neighbours were selected for removal. Frame trees no. 47 and 54 share one competitor marked for removal at the boundary of their influence zones. For the largest frame tree no 32 the respective forest manager did not select any competitor for removal, because he did not consider this necessary for the next five years

---

[1]Köstler (1956) described desirable frame tree characteristics in a commercial scenario as stable trees "with stems running right through with one definitely predominant axis. Such trees should be straight, erect and of circular cross-section. The crowns of frame trees should have a dominant leader. There should be a sufficient branch-free length of high-quality timber. The crown should be finely branched and should display a symmetrical structure, as with a symmetrical crown the stem grows concentrically."

Unfavourable tree characteristics in a commercial context include deeply forked stems, heavy and many branches, epicormic shoots, bent-over stems, cracks, spiral grain, broken leaders/tops, harvesting and extraction (bark abrasion) damage, insufficient root spread and anchorage in the soil, swellings, canker and other diseases.

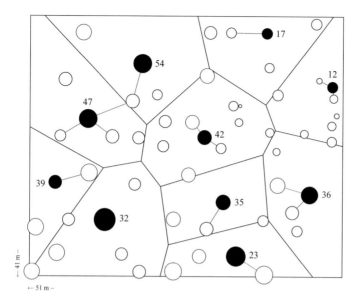

Fig. 3.7 Schematic example representation of how frame trees (filled circles) form local management units or frame-tree influence zones within a forest stand that include frame trees and their
nearest matrix neighbours (open circles). The red lines lead to frame-tree neighbours selected for
removal whilst, based on Dirichlet tessellation (see also Sect. 4.4.5), the black lines denote imagi-
nary boundaries of the local management units (frame-tree influence zones). The numbers next to
the frame trees are identification numbers and the circle diameters indicate tree size

to come. Figure 3.7 is reminiscent of spatial neighbourhood graphs as discussed in
Rajala and Illian (2012).

Dispersion is often referred to as slightly less important than vigour and quality
(Abetz and Klädtke 2002), however, distances and spatial patterns are not entirely
unimportant, since thinnings are only supposed to take place in the vicinity of frame
trees. A good spread of them across the whole stand area avoids creating pockets
of unthinned stand areas that may create problems later (e.g. in spruce (*Picea spp.*)
stands), but do not necessarily need to be a problem. However, in mountain forests
with heterogeneous localised site conditions (e.g. soil depth) and with certain species
in general, e.g. beech (*Fagus sylvatica* L.) a clustered arrangement of 2–3 frame trees
at close proximity and large distances between the groups may be a more appropriate
strategy for taking local, natural trends into account (Busse 1935; Mülder 1990),
where several trees at close proximity seemingly form a superorganism or biogroup,
see also Fig. 7.5.

Rittershofer (1999, p. 95f.) designed a detailed functional tree stratification system
for commercial woodland management based on the frame-tree method. A similar
system was also given by Assmann (1970, p. 89) who referred to it as the *Danish
tree classification*. Such systems are helpful for modern individual-based tree management where trees need to be identified for release and thinning in the field. A
classification system such as the one by Rittershofer may facilitate the decision making process (Fig. 3.8). In this and similar classifications, it is often recommended

that rubbing and whipping trees should be removed before competitors and wolf trees. The same priority applies to smaller neighbours growing into the crown space of frame trees from below. A good "rule of thumb" is to select approximately 100 frame trees per hectare. For conservation and for the transformation of plantations to CCF or when the selection process is delayed, 50 frame trees per hectare suffice. In broadleaved forests, where trees usually have larger crowns than conifers, 60–80 trees per hectare is appropriate whilst the number can range between 100 and 150 in conifer forests. Corresponding distances between frame trees of 10–12 m are also good, general advice (Wilhelm and Rieger 2018).

Frame trees (F)	Trees selected for their outstanding vigour, stem quality, productivity, stability and crown morphology. Usually not more than ± 100 trees/ha
Matrix trees (M)	All non-frame trees.
Hazard trees (H)	Diseased and damaged trees, trees potentially being a threat to frame trees:
Wolf trees (W)	Dominant, very competitive trees with poor stem quality.
Rubbing trees (R)	Sub-dominant and suppressed trees rubbing frame trees with larger branches or parts of their crown.
Whipping trees (Wh)	Sub- or co-dominant trees with slender stems and very small brush-like crowns. Whipping trees tend to move heavily in windy conditions and by doing so can seriously damage the crowns of their neighbours.
Competitors (C)	Neighbours of frame trees that potentially have a negative effect on the growth and development of frame trees.
Nurse trees (N)	Trees of the over-, mid- and understorey that are beneficial to frame trees, e.g. by providing shelter against climatic extremes, by preventing epicormic growth or the growth of invasive ground vegetation (bramble, bracken).
Indifferent trees (I)	Dominant or sub-dominant trees at sufficient distance to the frame trees that have no effect on them. Such trees can potentially replace damaged or diseased frame trees.

Fig. 3.8 Crown classes according to Rittershofer (1999) and result of a selective thinning in favour of frame trees followed by a growth process

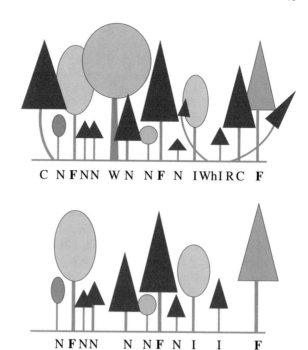

C N F NN W N N F N IWhI RC   F

N F NN   N N F N I   I   F

The more frame trees are selected the more difficult the selection (too few choices) and the more homogeneous the stand structure will become as a consequence. If the target diameter is low, more frame trees with short distances between them can be accommodated. Larger target diameters require smaller numbers of frame trees with large distances between them (see Fig. 3.9).

Frame trees can be selected and marked *permanently* or *temporarily*. A temporary selection implies that new frame trees are selected prior to every new thinning intervention. Generally it is advisable to mark frame trees permanently, because management success or failure can then be more easily identified and as a consequence treatments becomes more consistent. However, a temporary selection sometimes potentially offers more flexibility. Where possibilities for detailed tree marking in the field are limited (e.g. because of financial restrictions), permanent selection of frame trees is recommended. In some countries, silvicultural guidelines suggest appointing a large number (e.g. 200–300) of frame-tree candidates first and to reduce them to a smaller number (e.g. 100–150) of definite frame trees later, in case frame-tree candidates differentiate in unfavourable ways. In our experience, this is an unnecessary complication and usually leads to more confusion and inconsistent management compared to the benefits this concept offers. The same applies to keeping reserve frame trees (Röhrig et al. 2006). Simple modifications of the Rittershofer classification system could lead to an approach with primarily conservation or recreation objectives where valuable habitat and rare species trees are appointed as frame trees. Then the above-mentioned criteria of frame trees can be replaced by others, for example by:

- Morphology similar to open-grown trees (e.g. large stem diameter with considerable taper; long, wide crowns, large root plate, buttresses and forked stems, i.e, "fairy-tale trees").
- Leaves, bark etc. (easy to decompose, scenic, aesthetic value).
- Non-deciduous trees particularly with shallow root systems (e.g. spruce (*Picea spp.*)) should have a total height to stem diameter ratio (h/d ratio) which does not exceed a value of 80.
- Species (rare or offering many ecological niches).
- Dispersion (anything but uniform).

A larger number of frame trees is temporarily possible in mixed-species stands, when the frame trees of one or several component species are harvested much earlier than those of others (Wilhelm and Rieger 2018). Otherwise the number of species-specific frame trees in mixed forests is a reflection of the desired species composition.

When light is the most limiting factor, the maximum number of frame trees per hectare is determined by the final crown size of the trees at the time when target diameter harvesting commences. From relationships between stem and crown diameter required growing space for each tree of a certain size can be approximated. To simplify the calculation square spacing and equal growth rates can

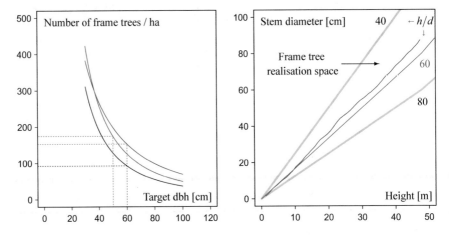

Fig. 3.9 Left: Number of frame trees per hectare approximated from crown diameter models published by Savill (1991) for British tree species. Square spacing was assumed. Black: European beech (*Fagus sylvatica* L.), red: Sitka spruce (*Picea sitchensis* (BONG.) CARR.), blue: Douglas fir (*Pseudotsuga menziesii* (MIRB.) FRANCO). The dashed lines indicate the number of frame trees per hectare given a target diameter of 50 cm for Sitka spruce and of 60 cm for both beech and Douglas fir. Right: Frame tree realisation space (within the grey boundary lines) defined by $h/d = 40$ and $h/d = 80$. Ideal h/d is 60 and the blue line gives the observed h/d development of dominant Sitka-spruce tree no. 1947 in Artist's Wood (Gwydyr Forest, North Wales, UK). Modified from Abetz and Klädtke (2002)

be assumed for determining the maximum number of trees per unit area, i.e. number of frame trees $= 10000/$crown diameter^2 (Abetz and Klädtke 2002). The example in Fig. 3.9 (left) follows the method suggested by Abetz and Klädtke (2002) for determining the number of frame trees per hectare. We recognise the aforementioned trend that broadleaved trees tend to have larger crowns and therefore fewer frame trees can be accommodated in broadleaved forests. Assuming a target diameter of 60 cm, the given site can only support a maximum number of 93 beech frame trees. For Sitka spruce with an average commercial target diameter of 50 cm this maximum number is 175. The Douglas fir curve is close to that of Sitka spruce, however, for the former species a target diameter of 60 cm is quite common. As a result the maximum number of frame trees per hectare is 153 trees for the given site (Fig. 3.9, left).

As indicated before, it is generally advisable to stay well below these maximum or potential frame tree numbers in order to achieve a more diverse horizontal and vertical woodland structure (Weihs 1999).

Reininger (2001) developed and tested a forest management method that he termed *structural thinning*. The core of this method involves selecting frame trees in two different canopy strata allowing the maintenance of two-storeyed high forests on a continuous basis. He tested his structural thinning method in pure or mixed Norway spruce (*Picea abies* (L.) KARST.) woodlands at the Schlägl estate in Austria. The method involves the simultaneous selection and permanent marking of frame trees from upper (F1) and lower canopies (F2) at a fairly early stage of stand development (see Fig. 3.10). As part of this method, F1 trees are selected from the most dominant trees in the stand.

All subsequent interventions are strict crown thinnings aiming at releasing F1 trees from the perceived competition of matrix trees in the same canopy layer. During these operations F2 trees are only released to such a degree that they can survive in a shaded "stand-by position" but do not emerge into the F1 stratum. However, the main stand canopy is never fully closed at any time and the number of frame trees is moderate. Depending on initial stand conditions, F2 trees are recruited either from natural regeneration or suppressed trees of the same age as the main canopy trees or from both. F2 trees are eventually released and allowed to progress into the main canopy when target diameter felling of the F1 trees commences. The new F2 trees are then recruited from natural regeneration. The selection and maintenance of F2 trees diversifies horizontal and particularly vertical forest structure. The idea of this management method is a continuous forest, where target-diameter trees are not finally removed within a short period of time but are harvested individually as part of continued thinning operations (Weihs 1999; Spiecker et al. 2004). The Tyfiant Coed team of Bangor University (North Wales, UK) successfully applied this method to Sitka spruce (*Picea sitchensis* (BONG.) CARR.) at Clocaenog Forest (plot 3).

In each local thinning, only the neighbourhood of frame trees is considered, hence the term "local thinning method". This is achieved either by selecting a certain number of competitive neighbour trees (in middle-aged to older forest stands) or by removing all other trees within a certain radius around each frame tree. The latter method is preferred in comparatively young stands, where trees have so far differentiated little. The selection of a number of apparent competitor trees around

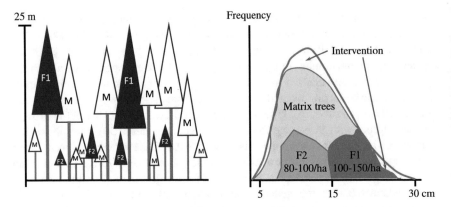

Fig. 3.10 Schematic illustration of the frame-tree method devised by Reininger (2001) aiming at a continuous two-storied conifer forest. Left: Vertical forest structure. Right: Empirical stem-diameter distribution. F1—frame trees recruited from the upper canopy, F2—frame trees representing lower canopies. The frame-tree numbers were modernised

each frame tree implies the crown thinning method. The fact that all thinnings are oriented towards frame trees and occur in their neighbourhood only leads to greater efficiency through a rationalisation of efforts. It is also easier to detect success or failure of an intervention, since only the frame trees need to be evaluated. Harvesting, extraction or bark stripping damage caused by animals only counts, if frame trees are affected.

Abetz and Klädtke (2002) recommended monitoring the h/d ratio (Eq. 2.6) of frame trees as a performance indicator (Fig. 3.9, right): Increasing h/d ratios imply that neighbouring tree crowns are closing in again and as a consequence—for mechanical reasons and because of increasing competition—the frame tree allocates more biomass to height than to diameter growth (see Sect. 2.2). The larger the h/d ratio the more the stem-diameters of frame-tree neighbours and potential competitors typically approach the stem diameter of the frame tree and reduce its diameter growth rate. For frame trees with $h/d > 80$ Abetz and Klädtke (2002) reckoned that it would take too long until trees reach their target diameters and individual-tree stability would be quite low. For frame trees with $h/d < 40$ on the other hand timber quality would be very low because of increased taper as a consequence of very open conditions. Therefore $h/d > 80$ and $h/d < 40$ define the realisation space of frame trees in the system devised by Abetz and Klädtke (2002). The h/d development of tree no. 1947 in Artist's Wood (Gwydyr Forest, North Wales, UK), for example, is well within the frame tree realisation space and close to the ideal line with $h/d = 60$ (Fig. 3.9, right). Instead of plotting the h/d development of individual frame trees it is also possible to plot the mean h/d development of all frame trees of a given forest stand instead. Naturally, in other climates different numbers and relationships may apply.

Based on growth trials and observational plots, Abetz and Klädtke (2002) also developed stem-diameter growth curves (so-called frame-tree norms) dependent on age or stand height for various species and sites to be used for comparison with field observations. However, it is also possible to use the growth records of nearby open-grown trees (Hasenauer 1997) instead. For stem-diameter growth they would form an upper boundary and one could define a suitable growth curve for frame trees through quantile regression (see Sect. 5.2.2; Cade and Noon 2003).

Frame-tree based thinnings are intended to benefit frame trees and this has the highest priority. A promotion of matrix trees can accidentally promote frame-tree competitors and can lead to homogeneous stand structures, thus this should be avoided.

Some guidelines suggest first marking frame trees and then to re-visit each frame tree by marking competitors for thinning among their nearest neighbours in a second step. However, the authors made the experience that it is easier and more natural to consider each management cell as a whole, i.e. each frame tree and its neighbourhood simultaneously, and only then to move on to the next. As a consequence frame trees and potentially competing neighbours are selected and marked at the same time. This approach also avoids falling back into the habit of global thinnings and it is easier to see how the different management units interact with each other. As previously discussed, low and crown thinnings in their pure form are global thinning methods where no particular distinction between trees of interest or intertree distances is made. However, it is possible to quantify in retrospect the results of local thinnings in terms of whether they led to a low or a crown thinning. Frame-tree based thinnings were originally designed to result in crown thinnings, because dominant neighbours of frame trees were supposed to be removed. Despite this original intention it is theoretically also possible and sometimes even necessary to evict neighbours that are sub-dominant relative to the frame trees, which then results in a thinning from below (see Chap. 7).

For identifying competing neighbours that potentially need to be removed, size, distance and species are the most important criteria. In practice, particularly crown measures (width and length) as well as total tree height and quality/habitat characteristics are considered. With increasing understanding of root systems and water/nutrient uptake from the soil some of the aforementioned variables may in the future be replaced by root measures. If, for example, water or nutrients are more limited than light, crown measures may fail to be good indicators of competitiveness and frame-tree influence zones need to be much bigger.

The frame-tree method can even be applied in intensively mechanised forest management. According to the authors' experience it suffices to mark frame trees permanently and clearly visible at an early stage of stand development. After initial training harvester drivers can be trusted to select frame-tree competitors whilst driving through a forest stand and carrying out the thinning. This has proved to be a good compromise between no tree marking at all and intensive tree marking that includes both frame trees and competitors prior to actual thinnings.

3.6.2 Thinning Intensity

Thinning intensity describes the planned or realised loss of stand volume, biomass or basal area at a particular time. The same concept, of course, also applies to natural disturbances in analogy (Fig. 3.11).

In many parts of central Europe, thinning intensity was historically defined in terms of so-called "thinning grades". Thinning grades were fuzzy qualitative descriptions of thinning intensity based on crown classes, i.e. forest managers relied on them to roughly define from which crown classes to recruit trees for global thinning methods. The selected classes coupled with some additional descriptions resulted in different grades or thinning intensities. These were largely combinations of thinning types and thinning intensities and received qualitative labels such as weak thinning from below (grade A), moderate thinning from below (grade B), heavy thinning from below (grade C), heavy release thinning (grade L), weak crown thinning (grade D) and heavy crown thinning (grade E) (Wenk et al. 1990; Röhrig et al. 2006). However, as with many qualitative definitions, tree selection for thinnings following these guidelines left much room for interpretation. Therefore residual basal area, i.e. basal area per hectare after thinning, was often considered as a quantitative criterion for thinning intensity to ensure certain standards. Basal area per hectare as a measure of stand density or crowding has the advantage of being negatively correlated with below-canopy light levels whilst being easier to measure (Burschel and Huss 1997). Many other guide-curve systems and silvicultural prescriptions were developed for both forest practice and forest simulators that worked on the basis of continuous residual-basal area dependent on tree size such as the quadratic mean diameter, d_g (Eq. C.1, Pretzsch 2009).

In individual-based frame-tree thinnings, thinning intensity is defined by the number of competitors to be removed in the vicinity of each frame tree. This number can

Fig. 3.11 Using a hypothetical "sawtooth" curve of stand basal over time to explain the concepts of thinning intensity and thinning cycle

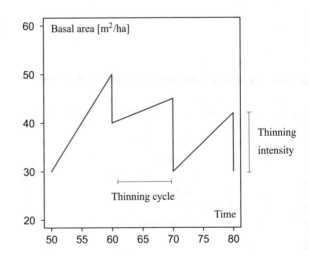

Fig. 3.12 Tree number guide curves depending on the crown spread ratio (assuming square spacing, see Table 2.4)

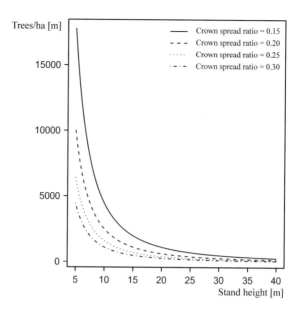

obviously differ from frame tree to frame tree depending on the local release requirements of the tree in question (see Fig. 3.7), however, mean numbers can be defined as targets: On average a removal of 0–2 frame-tree neighbours qualifies for a weak thinning, 2–3 neighbours for a moderate thinning and 3+ neighbours for a heavy thinning. In practice, some forest managers measure the stem diameters of the trees they mark for thinning to estimate the total basal area of the trees marked for removal. Local thinnings typically follow the growth dynamics of forest stands, particularly the tree crown-width development. Therefore thinning intensity in local thinnings is heavy early in stand development and weak towards mature, old-growth stages when tree growth is much reduced (Röhrig et al. 2006).

In global thinnings, the *crown spread ratio* (see Table 2.4) has often been used to describe growing space requirements of trees depending on stand height, because it does not change much in dominant trees of a given species with time. Based on these studies height-based tree-number guide curves have been developed for practical use in forest management (see Fig. 3.12). With square spacing, $N = 10000/\text{crown spread ratio}^2 \times H_o^2$ (where H_o is dominant stand height) and for other tree dispersion patterns this relationship can be adapted (Pretzsch 2009; Kramer 1988). A similar measure leading to guide curves is relative spacing, RS (Kramer 1988):

$$RS = \frac{\sqrt{\frac{10000}{N}}}{H_o}, \tag{3.1}$$

where $\sqrt{\frac{10000}{N}}$ calculates mean tree distance of regularly spaced trees, H_o is stand top height, e.g. the mean height of the 100 largest trees per hectare, and N is the number of trees per hectare. The *SDI* concept (Eqs. 2.1 and 2.5) can also be used to produce guide curves for deriving thinning intensities. However, using such general density guide curves contradicts the principle of local thinnings.

3.6.3 Thinning Cycle

Thinnings start at some point during stand development and need to be repeated at certain intervals. Starting point and time between two successive thinnings define the thinning cycle (see Fig. 3.11). Thinning cycles usually are a compromise between biological processes (e.g. growth) and economic restrictions. For practical reasons and convenience, silvicultural planning often operates on the basis of five-year intervals, however with fast-growing species such as *Eucalyptus spp.*, Sitka spruce (*Pinus sitchensis* (BONG.) CARR.) and *Pinus radiata* D. DON these can also be shorter. In accordance with species-specific growth patterns, it is also possible to apply shorter cycles of 3–5 years at young ages or early development stages and longer ones (8–10 years) in mature stands.

Thinning cycles can also be defined by intervals of stand height. If height intervals (usually stand top height is referred to) are used instead of time intervals, environmental conditions and changes in growth patterns are automatically taken into account. Height intervals of 2–4 m commonly apply to determine the timing of thinnings during early phases of stand development. When height growth eventually slows down in later stages of stand development, thinning cycles are more likely to be defined by the development of stand basal area, canopy closure or the competitive situation of frame trees. Light-demanding species generally require another thinning when the canopy has closed following the previous thinning, whereas shade-bearing species can usually tolerate a certain degree of crown pressure and need interventions only when the crowns start to intercept each other. Again, on sites where other environmental factors such as water are more limiting than light, tree crowns may be less suitable for deriving thinning requirements.

In areas of high wind risk it is generally preferable to apply lighter thinnings and repeat them more often. The necessity for thinning can be gauged from changes in allometric indicators, such as the h/d ratio (Eq. 2.6) or the crown ratio (Table 2.4) of frame trees (Davies et al. 2008).

Finally, thinning type, thinning intensity, thinning cycles and silvicultural systems (Sect. 3.7) can be aggregated in a silvicultural programme for a whole woodland community on a given site (Table 3.1). Using top height as reference ensures that the programme is comparatively site independent. The programme in Table 3.1 illustrates that even mixed-species forests, where the main species has quite different growth dynamics, can be successfully managed using local thinning methods. It also shows how methods of local individual-tree forest management can be integrated to form a silvicultural programme.

Such individual-based guidelines also have a normative character and therefore can act as references to compare observed forest stand development with that deviates

Table 3.1 Example of a full individual-based silvicultural programme for mixed Sitka spruce (SS, *Picea sitchensis* (BONG.) CARR.)—birch (BI, *Betula spp.*) woodlands at Coed y Brenin in North Wales (UK) based on the frame-tree concept and on results from a chronosequence. THT—top height (mean height of the 100 largest trees per hectare), h/d—height-diameter ratio, see Eq. 2.6, c/h—crown ratio, see Table 2.4

THT < 10–12 m	THT = 12–20 m	THT = 20–30 m	Harvesting	Regeneration
Reduction to 1500–2500 trees/ha	Installation of extraction racks	Removal of 1–2 co- to sub-dominant SS frame tree neighbours every 5–8 years	Selective target diameter harvest of SS > 40 cm, BI > 25 cm every 5–7 years but not before advance regeneration established	Final overstorey removal after 5–15 years
Selective removal preferred	Permanent marking: 50 SS frame trees every 15 m, 30 BI frame trees/ha in clusters		Regeneration method: Group/strip system	Allow for 10–15 BI standards/ha
Removal of BI wolf and whip trees	Removal of 2–3 dominant SS competitors per frame tree every 3–5 years or at least in 2 separate heavy selective crown thinnings	Target basal area: 30–35 m²/ha	Target basal area: 25 m²/ha	

No more than 5–8 m² BI and 50–80 m² SS to be removed in any intervention

SS: Max h/d = 80, min c/h = 50; BI: Promote clusters. Keep at least 1.5 m free space between BI and SS crowns from this norm. This helps to understand differences that may arise from special site conditions or other circumstances. Individual-based silvicultural programmes are usually developed from long-term observational research plots and/or from model simulations, see Sect. 5.2. Particularly the combination of observations and simulations leads to robust, generalisable results.

3.7 Regenerating Forest Stands and Silvicultural Systems

Adopting again a generic point of view, this section describes the main silvicultural systems that can be used to regenerate stands without resorting to clearfelling, i.e. they generally result in a smoother transition from one forest generation to the next and make extensive use of natural processes. Since all forests under normal circumstances eventually regenerate naturally, as with thinnings the idea of silvicultural systems is to accelerate processes and to optimise outcomes by providing favourable microclimatic conditions and neighbourhood relations (see Sect. 3.4). Therefore silvicultural systems are an important element of continuous cover forestry and apart from the advantages of working with natural ecosystem processes also help to save expensive planting costs.

Silvicultural systems are essentially methods used to mimic small- to medium-scale natural disturbances and to carefully manage light and microclimatic conditions. For an overview and quick orientation see Fig. 3.13. Here we present the main types only and many local and historical adaptations and combinations exist (Burschel and Huss 1997; Rittershofer 1999; Röhrig et al. 2006). The main distinction is between selection and shelterwood systems, with regeneration establishing continuously over the entire stand area in selection systems, whereas it is confined to a certain time or space in all other systems. Although the seed tree system is not, strictly speaking, a shelterwood approach, it shares many similarities with these systems and is therefore included here. Two or more regeneration methods may be applied in combination, and one of these combinations, the group/strip shelterwood system, is also described. Silvicultural systems are mainly characterised by the geometry of canopy openings, i.e. by the spatial gap structure applied (see Fig. 3.13). They also differ in the spatial pattern of residual trees, which can be analysed using the methods described in Chap. 4.

There are marked differences in the spatial and temporal scales of regeneration (Fig. 3.14). While the clearfelling system leads to a very rapid regeneration (usually through planting although natural regeneration is not uncommon, e.g. stands of maritime pine (*Pinus pinaster* AIT.) in Spain) that affects the whole area, the shelterwood systems retard regeneration and only affect parts of the stand area at any point in time (Ouden et al. 2010). The differences in the shelterwood systems can therefore be also well described by their difference in spatio-temporal regeneration patterns. The irregular shelterwood system, for example, caters for small-scale regeneration that unfolds very slowly. With these characteristics the irregular shelterwood system comes close to the selection system, where there is uninterrupted regeneration at

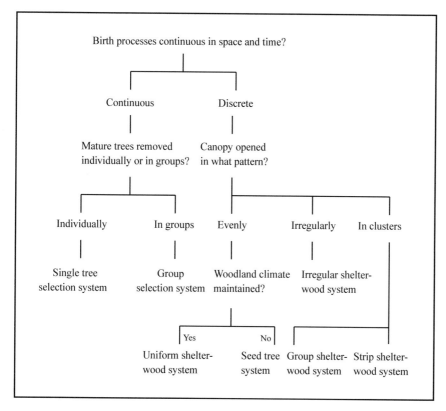

Fig. 3.13 Silvicultural or regeneration systems using natural birth processes (modified from Davies et al. 2008)

extremely small scale. On the other hand, the uniform shelterwood is not so far apart from the clearfelling and replanting system with regard to the spatio-temporal scales of regeneration.

There is no single optimal prescription for the regeneration of stands. When applied, each stand must be treated individually and an appropriate regeneration method should be chosen on the basis of a detailed stand analysis. In some cases, the advance natural development of regeneration may suggest a particular silvicultural system. For example, advance regeneration in small canopy gaps might suggest the group shelterwood system, provided the risk of wind damage is not too great, where the canopy trees are wind prone, or a stand edge exposed to side light by the felling of an adjacent stand might begin to regenerate in a manner similar to a strip shelterwood. Also "local accidents", where unintended and unprecedented interventions triggered the unexpected but promising development of diverse woodland structure, may give vital clues.

Ideally, the removal of mature trees proceeds in tandem with the establishment of the next tree generation and thinning/harvesting operations are designed to facilitate

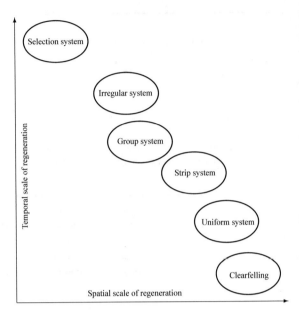

Fig. 3.14 Relationship between spatial and temporal scale of natural tree regeneration in different silvicultural systems. The systems denoted as irregular, group and strip also include their shelterwood variants and uniform system is short for uniform shelterwood system. Modified after Ouden et al. (2010, p. 327)

the regeneration process at the same time. As with CCF in general, the maximum value of individual trees should be preferred over the maximum volume production of a stand and this can be achieved through selective interventions. However, it is important that trees with desirable phenotypes have the opportunity to regenerate prior to their removal (Davies et al. 2008).

Shelterwood systems typically reduce precipitation reaching the forest floor due to the remaining main canopy trees. In group systems, more precipitation reaches the forest floor in the gaps, however, wind turbulences can be strong in large groups and can cause damage on residual main canopy trees at the edges. Large canopy openings can trigger localised waterlogged soils due to a lack of interception by main canopy trees and a lack of water consumption. They are also more susceptible to frost events.

In the past, the remaining main canopy trees were more or less simultaneously removed, when regeneration was sufficiently secured. This simple way of removing the remnants of the overstorey has increasingly given way to target-diameter harvesting (see Sect. 3.6.1) staggered in time: Once regeneration is established and safe, overstorey trees are individually removed depending on their size. The target size (usually judged by stem diameter) is species specific and in commercial scenarios mainly depends on the requirements of local and/or international markets. In a conservation context, more general ecological considerations such as habitat requirements apply.

3.7.1 Uniform Shelterwood System

This method involves a uniform, moderate opening of the crown canopy, either on the whole stand area or in parts of the stand, with the aim of establishing relatively even-aged, uniform regeneration underneath. The uniform shelterwood system is one of the oldest silvicultural systems going back to the 18th century, when it was designed for regenerating European beech (*Fagus sylvatica* L.). An initial seeding felling establishes understorey light conditions suitable for regeneration, although suitable conditions may already have been created by regular thinnings preceding the first shelterwood cut, particularly where less light-demanding species are involved. In stands where seeding is infrequent or irregular, or where admitting sufficient light for regeneration is likely to lead to strong growth of competing ground vegetation, the seeding felling should be timed to coincide with a good seed year. Following this, the remaining overstorey trees are removed in a series of interventions, the number of which depends upon the growth of regeneration, the stability of the overstorey trees, and, particularly for broadleaves, the time at which overstorey trees reach their target diameter. If initial regeneration is sparse or if the species to be regenerated is frost tender, it may be necessary to prolong the retention of the overstorey. Generally speaking, following the seeding felling, a broadleaved overstorey can be removed over 5–30 years in two to six interventions, and a conifer overstorey over 15–30 years in three to six interventions. In each shelterwood cutting, no more than 50–80 m^3 per ha for broadleaves or 50–100 m^3 per ha for conifers should be removed. Gap size and resulting light conditions in uniform shelterwood systems are uniform, hence the name of the system and there is hardly any direct sun light.

The uniform shelterwood approach is particularly suitable for intermediate or shade-tolerant species such as beech (*Fagus spp.*) or spruce (*Picea spp.*). More light-demanding species, such as ash (*Fraxinus spp.*), oak (*Quercus spp.*), Scots pine (*Pinus sylvestris* L.) and Japanese larch (*Larix kaempferi* (LAMB.) CARR.), require low canopy cover (<40%) and the rapid removal of the remaining overstorey if regeneration is to be successful. Of all the shelterwood systems, the uniform approach best retains woodland climate. A uniform opening of the canopy is comparatively easy to achieve as a natural consequence of ongoing, regular thinnings, and the establishment of even-aged regeneration promotes timber quality in the successor stand, particularly in broadleaves. However, if regeneration fellings are not managed carefully according to individual species requirements, frame trees may be exposed to sun scorch in some climates, to epicormic growth or to windthrow. As regeneration occurs throughout the stand, directional felling on to extraction racks is necessary to prevent damage to the successor stand. Uniform shelterwood systems provide optimal protection against frost and often an abundance of regeneration trees is produced, which can lead to increased respacing costs (Davies et al. 2008).

A uniform shelterwood system can also be combined with artificial regeneration: Under the light canopy of the overstorey another or the same species can be planted. This is often considered a good compromise, because the planted trees are nursed by the overstorey and the spacing between them can therefore be quite wide, i.e. less plants are needed compared to planting on bare land after clearfelling.

A special application of the uniform shelterwood system is the *nurse crop system.* The method is a way of establishing diverse woodlands from scratch on bare land and as such is used in afforestation and restocking. The idea is to establish a "nurse crop" of fast-growing early successional species such as common alder (*Alnus gluti-nosa* (L.) GAERTN.), birch (*Betula spp.*) or aspen (*Populus tremula* L.) by planting at a comparatively wide spacing. Usually at the same time or a little later, late successional species are introduced as target species by (under)planting. Because of the difference in growth dynamics, the early successional species grow rapidly and form an open, upper canopy that protects the slow-growing, late-successional target species (Pommerening and Murphy 2004).

3.7.2   Seed Tree System

The seed tree system lies part-way between clearfelling and the uniform shelterwood. It is but a small step from clearfelling and is often used to mitigate the negative environmental and aesthetic impacts of this more radical harvesting method. Like the uniform shelterwood system, the seed tree system involves a uniform reduction in canopy cover throughout a stand in order to stimulate regeneration. In the seed tree approach, however, the reduction is far more extreme, leaving no more than 50 seed trees (also referred to as standards) per hectare (Mason and Kerr, 2004) and the positive effects of canopy shelter are largely lost. The system is most suitable for hardy light-demanding species with wind-dispersed seeds, chiefly birch (*Betula spp.*), larch (*Larix spp.*) and pine (*Pinus spp.*) species. The prospective standards need to be trained a few years in advance to build up a sufficient degree of individual-tree stability. Depending on species and ground vegetation, it may be necessary to time the seeding felling to coincide with a seed year and ground preparation in the form of scarification may be required. In Scandinavia and North America, this system is also known as *green tree retention* and mainly applied for diversifying clearfelling sites but also for conservation (Rose and Muir 1997; Sullivan and Sullivan 2017). The sparsity of mature tree cover can potentially encourage competing ground vegetation to take hold for some time (Davies et al. 2008).

3.7.3   Strip Shelterwood

Another shelterwood approach in which regeneration is concentrated in specific areas is the strip shelterwood system. In this case, strips roughly one tree length (typically around 30 m) in width are either clearfelled (in which case this is properly referred to simply as the "strip system") or are subjected to heavy seed-tree fellings to leave only a small number of mature residual trees or standards. This silvicultural system is not far from clearfelling and the seed tree system, as the strip cuttings are either small clearfells or small seed tree systems staggered in time. The strips need not be straight and can be shaped to follow stand boundaries or topographical features, e.g. by forming bays and wedges. The strip shelterwood system creates two distinctive zones, each with some degree of woodland climate. The inner zone, between the new overstorey boundary and one tree length into the stand, is suitable for the regeneration of moderately shade-tolerant species. The outer zone, between the new overstorey frontier and the limit of noon shade in summer, is suitable for the regeneration of intermediate and light-demanding species. An adjacent strip is cut in the next intervention. In this way the strips advance across the stand at each intervention with the total regeneration period depending on the rate at which regeneration establishes and on the size of stand: In very large stands, more than one strip system can be established. The successor stand is even-aged in strip direction, and uneven-aged, with a clear age gradient, in the direction of strip progression (Davies et al. 2008).

The strip shelterwood system can be a secure approach in areas with higher wind hazard and wind prone species. Also, it is easy to apply even with little experience. Strips should be cut perpendicular to the prevailing wind direction, in the lee of the unopened part of the stand. Although well protected from prevailing winds, this arrangement of strips is still vulnerable to gales from other directions. Obviously, only the most stable trees in the stand should be retained as standards in each strip. After considering the prevailing wind direction, in the Northern Hemisphere south-facing strips should also be avoided in all but the most moist climates, because of the risk of drought and sunburn.

The strip shelterwood system is potentially very useful, being generally more robust to wind damage than the group shelterwood and also suitable for the regeneration of both light-demanding and shade-tolerant species, in pure stands or in mixtures. The side shelter provided by the adjacent unopened stand may be less effective than overhead shelter in limiting the effects of drought and frost (Matthews 1991). Light conditions vary a lot in strip shelterwood systems. Damage to regeneration can be avoided more easily than with most other systems, as there are fewer trees to be felled in regenerating areas, and these can be felled into and extracted through the unopened stand. However, the system tends to come with little flexibility.

3.7.4 Group Shelterwood

An alternative to the uniform opening of the main crown canopy is to arrange shelterwood cuts in groups, generally in order to encourage the development of existing regeneration or after a preparatory uniform shelterwood cut. For light-demanding species, the group overstorey may be removed entirely in this first felling. Sometimes this variant is referred to simply as the "group system". Otherwise, the successful establishment of regeneration is followed by the gradual removal of the group overstorey and in both cases groups are gradually widened. In each intervention, new groups may be created. Ultimately, the expanding cones of regeneration coalesce. The regeneration period is likely to be 20–50 years.

The opening of distinct gaps permits the regeneration of light-demanding species, and is also important for securing regeneration of very shade-tolerant species such as beech (*Fagus sylvatica* L.), hornbeam (*Carpinus betulus* L.), lime (*Tilia spp.*) or silver fir (*Abies alba* MILL.). For shade-tolerant and intermediate species, initial shelterwood groups should be no more than one tree length in width between the edges of the crowns of the surrounding trees. For light-demanding species, groups should be at least one tree length or 30 m wide. Group radius should be increased by 10–30 m in each subsequent intervention. North and north-east patches of groups can be prone to drought effects due to a combination of rain shelter and strong sun radiation in the Northern Hemisphere (Davies et al. 2008).

Groups are sometimes expanded elliptically towards the south or south-west to provide more suitable microclimatic conditions for the target species. In mountain forests, ellipses are generally favoured to groups. They are a compromise between light and cover requirements. For example for regenerating Norway spruce (*Picea abies* L.) in the Swiss Alps 50–70 m long and 15–20 m wide elliptic openings were recommended for north-facing sites, whilst smaller gaps were proposed on south-facing slopes where light is widely available to avoid drought effects. The main considerations for the design of elliptic groups in mountain forests are to grant seedlings sufficient light, to reduce snow cover and not to trigger avalanches in winter. The best orientation of elliptic groups in the Swiss Alps was found to be north-east to south-west (Streit et al. 2009).

In some cases the spacing of groups is determined by the occurrence of patchy advance regeneration. In other cases, where advance regeneration is more uniform, the spacing of groups may be optimised so that when they expand they eventually cover the entire stand area with minimal overlap. The ideal spacing depends on initial gap radius, the increase in radius with each intervention, the number of interventions and the intended regeneration period.

The group shelterwood approach is potentially very useful as it creates a range of microclimates and light regimes suitable for species with different light and climate requirements and has therefore often been considered for regenerating mixed-species forests. Gaps give rise to turbulent air flow over the canopy surface and also allow wind entry into the stand leading to increased wind hazard. Although damage to regeneration is easily avoided in the early stages by felling away from the centre of gaps, it becomes increasingly challenging as the last overstorey trees are felled and extracted.

Group systems are close to regeneration processes in natural Central European forests involving small disturbance patches.

3.7.5   Irregular Shelterwood

In some cases it may be desirable or necessary to open the crown canopy of a stand in an irregular fashion, thus producing a more uneven-aged successor stand than in the uniform shelterwood system. This irregular approach may be adopted because of variations in ground conditions, the occurrence of groups of advance regeneration or the particular requirements of desired species. The system usually leads to a more diverse stand structure than the shelterwood systems described previously. The removal of the overstorey is considerably more gradual than in the uniform shelterwood system. As with the uniform system much depends on the stability and target diameter of the remaining trees. A perceived advantage of this system compared to the uniform shelterwood system is that resulting natural regeneration is usually less abundant with sparser and thinner branches thus decreasing the need for costly respacings/pre-commercial thinnings and artificial pruning.

The irregular shelterwood system is preferable to the uniform system for mixed stands, particularly mixtures of species with different light requirements, as it allows greater flexibility in the management of understorey light conditions. Without careful control, however, shade-tolerant species will be favoured at the expense of light demanders. Resulting stands tend to be complex with a wider range of sizes and offer potential benefits for amenity and habitat creation. However, the dispersed nature of thinning/harvesting and regeneration mean that operations require more effort to manage. Skill is required in all operations to avoid damage to trees of all sizes. An irregular shelterwood system in progress is often hard to distinguish from a group selection system (Davies et al. 2008).

3.7.6   Shelterwood Combinations

It is possible to combine shelterwood approaches and Rittershofer (1999) referred to these combinations as "additive methods". The most common case is the group-strip shelterwood system (see Fig. 3.15). In this system, shelterwood groups are opened up to 100–150 m into the stand from the leeward edge. A strip shelterwood is then initiated from the same sheltered edge. As the strips advance towards the windward edge of the stand, existing groups are expanded and new groups are cut up to 100–150 m ahead of the strips. Although canopy gaps are opened and enlarged, potentially risking turbulence and wind damage are kept towards the relatively well-protected leeward side of the stand, where in any case the advancing strip shelterwood feelings remove all but the most stable individuals. This combination of methods provides a wide range of growing conditions for tree species with differing demands and can give rise to very heterogeneous stands.

Essentially there is no limit to experimenting with various combinations of silvicultural systems and this is clearly encouraged in an attempt to identify the best method for a given site and tree population.

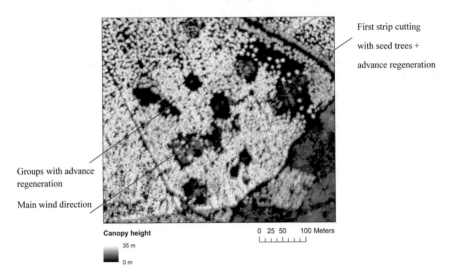

Fig. 3.15 Example of a group-strip shelterwood system with Sitka spruce (*Pinus sitchensis* (BONG.) CARR.) in progress. LiDAR-derived canopy height model (1 m spatial resolution) for block 3, Cefn Du, Clocaenog Forest, North Wales, UK in 2006. Data courtesy of Rachel Gaulton

3.7.7   Single-Tree and Group Selection

Originally invented by farmers with small forest ownerships (Schütz 2001b), the single-tree selection system is characterised by felling and regeneration spread throughout the stand and occurring simultaneously. The system represents a kind of process conservation, where a forest stand is permanently kept in a disturbance and regeneration phase. Ideally, individual trees are harvested when they reach their target dimensions and regeneration occurs in the gaps created by their removal leading to a completely uneven-aged stand in which many tree sizes and cohorts are intimately mixed. Target diameter harvesting alone, however, will not preserve the desired stand structure or ensure sustained yields of timber. All of the operations typical of the management of an even-aged stand such as thinnings must be carried out in the various cohorts and canopy layers spread throughout the stand, although this is often taken care of by biological automation, i.e. natural processes. Diffuse operations can be challenging to plan, execute and control. Thinnings are generally carried out at the same time as the harvesting of large trees (Davies et al. 2008).

Single-tree selection is particularly suitable for relatively shade-tolerant species, as regeneration is often obliged to germinate and grow in comparatively small gaps created by the removal of individual trees, where light is extremely limited. If harvesting is carried out frequently, it is possible to take advantage of all seed years. It is also possible to keep particularly promising trees growing for as long as they continue to grow, without compromising the regeneration of the stand. The presence of many canopy strata helps to suppress branching on the lower parts of stems, although heavy branching in well-developed crowns leads to large knots in upper stem parts. Selection forests can be extremely aesthetically pleasing, are very suitable to community and recreational forests because they conform to many common conceptions of the appearance of natural forests with trees of all sizes standing side by side. Considerable skill is needed for the marking of thinnings and the execution of felling and extraction operations, and yields are less easy to forecast than in even-aged stands. Thinnings in selection systems are mainly selective crown thinnings aimed at predominant trees, however, they are carried out to maintain the particular equilibrium of tree sizes that retains a forest stand in the aforementioned permanent disturbance and regeneration phase. Since this thinning approach is quite special, thinnings in selection systems are termed *selection thinnings* to distinguish them from the more general selective thinnings (Schütz 2001b).

The classic Norway spruce, European silver fir and beech selection forests of Central Europe are confined to the mountainous regions of the Vosges, Jura, Alps and Carpathians, where permanent forest cover on steep valley sides is vital to guard against avalanche and rock fall (Matthews 1991). This combination of species seems ideally suited to management by single-tree selection (Anderson 1960), however, the selection system is certainly not limited to this combination of species (see for example Schütz and Pommerening (2013) for experience with a Douglas fir (*Pseudotsuga menziesii* (MIRB.) FRANCO) selection forest in North Wales).

The group selection system is an alternative to single-tree selection that makes allowances for the regeneration of light-demanding species. Here the unit of harvesting is a group of trees rather than an individual. The size of groups depends on the shade tolerance of the species to be regenerated, and also on the predicted crown size of trees of target dimensions (Matthews 1991). Wind risk may be increased by the cutting of definite gaps, but surrounding groups are likely to have been exposed to the wind at some stage during their development and, if well managed, should be relatively windfirm.

The fascination with the single-tree selection system has tempted many researchers to develop guideline models describing a supposedly ideal exponential stem-diameter distribution. The idea of these demographic models was to assist forest managers in deriving thinning intensity and thinning cycles. O'Hara (2014) gives an overview and detailed, dynamic models are described in Schütz (2001b), Schütz and Pommerening (2013) and Brzeziecki et al. (2016). However, individual-based models such as those discussed in Sect. 5.2 are more likely to give better guidance.

3.7.8 Managing Regeneration and Juvenile Trees

After successful regeneration, the cohorts of small trees were traditionally subjected to a series of *respacings* and *pre-commercial thinnings* for reducing stem numbers in several steps. These usually started earlier in conifers (particularly when spruce (*Picea spp.*) was involved) and later in broadleaves to allow the development of straight, single stems in commercial scenarios (Röhrig et al. 2006; Smith et al. 1997). Since these types of thinnings are very costly and the results have not always been satisfying, the concept of *biological rationalisation* has recently been pioneered by Peter Ammann (Silvicultural Competence Centre, Lyss) and others in Switzerland to cut costs. The fundamental idea of this approach is to leave naturally regenerated forest stands for about 20–25 years (or up to a top height of 15–20 m) completely to natural devices including processes such as self-thinning, natural pruning and self-differentiation. Wilhelm and Rieger (2018) referred to this period as *qualification phase* (Q), since during this time some trees naturally improve in timber quality and size dominance so that they eventually qualify as frame trees. Once young stands have reached this target, frame tree selection among dominant, good quality trees would kick in as described in Sect. 3.6.1 and frame trees would be released by initially removing all other trees within a radius of for example 7 m and then by selectively removing 1–3 competitors in 2–3 subsequent interventions (Schütz et al. 2015). The initial intervention would also include the cutting of extraction racks. Wilhelm and Rieger (2018) referred to this period of successive selective, frame-tree based thinnings as *dimensioning phase* (D), where they place particular importance on the crown development of frame trees. This Q-D method of biological rationalisation not only markedly reduces management costs, but also consistently applies the principles of individual-based forest management (Wilhelm and Rieger 2018).

References

Abetz P, Klädtke J (2002) The target tree management system. Forstwissenschaftliches Centralblatt 121:73–82

Anderson ML (1953) Plea for the adoption of the standing control or check in woodland management. Scott For 7:38–47

Anderson ML (1960) Norway spruce - silver fir - beech mixed selection forest. Scott For 14:87–93

Aplet GH, Johnson H, Olson JT, Sample VA (1993) Defining sustainable forestry. Island Press, Washington, 320 p

Assmann E (1970) The principles of forest yield study. Studies in the organic production, structure, increment and yield of forest stands. Pergamon Press. Oxford, 506 p

Bettinger P, Boston K, Siry JP, Grebner DL (2009) Forest management and planning. Academic Press, Elsevier Inc., Burlington, 331 p

Bončina A (2011) Conceptual approaches to integrate nature conservation into forest management: a central European perspective. Int For Rev 13:13–22

Bruciamacchie M, Pierrat J-C, Tomasini J (2005) Modèles explicatif et marginal de la stratégie de martelage d'une parcelle irrégulière. [Explicative and marginal models for a marking strategy of an unevenaged stand.] Ann For Sci 62:727–736

Brzeziecki B, Pommerening A, Miścicki S, Drozdowski S, Żybura H (2016) A common lack of demographic equilibrium among tree species in Białowieża National Park (NE Poland): evidence from long-term plots. J Veg Sci 27:460–469

Burschel P, Huss J (1997) Grundriss des Waldbaus. [Outline of silviculture.] Parey Buchverlag, Berlin, 488 p

Busse J (1935) Gruppendurchforstung. [Group thinning.] Silva 19:145–147

Cade BS, Noon BR (2003) A gentle introduction to quantile regression for ecologists. Front Ecol Environ 8:412–420

Churchill DC, Larson AJ, Dahlgreen MC, Franklin JF, Hessburg PF, Lutz JA (2013) Restoring forest resilience: from reference spatial patterns to silvicultural prescriptions and monitoring. For Ecol Manag 291:442–457

Coates KD, Canham CD, Beaudet M, Sachs DL, Messier C (2003) Use of a spatially explicit individual-tree model (SORTIE/BC) to explore the implications of patchiness in structurally complex forests. For Ecol Manag 186:297–310

Davies O, Haufe J, Pommerening A (2008) Silvicultural principles of continuous cover forestry - a guide to best practice. Bangor University, Bangor, 111 p

de Groot RS, Wilson MA, Boumans RMJ (2002) A typology for the classification, description and valuation of ecosystem functions, goods and services. Ecol Econ 41:393–408

Dengler A (1944) Waldbau auf ökologischer Grundlage. [Silviculture on an ecological basis.], 3rd edn. Berlin, 560 p

Dodson EK, Ares A, Puettmann KJ (2012) Early responses to thinning treatments designed to accelerate late successional forest structure in young coniferous stands of western Oregon, USA. Can J For Res 42:345–355

Gadow Kv (2005) Forsteinrichtung – Analyse und Entwurf der Waldentwicklung. [Forest planning – analysis and outline of forest development.] Universitätsverlag Göttingen. Göttingen, 342 p

Gadow Kv, Bredenkamp B (1992) Forest management. Academia, Pretoria, 151 p

Gadow Kv, Stüber V (1994) Die Inventuren der Forsteinrichtung. [Forest management inventories.] Forst und Holz 49:129–131

Garfitt JE (1994) Natural managements of woods - continuous cover forestry. Research Studies Press LTD, Taunton, 152 p

Hart H (1991) Practical forestry for the agent and surveyor, 3rd edn. Sutton Publishing, Thrupp Stroud, 658 p

Hasel K (1985) Forstgeschichte. [Forestry History.] Ein Grundriss für Studium und Praxis. Verlag Paul Parey, Berlin, 258 p

Hasenauer H (1997) Dimensional relationships of open-grown trees in Austria. For Ecol Manag 96:197–206

Helms JA (ed) (1998) The dictionary of forestry. Society of American foresters. Bethesda, 210 p

Kimmins JP (2004) Forest ecology - a foundation for sustainable management, 3rd edn. Pearson Education Prentice Hall, Upper Saddle River, 700 p

Köstler J (1956) Silviculture. Oliver and Boyd, Edinburgh, 416 p

Kraft G (1884) Beiträge zur Lehre von Durchforstungen, Schlagstellungen und Lichtungshieben. [On the methodology of thinnings, shelterwood cuttings and heavy release operations.] Hanover, 154 p

Kramer H (1988) Waldwachstumslehre. [Forest growth and yield science.] Verlag Paul Parey, Hamburg and Berlin, 374 p

Li Y, Ye S, Hui G, Hu Y, Zhao Z (2014) Spatial structure of timber harvested according to structure-based forest management. For Ecol Manag 322:106–116

Mason WL, Kerr G (2001) Transforming even-aged conifer stands to continuous cover management. Forestry commission information note, vol 40. Forestry Commission, Edinburgh, 8 p

Matthews JD (1991) Silvicultural sytems. Clarendon Press, Oxford, 284 p

Mayer H (1984) Waldbau auf soziologisch-ökologischer Grundlage. [Silviculture on a sociological-ecological basis.], 3rd edn. Gustav Fischer Verlag, Stuttgart, 514 p

Messier C, Puettmann KJ, Coates KD (2013) Managing forests as complex adaptive systems. Building resilience to the challenge of global change, Routledge, Oxon, 353 p

Mülder D (1990) Nur Individuenauswahl oder auch Gruppenauswahl?. [Selection of individuals only or group selection as well?] Schriften aus der Forstlichen Fakultät der Universität Göttingen und der Niedersächsischen Forstlichen Versuchsanstalt, vol 96. Göttingen, 53 p

Nyland RD (2002) Silviculture. Concepts and applications, 2nd edn. Waveland Press, Long Grove, 682 p

O'Hara KL (2014) Multiaged silviculture. Managing for complex forest stand structures. Oxford University Press, Oxford, 213 p

Ouden Jd, Muys B, Mohren F, Verheyen K (2010) Bosecologie en bosbeheer [Forest ecology and silviculture.] Acco, Leuven, 674 p

Pommerening A, Murphy ST (2004) A review of the history, definitions and methods of continuous cover forestry with special attention to afforestation and restocking. Forestry 77:27–44

Poore A (2011) The marteloscope - a training aid for continuous cover forest management. Woodl Herit 2011:28–29

Pretzsch H (1996) Erfassung des Pflegezustandes von Waldbeständen bei der zweiten Bundeswald-inventur. [Monitoring forest management in the second national forest inventory of Germany.] AFZ/DerWald 15:820–823

Pretzsch H (2009) Forest dynamics, growth and yield. From measurement to model. Springer, Heidelberg, 664 p

Price M, Price C (2006) Creaming the best, or creatively transforming? Might felling the biggest trees first be a win-win strategy? For Ecol Manag 224:297–303

Puettmann K, Coates KD, Messier C (2009) A critique of silviculture. Island Press, Washington, 204 p

Pukkala T, Gadow Kv (eds) (2012) Continuous cover forestry, 2nd edn. Springer, Dordrecht, 296 p

Putz FE, Zuidema PA, Synnott T, Peña-Claros M, Pinard MA, Sheil D, Vanclay JK, Sist P, Gourlet-Fleury S, Griscom B, Palmer J, Zagt R (2012) A typology for the classification, description and valuation of ecosystem functions, goods and services. Conserv Lett 5:296–303

Rajala T, Illian J (2012) A family of spatial biodiversity measures based on graphs. Environ Ecol Stat 19:545–572

Reininger H (2001) Das Plenterprinzip. [The selection principle.] Leopold Stocker Verlag, Graz, 238 p

Rittershofer F (1999) Waldpflege und Waldbau. Gisela Rittershofer Verlag, Freising, 492 p

Roberts SD, Harrington CA (2008) Individual tree growth response to variable-density thinning in coastal Pacific Northwest forests. For Ecol Manag 255:2771–2781

Röhrig E, Bartsch N, Lüpke Bv, (2006) Waldbau auf ökologischer Grundlage. [Silviculture on an ecological basis]. Verlag Eugen Ulmer Stuttgart. Stuttgart, 479 p

Rose TP, Muir D (1997) Consequences for timber production in forests of the Western Cascades, Oregon. Ecol Appl 7:209–217

Rozsnyay Z (1979) Forstgeschichtliche Betrachtungen zur Entstehung der Kraftschen Baumklassen. [Historical reflections on the origin of crown classes]. Allgemeine Forst- und Jagdzeitung 150:65–72

Savill PS (1991) The silviculture of trees used in British forestry. CAB International, Wallingford, 143 p

Schädelin W (1934) Die Durchforstung als Auslese- und Veredlungsbetrieb höchster Wertleistung. [Selective thinnings for achieving high-quality timber.] Haupt, Bern, 96 p

Schütz JP (2001a) Opportunities and strategies of transforming regular forests to irregular forests. For Ecol Manag 151:87–94

Schütz JP (2001b) Der Plenterwald und weitere Formen strukturierter und gemischter Wälder. [The selection forest and other types of structured and mixed species forests.] Parey Buchverlag, Berlin, 207 p

Schütz JP (2003) Waldbau I. Die Prinzipien der Waldnutzung und der Waldbehandlung. Skript zur Vorlesung Waldbau I. [Silviculture I. The principles of forest exploitation and forest management. Notes accompanying the lectures in silviculture I.] Unpublished manuscript. ETH Zürich, 212 p

Schütz JP, Pommerening A (2013) Can Douglas fir (Pseudotsuga menziesii (Mirb.) Franco) sustainably grow in complex forest structures? For Ecol Manag 303:175–183

Schütz JP, Ammann PL, Zingg A (2015) Optimising the yield of Douglas-fir with an appropriate thinning regime. Eur J For Res 134:469–480

Schweizerischer F (1925) Die forstlichen Verhältnisse der Schweiz. [Forestry in Switzerland.], 2nd edn. Kommissionsverlag von Beer & Cie, Zürich, 276 p

Smith DM, Larson BC, Kelty MJ, Ashton PMS (1997) The practice of silviculture: applied forest ecology, 9th edn. Wiley, New York, 537 p

Speidel G (1972) Planung im Forstbetrieb. Grundlagen und Methoden der Forsteinrichtung. [Planning in a forest enterprise. Basics and Methods of forest planning.] Parey Buchverlag, Berlin, 267 p

Spiecker H, Hansen J, Klimo E, Skovsgaard JP, Sterba H, Teuffel Kv (2004) Norway spruce conversion – options, and consequences. European forest institute research report, vol 18. Koninklijke Brill NV, Leiden, 269 p

Sterba H, Zingg A (2001) Target diameter harvesting - a strategy to convert even-aged forests. For Ecol Manag 151:95–105

Streit K, Wunder J, Brang P (2009) Slit-shaped gaps are a successful silvicultural technique to promote Picea abies regeneration in mountain forests of the Swiss Alps. For Ecol Manag 257:1902–1909

Sullivan TP, Sullivan D (2017) Green-tree retention and recovery of an old-forest specialist, the southern red-backed vole (Myodes gapperi), 20 years after harvest. Wildl Res 44:669–680

Susse R, Allegrini C, Bruciamacchie M, Burrus R (2011) Management of irregular forests. Developing the full potential of the forest. Azur Multimedia, Saint Maime, 144 p

Thomasius H (1990) Waldbau 1. Allgemeine Grundlagen. Hochschulstudium Forstingenieurwesen. [Silviculture 1. General basics.] Leisnig, 180 p

Toman MA, Ashton PM (1996) Sustainable forest ecosystems and management: a review article. For Sci 42:366–377

Troup RS (1928) Silvicultural systems. Oxford University Press, Oxford, 199 p

United Nations, 2001 United Nations sustainable development – agenda 21. http://www.un.org/esa/sustdev/documents/index.htm

Vítková L, Ní Dhubháin Á (2013) Transformation to continuous cover forestry: a review Irish. Forestry 70:119–140

Weihs U (1999) Waldpflege. Ein geeignetes Instrument zur nachhaltigen Sicherung der vielfältigen Waldfunktionen. [Forest management. A suitable method for sustaining multiple forest functions.] Förderverein des Fachbereichs Forstwirtschaft und Umweltmanagement. Göttingen, 308 p

Wenk G, Antanaitis V, Šmelko Š (1990) Waldertragslehre. [Forest growth and yield science.] Deutscher Landwirtschaftsverlag. Berlin, 448 p

Whitefield P (2004) The earth care manual: a permaculture handbook for Britain and other temperate climates. Hyden House Limited, East Meon, 381p

Wikström P, Edenius L, Elfving B, Eriksson LO, Lämås T, Sonesson J, Öhman K, Wallerman J, Waller C, Klintebäck F (2011) The Heureka forestry decision support system: an overview. Math Comput For Nat-Resour Sci 3:87–94

Wilhelm GJ, Rieger H (2018) Naturnahe Waldwirtschaft mit der QD-Strategie. [Near-natural forest management based on the QD strategy.] Eugen Ulmer, Stuttgart, 217 p

Willis JL, Roberts SD, Harrington CA (2018) Variable density thinning promotes variable structural responses 14 years after treatment in the Pacific Northwest. For Ecol Manag 410:114–125

Chapter 4
Spatial Methods of Tree Interaction Analysis

Abstract In this chapter, spatial methods, particularly in the field of point process statistics are introduced. These methods have markedly improved our ability to study and measure statistical tree interactions in the last twenty to thirty years. Point process statistics is a universal theory, which is not unique to forest ecology and management but has been developed in mathematical statistics and successfully applied in various fields of natural sciences. Specifically the methods described in this chapter assist in uncovering the underlying ecological and management processes that have caused the studied pattern and prepare modelling. Following the presentation of the most important concepts, recent research results achieved with these methods are demonstrated. The R code provided helps to understand and to reproduce the concepts. Towards the end of the chapter we discuss important technical issues relating to edge-bias compensation and hypothesis testing.

4.1 Spatial Statistics for Plant Pattern Analysis

During the last 50 years spatial statistics has emerged as a special branch of statistics with a wide range of methods that have considerably improved our ability to identify and quantify spatial plant patterns and opened the possibility of linking them to environmental processes. Most of these methods were first devised in mathematical statistics and later found applications in various fields of natural sciences. Eminent statistical scientists such as Bartlett, Matérn, Matheron and their successors Cressie, Diggle, Penttinen, Ripley and Stoyan have laid the foundations of modern spatial statistics and the analysis of forest data has become a natural field for application of spatial statistics. This development has been paralleled with significant progress in mapping and surveying as well as in general computer technology. During the same period ecologists and forest scientists have often independently developed various unrelated quantitative concepts to describe and to model spatial plant patterns and based on them measures of structure, diversity and competition.

In a nutshell, spatial statistics is a methodology for describing and modelling the uncertainty of the spatial dimension in data. More explicitly spatial statistics aims to provide quantitative descriptions of natural variables distributed in space or in time

© Springer Nature Switzerland AG 2019

A. Pommerening and P. Grabarnik, *Individual-based Methods*
in Forest Ecology and Management, https://doi.org/10.1007/978-3-030-24528-3_4

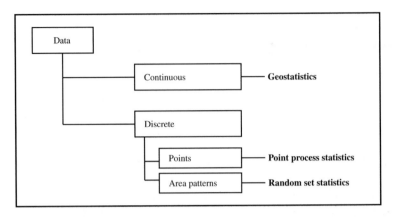

Fig. 4.1 Spatial data in forest ecology and management

and space. The nature of spatial data, however, can differ considerably. There are two main spatial data types, i.e. those that have a *continuous* nature and those that are naturally *discrete*. The former are at least theoretically defined at any location in forest ecosystems. This data group includes environmental variables such as wind, temperature and precipitation. Continuous data are considered in *geostatistics* (see Sect. 4.2), a very prominent field of spatial statistics (Fig. 4.1).

Discrete data are not defined at all possible locations in space. Tree locations, for example, are often determined by stem or crown centre locations and it is sufficient to describe such study objects as points. Similar applications include fox dens, bird nests and springs. These are typical applications of point process statistics.

Sometimes study objects cannot be well represented by single points, but rather by sets of points where individual points have merged. Image data from terrestrial or airborne laser scans, digital cameras or aerial photography often provide such information, where it is impossible, unnatural or very difficult to distinguish between individual objects such as individual trees. These are typical applications of *random-set statistics*. In the simplest case the interaction of sets of black and white pixels are studied (see Sect. 4.3).

This chapter focusses on *point process statistics* (see Sect. 4.4) because this field is best suited for studying tree interactions as part of individual-based forest ecology and management. For completeness we included brief characterisations of geostatistics and random set statistics as well.

4.2 Geostatistics

Geostatistics is that branch of statistics which studies the variability and prediction of *regionalised* variables (Chilès and Delfiner 1999; Wackernagel 2003). Such variables can take values anywhere in the two- or three-dimensional space under study, for example in a forest stand or forest block. Examples are precipitation and pollution.

Stem diameter is not a regionalised variable, since it can be defined only at tree locations. Geostatistics has found a wide range of applications in forest science (see for example Jansen et al. 2002), typically in the analysis of covariates of forest point patterns (see Sect. 4.4). Sample data for a regionalised variable $Z(\xi)$ are gathered at discrete points, ω_i, which are chosen by the investigator, often following a systematic grid or lattice.

One of the key applications in geostatistics is *spatial interpolation*. The value $Z(\xi)$ at a location of interest, ξ, different from the sampling locations, ω_i, can be estimated through a number of interpolation methods which include kriging, splines and weighted moving averages as well as regression techniques (Cressie 1993; Chilès and Delfiner 1999; Jansen et al. 2002), see Fig. 4.2. Spatial interpolation is an important pre-requisite for producing maps of the whole study area and some of these methods are implemented in Geographic Information Systems (GIS). Kriging is a least squares prediction method using a special second-order summary characteristic, the *(semi)variogram*, $\gamma(\mathbf{r})$. It is the mean squared difference of the values of the regionalised variable at ξ and $\xi + \mathbf{r}$ divided by 2, where $\mathbf{r}$ is a difference vector of length r:

$$\gamma(\mathbf{r}) = \frac{1}{2}\mathrm{E}(Z(\xi) - Z(\xi + \mathbf{r}))^2 \qquad (4.1)$$

The variogram characterises the spatial variability of a given regionalised variable $Z(\xi)$ at points ξ and $\xi + \mathbf{r}$ (Wackernagel 2003; Illian et al. 2008). Its values for different $\mathbf{r}$ give information on the behaviour of $Z(\xi)$ for arbitrary spatial scales.

Two important assumptions in the realm of geostatistics are that 1. the sample points, ω_i, are independent of the regionalised variable and 2. values measured at points close together in space tend to be similar. Violations against the first assumption can lead to estimation bias.

Three examples of many applications in forest science are given here. In a case study Jansen et al. (2002) used geostatistical methods to improve the ecological site description for forest plannning in the Harz mountains (Lower Saxony, Germany). Humus content, rooting depth and mean annual air temperature were some of the regionalised variables estimated for the whole mountain range from sample points. In New Zealand, Payn et al. (1999) applied variogram and kriging methods to monitor changes in forest productivity and nutrition using site index and basal area index as regionalised variables. Finally, Zawadzki et al. (2005) reviewed the application of geostatistics for investigations into forest ecosystems using remote sensing imagery. These authors concentrated on three main aspects, 1. the spatial variability of features identified from digital images, 2. the estimation of biophysical forest parameters and of variables of forest ecosystem structure and 3. forest classification methods.

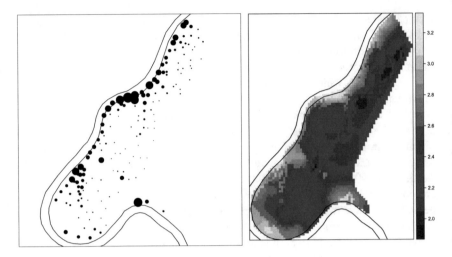

Fig. 4.2 The publicly available "Meuse" dataset (R package sp, Burrough and McDonnell 1998) includes 155 observations taken from the top 0–20 cm of alluvial soils in a 5 × 2 km part of the right bank of the floodplain of the river Meuse near Stein in Limburg province (NL). Sampling locations weighted by zink concentration (left) and spatial interpolation using the spherical variogram model and universal kriging (zink concentration given in logarithmic scale)

4.3 Random Set Statistics

Random sets serve as mathematical models for irregular geometrical patterns. Simple examples of random sets, denoted for example by X, include the part of a landscape covered with forest or the part of the forest floor occupied by vascular plants and shrubs. In some sense, a random set is simply a special case of a regionalised variable, one that takes only the values 0 or 1, where values of 0 are depicted as white (vacant) and values of 1 as black (occupied) pixels. Fundamentals of the theory of random sets are given in Chiu et al. (2013).

A random set model featuring in many publications is the *germ-grain model*, the simplest case of which is the Boolean model (also known as Boolean scheme, Poisson germ-grain model, Poissonian penetrable grain model, fully penetrable grain system or homogeneous system of overlapping particles), see Fig. 4.3. The "germs" of this model are points that form a Poisson point process and the grains are discs with radius r around each point. The Boolean model considers the set-theoretic union of all these discs that includes the possibility that the sets overlap and leads to patches. For this theoretical model formulae are known for all important summary characteristics, see the equation in Fig. 4.5. Boolean-type models are very suitable for describing irregular patterns observed in nature. The model was, for example, applied to the pattern of lichens on a stone in Chiu et al. (2013). Diggle (1981) used the Boolean model for describing the spatial distribution of heather (*Calluna vulgaris* (L.) HULL) in a forest.

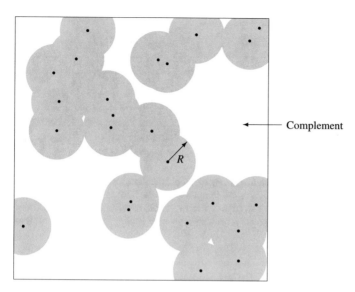

Fig. 4.3 Mosaic of overlapping and non-overlapping grains and empty space resulting from the Boolean model assuming a constant disc radius R. The union of grains is the set X_R shown in grey and the complement in white. This is a natural model for randomly distributed events and irregular patterns

Random sets can be described by various summary characteristics. Practical examples are characteristics which statistically describe the components or objects forming X, such as mean area or perimeter, which were used for example by Kleinn (2000). If such components are difficult to define, set-theoretic characteristics show their power. Simple numerical characteristics of a set-theoretic nature describing a random set X are area fraction (i.e. the percentage of area covered by X) and specific boundary length (i.e. the total boundary length of X per unit area).

A more sophisticated characteristic is the *spherical contact distribution function*,[1] $H_{s,\xi}$:

$$H_{s,\xi}(r) = 1 - \frac{P(X \cap b(\xi, r) = \emptyset)}{1 - p} \quad \text{for } r \geq 0 \quad (4.2)$$

Here $P(X \cap b(\xi, r) = \emptyset)$ is the probability that a sphere or disc with radius r centred at ξ does not intersect with a random set X. p is the area fraction of a random set X, i.e. the percentage of area covered by X. In random-set applications, characteristic $H_{s,\xi}(r)$ gives the distribution of the distance from an arbitrary test location outside X to the nearest point of X. In a sense this function describes the size of gaps (white space) within a pattern. Diggle (1981) used this function in an ecological context to study the spatial pattern of heather (*Calluna vulgaris* (L.) Hull). The potential of

---

[1]The spherical contact distribution function is also known as *empty-space function* or the *law of first contact* (Chiu et al. 2013).

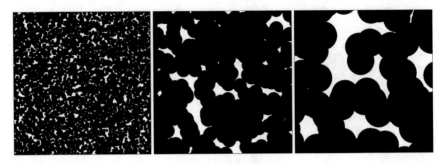

Fig. 4.4 Realisations of simulations using the Boolean model for mimicking patterns of tree canopy (black) interspersed by gaps (white, the complement of the Boolean model, see Fig. 4.3) with $R = 1$ (left), $R = 5$ (centre) and $R = 10$ (right). The size of the observation window is 100×100 m and the area fraction p of black pixels representing the tree canopy is the same in all three cases, i.e. $p = 0.9$

this characteristic for applications in ecology and forest science is not yet exhausted, particularly in the field of remote sensing.

Random set statistics includes methods that are very appropriate to the analysis of digital images and data obtained from laser scanning techniques (e.g. Moffiet et al. 2005; Riaño et al. 2003; Næsset and Økland 2002). These typically do not produce point process data, but data similar to those from high-resolution digital cameras.

Figure 4.4, for example, shows an application of the Boolean model to simulating the tree canopy of a young (left), middle-aged (centre) and old (right) plantation forest. Although the proportion of tree-canopy pixels is the same in all three simulations, the gap structure differs markedly: The number of gaps decrease from left to right in Fig. 4.4 whilst gap size increases.

This observation is well characterised by the density variant of the spherical contact distribution function, $h_s(r)$. Since the Boolean model was applied, this function can be calculated directly from a formula related to this model, see Fig. 4.5. In this case, λ is the density of the germs and R again is the radius of the grains. Patterns with small canopy gaps are indicated by large values of $h_s(r)$ at small r and smaller maximum distances. By contrast, larger maximum distances result from larger, continuous canopy gaps.

A typical field of application of set-theoretic methods are those problems which are analysed by *landscape metrics*. Landscape metrics is a collection of summary characteristics for describing the pattern of irregularly shaped landscape elements, such as forests and forest patches, which are assumed to be correlated with ecological processes. While these statistics were originally devised to deal with scales of kilometres or more, they are really scale independent and can also be applied to plant mosaics at smaller scales, like the pattern of canopy gaps of a forest stand or the pattern of lichens on a rock face or of the aforementioned heather (Dale and Fortin 2014; Chiu et al. 2013; Diggle 1981).

Fig. 4.5 Spherical contact distribution functions $h_s(r)$ corresponding to the forest canopy simulations shown in Fig. 4.4

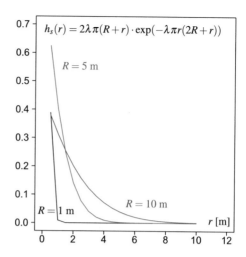

$$h_s(r) = 2\lambda\pi(R+r)\cdot\exp(-\lambda\pi r(2R+r))$$

4.4 Point Process Statistics

Point process methods are applied to the statistical analysis of point patterns aiming to analyse their structural variability. Of particular interest in the analysis are short-range interactions between points (Baddeley et al. 2016; Diggle 2014; Illian et al. 2008; Wiegand and Moloney 2014), in order to obtain information on underlying ecological processes. Spatial point processes are mathematical models for point patterns in two-dimensional or in three-dimensional space. Observed spatial patterns can be considered as realisations or samples of point processes.

In contrast to geostatistics, point process methods are concerned with points, which are determined and measured at discrete objects, e.g. plant locations. In geostatistics points are sampling locations and selected by the investigator. Often they follow a systematic grid or lattice. Also in point process statistics, marks—further information on points—only occur at discrete objects, i.e. the points of a point pattern, and cannot be apart from a point. Point process methods often investigate patterns where points and marks may be dependent whilst in geostatistics sample points should be independent of marks.

Publications involving point process statistics in forest ecology include Matérn (1960), Penttinen et al. (1992), Moeur (1993), Gavrikov and Stoyan (1995) and Pommerening (2002), which gave various examples using tree locations and tree attributes as points and marks, respectively. Comas and Mateu (2007) provided an overview of recent applications of point process methods in forest ecology and management including modelling.

To make things easy for the reader and to save lengthy code lines in this book we have extensively made use of the R spatstat package in this chapter. The package is well described and introduced in the book by Baddeley et al. (2016) and we refer the reader to this substantial text for details. Also, spatstat is well documented in the internet and easily accessible by Google searches. When using spatstat for

Fig. 4.6 Custom orientation of point process data and the observation window as used throughout this chapter

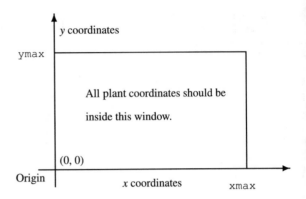

the first time, the package needs to be installed including all dependencies. Then you need to load the package in every new R session (second code line). For using your data in `spatstat` you first need to convert the data frame containing your data, which is assumed to have the name `myData` throughout this chapter, to a `spatstat` point process object referred to as `myDataP` in this book.

For ease of computing the code in this chapter, we further assumed that the boundaries of rectangular sample plots are true and parallel to the *x* and *y* axes of the system of coordinates. If your data do not satisfy this requirement, you can rotate the coordinates by applying the `spatstat` function `rotate()` to the point pattern (`myDataP`). Once the plant locations are correctly aligned, the boundaries of your rectangular research plot are defined by `xmax` and `ymax` assuming that the left bottom corner coincides with the origin (0, 0) of the system of coordinates (Fig. 4.6), which is not required by `spatstat`, but is good practice. This is achieved by transforming the original coordinates. The transformation of coordinates is easily done in R by applying the `range()` function to find the minimum and maximum *x* and *y* coordinates of the data set. Should the minima be much larger than 0, round them down and subtract them from all coordinates. This places the bottom left corner of the plot at the origin (0, 0). All coordinates should then be within the observation window defined by `xmax` and `ymax`, i.e. not outside and not even on the boundaries, see Fig. 4.6.

The code lines below tell you how to create a `spatstat` point process object (without marks) and they precede all following code snippets in this chapter.

```
> install.packages("spatstat", dep = T)
> library(spatstat)
> xwindow <- owin(c(0, xmax), c(0, ymax))
> myDataP <- ppp(myData$x, myData$y, window = xwindow)
```

4.4.1 Point Pattern Components

There are four major components of point patterns, i.e. *points*, *marks*, the *observation window* and *covariates*. The objects of study are mainly defined by points, which can be any ecologically meaningful set of locations, e.g. the locations of plants, of fruiting bodies of fungi, of animal dens or basking sites of reptiles. There is no limit to any researcher's creativity of defining points. Drawing on the nature of random variables (Diggle 2014) used the term *events* instead of points. Traditionally the most common example applications in forest ecology and management include patterns created by tree stem centre locations. This definition has been a convention originally stemming from forest inventory, where the decision whether a tree is inside or outside a sample plot, was based on the stem-centre location, but these locations are rather conservative. Crown-based tree locations better reflect interactions, particularly in light-demanding species (Uria-Diez and Pommerening 2017).

1. Points → e.g. tree locations ξ_i with Cartesian coordinates x_i and y_i,
2. Marks → e.g. tree attributes m_i,

   - quantitative (or real-valued e.g. tree stem diameter, height, biomass, leaf area index, growth rate),
   - qualitative (leading to a multivariate pattern e.g. species, age, crown class),
   - original (from in-situ individual measurements),
   - constructed (combining several measurements).

3. Covariates (e.g. environmental variables such as soil moisture or soil nutrient regimes).

It is also possible to survey two sets of plant locations and then to compare the results of the point pattern analysis for a better understanding of the ecological processes involved (Gavrikov and Stoyan 1995; Uria-Diez and Pommerening 2017).

In point process statistics, marks are attributes of points and the analysis of marked point patterns can provide greater insight into the processes underlying the pattern than an analysis of the points alone (Illian et al. 2008). For instance these additional attributes may describe the species or size of a tree and are usually referred to as *marks*, m_i (Diggle 2014; Illian et al. 2008). The analysis of marked point patterns usually provides deeper insights on the processes that caused the patterns than an analysis of unmarked point patterns. In many cases the marks are dependent on the points or vice versa, e.g. in areas of high point density, marks may tend to be smaller than in areas with low point density (Illian et al. 2008).

Marks can be *quantitative* or *qualitative*. Quantitative marks are real-valued and include plant attributes that can be measured, e.g. tree stem diameter, total height, biomass, growth rate and leaf area index. Qualitative marks such as species, age or crown class of trees can also be accommodated in the analysis leading to different types of points and multivariate patterns. Finally we consider *original* or natural marks, which are usually recorded in-situ in the field and involve the inherent attribute of a single tree only. By contrast, *constructed* or artificial marks are usually calculated from field data and combine several measurements including those related to other points such as nearest neighbours. Spatial nearest-neighbour indices are for example constructed marks. It is very important to realise that not only original marks but also constructed marks may be used in marked point pattern analysis.

Observed point patterns typically are samples in confined areas, i.e. the *observation window* is taken from theoretically infinite point processes. In some textbooks, the observation window is referred to as study area, region or domain. Observation windows define the spatial subset or sample included in the analysis and are often equivalent with research or experimental plots in field ecology and forest science. The boundaries of the observation window can follow simple geometric shapes such as squares, rectangles or circles but irregular shapes are possible, too. The development of unbiased estimators is, however, easier with boundaries complying with simple geometric shapes. The choice of size and location of an observation window is crucial, since it substantially influences the results of the statistical analysis.

In some studies point process and geostatistical methods are combined, for example when regionalised variables influence point patterns as so-called *covariates*, e.g. elevation, precipitation or soil properties (Møller and Waagepetersen 2007). Covariates are used in such studies to explore their influence on the variability of tree locations.

4.4.2 Point Pattern and Marked Point Pattern Types

There are three fundamental types of point patterns (Fig. 4.7, from left to right), i.e. *clustered, random* (quasi-synonyms are Poisson and complete spatial randomness [CSR], see Sect. 4.4.9) and *regular* patterns. These are believed to be the result of processes shaping them. *Attraction* or *clustering* or *clumping* of points leads to clustered or patchy patterns while *repulsion* or *inhibition* cause points to be regularly or uniformly spaced. Dale and Fortin (2014) referred to clustered point configurations as *underdispersion* and to regular ones as *overdispersion*. In patterns simulated from CSR, there is no correlation between the points and therefore it is assumed that there are also no ecological interactions. Departures from the CSR null hypothesis or null model are often considered as evidence of past or present interaction between the study objects, e.g. plants. In clustered patterns, nearest-neighbour distances are on average shorter compared to random patterns whilst in regular patterns the same distances are on average larger than in a comparable random pattern.

The three fundamental point pattern types can also be interpreted as patterns in the successional development of natural forests: Particularly in forests with trees of heavy seeds, offspring may regenerate and grow in clusters during early stages of development. Later, competition for resources kicks in as well as herbivores and diseases causing the death of many trees. This natural thinning leads to a more random dispersion of trees. In later, old-growth stages mature trees have a considerable demand on space for physical and physiological reasons, which is reflected by a regular or overdispersed pattern.

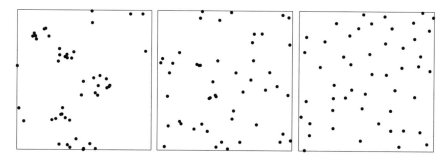

Fig. 4.7 The three fundamental point pattern types illustrated by samples from the Matérn cluster (left), the Poisson (centre) and the Matérn hard-core (right) processes in 25 m × 25 m observation windows and a point density $\lambda = 0.08$ points/m^2. The cluster radius is $R = 2$ m and the hard-core distance $r_0 = 1.8$ m (see Sect. 5.1.1)

There are also three basic mark patterns (Fig. 4.8): *Aggregated, random* and *segregated.* The aggregated case is also referred to as *positive correlation* and segregation as *negative correlation*. In the random case there is no correlation between the marks, i.e. they are *spatially uncorrelated.* Modellers often use the term *dependent marks* for the aggregated and segregated case and *independent marks* for a situation where the marks are randomly assigned to points.

The types of marked point patterns are harder to identify visually than the types of point patterns, see Fig. 4.8. Spatial summary characteristics are then particularly helpful to tell the difference.

The central role of the (marked) Poisson point process (with independent marks) explains why this case is often used as a reference or null model when analysing observed natural patterns. Testing for spatial randomness is therefore one of the first steps in data analysis (Dale and Fortin 2014; Illian et al. 2008). The dispersal of plants in natural vegetation is often not random and plant interactions are frequently involved in the causes. Once deviation from randomness has been established further

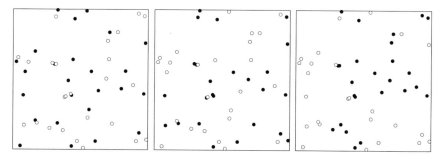

Fig. 4.8 The three fundamental bivariate marked pattern types illustrated by the same sample from a Poisson process as in Fig. 4.7 (centre) with aggregated marks (left), randomly dispersed marks (centre) and segregated marks (right) in 25 m × 25 m observation windows and a point density $\lambda = 0.08$ points/m^2. The marks are qualitative and type 1 points are indicated by open and type 2 points by filled circles. Both types have the same relative frequency

tests and models can help to identify the causes for the formation of a particular observed spatial patterns (see Sect. 4.4.9).

4.4.3   Stationarity and Isotropy

In the statistical analysis of point patterns it is often assumed that the pattern is sampled from an underlying point process which is *homogeneous* (or *stationary*) and *isotropic*, i.e. its probability distribution is invariant to translations and rotations (Diggle 2014; Illian et al. 2008, p. 64 and p. 35ff., respectively). In contrast, inhomogeneous point processes can, for example, have point densities that vary systematically, see also Fig. 5.2 in Chap. 5.

Although methods have also been developed for inhomogeneous point processes (see e.g. Møller and Waagepetersen 2007), patterns are often preferred in the analysis for which the stationarity and isotropy assumptions hold. These markedly simplify the methodology and allow a focused analysis of interactions between trees by ruling out additional factors such as, for example, varying site conditions. The stationary and isotropic case therefore currently forms the main domain of the application of point process methods in individual-based forest ecology and management. In this context the choice of size and location of an observation is crucial, because stationarity and isotropy are scale dependent concepts (Dungan et al. 2002). Both concepts are also often used in the other two fields of spatial statistics, i.e. geostatistics and random set statistics.

For illustrating this problem, Fig. 4.9 (left) shows a map of the shooting locations during six successive years of red foxes (*Vulpes vulpes* L.) in a mixed landscape in East Germany. Here the shooting by stalkers can be considered as sampling and autopsies were performed on each carcass to determine whether it was infected by the tapeworm *Echinococcus multilocularis* LEUCKART or not. Due to successful rabies vaccination of red foxes in the 1990s the populations of this species had much increased. Indirectly the tapeworm benefitted from this veterinarian success as well, since red fox is a definitive host of the adult stage of this parasite.

The left-hand map in Fig. 4.9 reveals that infected animals were clustered particularly in the bottom-right section of the observation window. This would potentially introduce inhomogeneity to what otherwise can be considered a homogeneous point pattern. In order to analyse the relationship between the shooting locations of infected and not infected animals it seemed a good idea to zoom into a 30 × 23 km subwindow (Fig. 4.9, right) to study interactions.

In other situations it can be necessary to increase the size of the observation window, since local inhomogeneities can turn out to be part of a homogeneous pattern at larger scale. This shows that the choice of size and location of an observation window is crucial, since it substantially influences the results of the statistical analysis. It requires both statistical knowledge and knowledge of the subject matter.

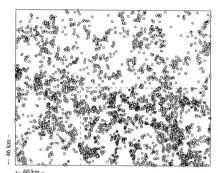
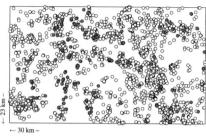

Fig. 4.9 Left: Shooting locations of 4319 red foxes (*Vulpes vulpes* L.) in Germany. Open circles indicate shooting locations where red foxes were not infected and filled red circles those where the animals were infected by the tapeworm (*Echinococcus multilocularis* LEUCKART). The blue dashed lines show the location of the subwindow. Right: The same shooting locations where infected and not infected red foxes were found for the subwindow $20 < x < 60$ km and $0 < y < 23$ km with a total of 2308 animals. Data courtesy of Dietrich Stoyan

4.4.4 Test-Location and Point-Related Summary Characteristics

Two different types of summary characteristics can be defined by the type of points at which they are measured: *test location* or *point related* summary characteristics[2] (Illian et al. 2008, p. 195).

   Test location related summary characteristics like the spherical contact distribution function mentioned in Sect. 4.3 are estimated with reference to deterministic test locations or sample points, which are chosen independently of the points of the point pattern. They describe the relationship between test locations and the points of the spatial pattern under study. Test locations can be based on a systematic grid or randomly placed throughout the observation window and are used particularly in geostatistics and random set statistics. In geostatistics, the sample points, ψ_i, where the sample data were gathered, are such test locations.

   In contrast, point related summary characteristics relate only to the points of the point pattern, i.e. they yield information on the ith point in the observation window.

   These two concepts of summary statistics were also discussed in relation to structural indices by Gadow and Hui (2002) and Staupendahl and Zucchini (2006). These authors used the terms *point-based* and *tree-based* which originate from *distance methods* used in forest inventory in which Loetsch et al. (1973, p. 369f.) distinguished between point-tree and tree-tree sampling methods. Point-tree (= test location related) sampling methods are more common in forest inventory, since tree-tree

---

[2]Diggle (2014, p. 26ff.) used a slightly different terminology and distinguishes between *point-to-nearest-event* and *inter-event* distances.

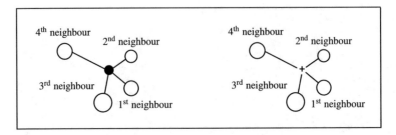

Fig. 4.10 Point- (left) and test-location (right) related groups of four neighbour trees

methods (= point related), also referred to as distance sampling, can lead to biased estimations (Diggle 2014; Krebs 1999, p. 45f. and p. 170, respectively).

Figure 4.10 shows two identical groups of four neighbours, which can be considered parts of the point pattern under study. In the first case (left), the mark is constructed for a typical point of the point pattern, whilst in the second case (right) the four points are nearest neighbours of a test location, e.g. a sample point, and the mark is constructed for this sample point. The majority of summary characteristics in point process statistics is point related.

4.4.5 Defining Local Neigbourhood

Quantifying microstructural information from a localised environment of points is central to individual-based forest ecology. It is also a common theme in spatial statistics with applications in all three aforementioned areas (see for example Chilès and Delfiner 1999; Wackernagel 2003; Illian et al. 2008). The estimation of nearest neighbour summary characteristics requires the selection of a set of neighbouring trees before the principles of constructing marks of Sect. 4.4.6 can be applied.

Local neighbourhood can be defined in many ways and the most common of these are given below.

(1) Simple distances. Most frequently measures of distance (Euclidean, Euclidean squared, Euclidean weighted, etc.) are used, i.e. neighbouring trees are defined by their distances to the reference tree or point. Sometimes these distances are weighted by the original marks (e.g. stem diameter, total height) of the trees involved (see for example the Hegyi competition index in Table 4.1). Early methods of using simple Euclidean distances implied that the number k of nearest neighbours was fixed. More advanced methods now include approaches, where k is made dependent on the size of the target tree or on local density (Rajala and Illian 2012), so that k varies from tree to tree.

(2) Mark-distance relationships. They are based on the concept that interaction is greater as neighbouring trees increase in size and proximity (Weiskittel et al. 2011).

Table 4.1 Construction principles for marks/test functions $t_i(m_i, m_j)$ used for estimating nearest neighbour and second-order summary characteristics. i denotes the typical point or reference tree and j a NN (nearest neighbour) or another point/tree separated by distance r. The principles are explained in the text. Modified from Pommerening and Sánchez Meador (2018)

Construction principle	Example(s)
Mark ratio	$t_i(m_i, m_j) = \sum_{j=1}^{k} \frac{m_j}{m_i} \cdot \frac{1}{r}$ Hegyi (1974) $t_i(m_i, m_j) = 1 - \frac{1}{k} \sum_{j=1}^{k} \frac{\min(m_i, m_j)}{\max(m_i, m_j)}$ Gadow (1993)
Mark comparison	$t_i(m_i, m_j) = \frac{1}{k} \sum_{j=1}^{k} \mathbf{1}(m_i > m_j)$ Hui et al. (1998) $t_i(m_i, m_j) = \frac{1}{k} \sum_{j=1}^{k} \mathbf{1}(m_i \neq m_j)$ Gadow (1993)
Mark difference	$t_i(m_i, m_j) = \sum_{j=1}^{k}(m_j - m_i) \cdot \frac{1}{r}$ Tomé and Burkhart (1989) $t_i(m_i, m_j) = \frac{1}{2} \sum_{j=1}^{k}(m_i - m_j)^2$ Stoyan and Stoyan (1994)
Mark product	$t_i(m_i, m_j) = m_i \sum_{j=1}^{k} m_j$ Stoyan and Stoyan (1994), Davies and Pommerening (2008)
Weighted geometric mean	$t_i(m_i) = \sqrt[\sum_{i=1}^{z} \lambda_i]{\prod_{i=1}^{z} m_i^{\lambda_i}}$ After Hui et al. (2018)

where

$t_i(m_i, m_j)$	Mark/test function of typical point/ reference tree i
k	Number of NN or other point(s)
m_i	Original mark(s) of typical point/reference tree i
m_j	Original mark(s) of NN or other point(s), $j = 1, \ldots, n$
r	Euclidean distance between the typical point/reference tree i and neighbour/other point(s) j
z	Number of marks m_i associated with point/tree i considered
λ_i	Weight associated with mark m_i
$\mathbf{1}(A) = 1$	If A is true, otherwise $\mathbf{1}(A) = 0$

Summary statistics using this method of defining neighbourhood can be related to both the horizontal and vertical plane. Such neighbourhood definitions may for example include a competitor selection that is based on an angular threshold (e.g. according to relascope sampling proposed by Bitterlich (1984)). Basal area factors (BAF) have been identified as good criteria for selecting nearest neighbours in conjunction with measures of competition (Pretzsch 2009). Equation (4.3) formalises the principle of this neighbour selection method: Neighbouring trees j (represented by ξ_j) with a distance to the reference tree i (represented by ξ_i) shorter than a critical distance or threshold are included in the local neighbourhood of reference tree i, otherwise they are rejected. Euclidean distance between ξ_i and ξ_j is denoted by $\|\xi_i - \xi_j\|$. Depending on the basal area factor this method tends to select larger (more competitive) neighbours and ignores smaller ones (in terms of stem diameter, d).

$$\|\xi_i - \xi_j\| < \frac{50}{\sqrt{BAF}} \cdot d_j \tag{4.3}$$

(3) Area potentially available (APA). In Dirichlet tesselations or two-dimensional Voronoi tesselations (Chiu et al. 2013; Dale and Fortin 2014) each tree holds a territory consisting of the part of the observation window which is closer to that particular tree location than to any other tree location. This method recruits neighbours whose Dirichlet domains share a common boundary with the reference tree and are therefore likely to have some kind of interaction with the tree under study. Spatial proximity is less important in this approach and direction is given more emphasis. Rajala and Illian (2012) referred to this method as Delaunay triangulation and it ensures that neighbours are selected from all possible directions around the reference tree (see Fig. 4.11). In the code listing below we made use of the spatstat package. The Dirichlet tesselation is computed based on function dirichlet() and the point process object myDataP including our data. Then the tesselation can be plotted and finally the points of the point process are added using the points() function.

```
> u <- dirichlet(myDataP)
> par(mar = c(0, 0, 0, 0))
> plot(u, main = "")
> points(myData$x, myData$y, col = "black", bg = "grey",
+ pch = 16, cex = 0.5)
```

In forest ecology and management, tesselation-based concepts are also referred to as *area potentially available* (APA) and have been used to model the growing space of trees (Weiskittel et al. 2011). To improve the estimation of APA tesselations tree sizes were later used as weights for defining the boundaries of individual areas (Abellanas et al. 2011; Gspaltl et al. 2012).

A similar method of identifying neighbours is based on the *Gabriel graph* leading to a *Gabriel neighbourhood*: Two points ξ_i and ξ_j are neighbours if the circular area between them is empty and the diameter of the circle is $\|\xi_i - \xi_j\|$, i.e. both points are located exactly on the circle boundary (see Fig. 2 in Rajala and Illian 2012). All points are neighbours of a focus point that fulfil this condition and the APA is the union of circular areas or the polygon resulting from connecting adjacent neighbour points. Dirichlet, Voronoi or Delaunay neighbourhoods are a special form of Gabriel neighbourhoods, where the empty circular space is defined by three points instead of two. Rajala and Illian (2012) found that Gabriel and Dirichlet neighbourhoods lead to more realistic estimations of spatial species mingling, see Sect. 4.4.7.1, because these are less sensitive to the underlying point pattern in the observation window.

(4) Zone of influence (ZOI). According to this method a two- or three-dimensional influence zone around the reference tree is defined and every other tree which directly intersects this influence zone or whose own influence zone overlaps it is considered to be a neighbour (Bella 1971; Biging and Dobbertin 1992, 1995; Berger

Fig. 4.11 Dirichlet
tesselation using the tree
locations of a mixed sessile
oak (*Quercus petraea* MATT.,
black filled
circles)—European beech
(*Fagus sylvatica* L., red filled
circles) forest stand at
Manderscheid
(Rhineland-Palatinate,
Germany)

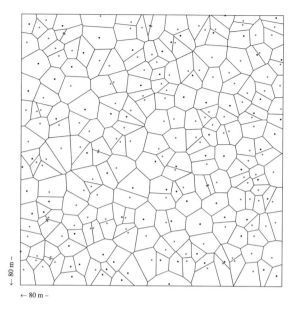

↕ 80 m

← 80 m →

and Hildenbrandt 2000). Usually influence zones are defined as more or less simple
geometric structures, e.g. circles, cylinders, inverted cones and can have their size
fixed or varied depending on an attribute of the reference tree. Initially circular zones
with fixed radii centred at the target trees were used and this concept is said to be
based on studies of gap size in forests and its implications (Burton 1993). The idea
was improved by modelling variable radii based on the size of the target tree, i.e.
as a result large subject trees have large ZOIs and small subject trees have small
ZOIs. Often the radii are a function of stem diameter or crown size and sometimes
related to the size of open-grown trees in comparable situations. Initially all other
trees within such circular ZOI were considered potential competitors, but it seems
a consensus has been reached that it is the trees in the overlap areas that are more
commonly regarded as competitors *sensu strictu*. In the work by Gerrard (1969) and
Bella (1971), the principle of index construction and the neighbourhood definition
are closely related: Trees whose ZOIs overlap are considered competitors and the
overlap areas between the competitors and the target tree are summed up and divided
by the ZOI area of the target tree, see also Sect. 5.2.2. Burton (1993) suggested dis-
tinguishing between "zone of influence" and "zone of perception". While the former
refers to a zone which is influenced by a given tree, the latter denotes an area within
which this tree can perceive its neighbours.

(5) Sky-view and light-interception approaches. These methods can in principle be
considered a sub-set of the ZOI concept. Sky-view and light-interception approaches
of defining neighbourhoods relate to the consideration that light is an important shared
resource that is not abundantly available in forest stands. In such models, inverted,
vertical light cones are often constructed at a certain height at the location of the target

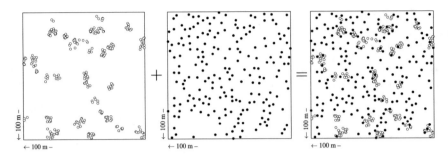

Fig. 4.12 The principle of superposition using a Matérn cluster process for species 1 (open circles) and a Matérn hard-core process for species (filled circles) for modelling the evolution of a bivariate spatial species pattern

trees and all trees whose crowns overlap the search cone are considered competitors (Burkhart and Tomé 2012; Pretzsch 2009). More mechanistic approaches explicitly model hemispherical photographs (Coates et al. 2003) and light penetration (Brunner 1998). However, in arid and semi-arid systems characterized by either water-limited resources and/or nutrient-poor soils, these approaches (e.g. ZOI or inverted cone approaches) may have limited capacity.

(6) Mark types. In combination with the aforementioned principles different types of qualitative marks, e.g. the species attributes or health classes, add to the complexity of defining local neighbourhoods. For example in a mixed woodland involving two species (bivariate pattern) it is useful to estimate summary characteristics separately for each of the two species groups and for the interaction of trees with different species marks. Statistically this kind of point pattern data may be regarded as a *superposition* or union of single-type point patterns (Chiu et al. 2013; Diggle 2014; Illian et al. 2008, see Fig. 4.12), where two or more component processes are superimposed, and some authors referred to the corresponding analysis of such patterns as *intra-* and *intertype* analysis (Lotwick and Silverman 1982; Diggle 2014; Moeur 1993; Goreaud and Pélissier 2003).

The concept is based on the hypothesis that most interactions between trees take place within species populations, i.e. between conspecific individuals. The composite pattern of the whole forest stand is then mainly the result of merging the point patterns of the component species, which are described by independent point process models (Goreaud and Pélissier 2003; Grabarnik et al. 2011). If, for example, two species have very different seed dispersal mechanisms (e.g. animal dispersal versus wind dispersal) and the currently observed plant locations are largely determined by the seed dispersal mechanisms involved, superposition of random point patterns is a suitable approach (Howe 1989; Wiegand et al. 2009). Also, recent research has suggested that intraspecific competition plays a greater role in terms of growth and survival than interspecific competition (Anderson and Whiteman 2015).

Intra- and intertype analysis is analogous to intra- and interspecific competition as defined in forest ecology and has important implications in sampling and analysis of structural indices and second-order summary statistics. Neighbours of points belonging to one type should either always be recruited from the same type set (intratype analysis: e.g. reference point of type 1—neighbour of type 1, reference point of type 2—neighbour of type 2) or from a specified other type to investigate for example the interaction of type 1 and type 2 points (intertype analysis). With s different qualitative marks, e.g. tree species, there are $\binom{s+1}{2}$ combinations of defining nearest neighbours. Two tree species would lead to $\binom{3}{2} = 3$ and three tree species to $\binom{4}{2} = 6$ combinations of defining nearest neighbours.

With nearest neighbour summary characteristics (NNSS) used for measuring competition research has shown that the inverted cone and the horizontal basal area factor methods are successful methods of defining nearest neighbours (see Pretzsch 2009). As a consequence the number of neighbours selected randomly varies from reference tree to reference tree depending on the neighbourhood selection method and the point pattern.

In contrast, although similar to measures of competition and vice versa, with NNSS used to quantify structure the number of neighbours is usually fixed for all trees and are determined arbitrarily. Little research has been done to identify an optimal number of nearest neighbours, see for example Pommerening (2006).

4.4.6 Principles for Constructing Marks and Test Functions

Principles of constructing marks (which includes both structural and competition indices, see Sect. 4.4.7.1) and constructing so-called test functions for second-order characteristics (see Sect. 4.4.7.2) are very similar in point process statistics, see Table 4.1. Test functions form an important element of second-order characteristics and largely define their behaviour and working principle (Illian et al. 2008; Diggle 2014; Baddeley et al. 2016). Constructed marks or NNSS are based on the mark of subject tree i, m_i, and m_j, the mark(s) of nearest neighbour j. Test functions are similar but depend on two marks m_i and m_j, where i and j are two points that are separated by distance r in the case of second-order characteristics. The test functions of Table 4.1 can typically be applied as part of a general type of mark correlation function (Illian et al. 2008; Baddeley et al. 2016, p. 342f. and p. 644f., respectively) that can take any kind of test function and mark type. At the same time the construction principles of Table 4.1 have also been applied to construct NNSS (Pommerening and Sánchez Meador 2018). Structural and competition indices are both constructed marks and NNSS that have been used to model plant interaction in the past.

Representatives of the *mark ratio* principle are the Hegyi competition (Hegyi 1974) and the diameter differentiation index (Gadow 1993) in which the ratio of the marks of the reference point and neighbouring points are summed. The ratios are sometimes multiplied by a weight such as the reciprocal distance in the case of the Hegyi index. Incidentally, Martin and Ek (1984) used an exponential function of distance and quantitative mark to construct weights for the mark ratio. The mark ratio can have an exponent, which changes the relative importance of the neighbour compared to the reference tree (Eq. 9, Boyden et al. 2005).

The *mark comparison* principle is used in the size dominance (Hui et al. 1998) and the species mingling index (Gadow 1993). This principle involves a qualitative comparison of marks and the result is of a boolean type, 0 or 1. The size dominance index is defined as the proportion of the k nearest neighbours that are smaller than reference tree i. The species mingling index is defined as the proportion of the k nearest neighbours that are of a species different to that of the reference tree i. Naturally it is also possible to consider situations instead, where the categorial marks m_i and m_j are equal, see Baddeley et al. (2016, p. 645).

Tomé and Burkhart (1989) published a modelling approach rare in forest science that included both competition and facilitation. In their practical application to *Eucalyptus globulus* plantations, it became evident that mark differences were well suited, because the differences result in signed values so that positive and negative interaction effects were automatically taken care of and produced asymmetric competition effects. The principle of *mark difference* is also demonstrated by the diameter variogram index (Stoyan and Stoyan 1994) in which half the squared difference of the marks of neighbouring trees is related to the test function used in mark variograms. These are related to geostatistical variograms (see Sect. 4.2) and the mark variogram index characterises the variability of quantitative tree marks at close proximity (Pommerening et al. 2011).

The mark correlation index is an example of the *mark product* principle (Davies and Pommerening 2008). It is the principle of the test function of the classical mark correlation function (Stoyan and Stoyan 1994). Here the mean product of the marks of the typical point or reference tree and the k nearest neighbours is considered.

Finally, the principle of weighted geometric mean was inspired by work recently published by Hui et al. (2018). The idea here is that multiple quantitative marks m_i are aggregated in a multiplicative way and each of them is weighted by λ_i. This is one way of simultaneously using multiple marks of the same points.

Baddeley et al. (2016), Illian et al. (2008) also introduced test functions for situations, where the original marks of points are angles.

4.4.7   Summary Characteristics

A basic principle of pattern analysis is to reduce raw data to a useful summary form Torquato (2002). This is often the key objective of the analysis of plant interactions and habitat structure. For this purpose a suitable sampling design is selected, which, in the context of individual-based forest ecology and management, often involves comparatively large, replicated rectangular observation windows that include at least 150 points (see also Sect. 1.4). The data collected in these observation windows are used to estimate summary characteristics, which help to understand the spatial patterns and the processes that shaped them. This book focuses on two major methods of statistical inference based on point process statistics that play an important role in forest ecology and management, i.e. *nearest neighbour* (NNSS) and *second-order* summary statistics.

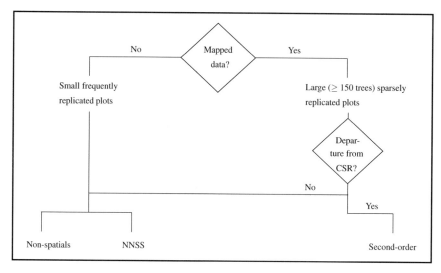

Fig. 4.13 The decision which summary characteristics to use often depends on the availability of data and on the point pattern in question. Modified from Gadow et al. (2012)

NNSS are usually applied when observation windows are fairly small and the number of points available is limited (<150 points). As part of forest inventories, for example, trees are sampled in small clusters (referred to as sample plots) and often only include 5–20 trees per plot. However, NNSS can also be helpful in explorative data analysis. If observation windows are sufficiently large to provide at least 150 points, the use of more powerful second-order characteristics is justified, but NNSS can also be applied in that situation (see Fig. 4.13).

All spatial summary characteristics require edge-correction methods to account for off-plot points and marks that have not been recorded. Without these corrections, edge effects can cause serious bias, particularly if the number of points in the observation window is small (see Sect. 4.4.8).

4.4.7.1 Nearest Neighbour Summary Statistics

Nearest neighbour summary statistics (NNSS) describe relationships between a test location or a point of the point pattern and the k nearest neighbours and statistically NNSS can be interpreted as means and probability density functions of constructed marks. As such they belong to the group of first-order characteristics, such as tree intensity or density λ. They take the individual's perception of local diversity into account (Pommerening et al. 2019), see also Pommerening and Uria-Diez (2017). NNSS are often called short-sighted methods because they quantify only the relationship between a point and its k nearest neighbours and ignore what is beyond the nearest neighbours (Pommerening 2002). Also, the distances between nearest neighbours depend on the point pattern and can therefore vary considerably from reference tree to reference tree.

Although we have mainly used simple Euclidean distances for defining nearest neighbours in our examples, any of the neighbourhoods described in Sect. 4.4.5 can be applied. The selection depends on the purpose of the study, the hypotheses, and often a comparison of the results of the same NNSS estimated based on different neighbourhoods is helpful in understanding patterns and eventually the ecological processes involved (Rajala and Illian 2012).

In forest ecology, these summary characteristics include *competition indices* (e.g. Biging and Dobbertin 1992, 1995) and *structural* or *diversity indices* (e.g. Krebs 1999; Gadow and Hui 2002; Pommerening 2002). The two types of NNSS are in fact very similar and share a common estimation process, (1.) the definition of the local neighbourhood (Sect. 4.4.5), i.e. the nearest neighbours, and (2.) the construction of the mark (Sect. 4.4.6).

Measures of Competition

In general plant science, measures of interaction have more commonly been used for analysing data, particularly from experiments (Weigelt and Jolliffe 2003; Damgaard 2011).

Testing hypotheses in community ecology often requires the quantification of the magnitude of interactions between individuals (Armas et al. 2004). In general plant science, competition is often studied in controlled experiments (Montgomery 2013) involving artificial environments where density and/or the proportion of different species are varied and the biomass or fecundity of the competing species are measured. Increasingly, such experiments are now performed in natural plant communities, where densities are manipulated (Damgaard 2011).

In general plant science, interaction is usually measured using performance indicators of single plants or of plant communities with and without considering neighbouring plants. Performance indicators can be yield, biomass, growth rates, mortality and recruitment (Weigelt and Jolliffe 2003; Armas et al. 2004; Díaz-Sierra et al. 2012) expressed as absolute and relative growth rates or size variables. The performance measures are then arranged in ratios and differences to compare the performance in monocultures and mixtures or between different species in pairs. The notion of "control" can include monoculture or open-grown conditions (no neighbours) whilst "treatment" can mean mixture-grown etc. A detailed discussion of the advantages and disadvantages of these indices can be found in Weigelt and Jolliffe (2003). These indices, however, quantify the net balance of interaction, i.e. the sum of all positive and negative factors that influence plant growth.

Interaction indices in general plant science either relate to the *intensity* or the *importance* of interactions. Intensity in this context describes the absolute impact of interactions on plant performance irrespective of other factors, with importance as a relative measure describing the performance of an organism relative to the impact of factors other than interaction, e.g. climate, soil properties or herbivory (Keddy 1989;

Burton 1993; Seifan et al. 2010; Seifan and Seifan 2015; Pommerening and Sánchez Meador 2018).

In forest science, modelling applications of competition prevail, where the effect of competition on the growth of individual trees has been studied to more accurately predict the performance of trees in terms of growth rates, mortality and birth processes. Measures of competition have therefore traditionally been key elements of individual-oriented forest growth models used to estimate the *response variable*[3] growth rate, e.g. diameter or basal area absolute growth rate, and quantify the *competition load* or *competition intensity* on individual trees (Weigelt and Jolliffe 2003). Response variable and performance indicator are similar concepts.

It has also been argued that indices of competition help to generalise forest models across a wide range of stand densities and species compositions in a larger geographic area, because they contribute information on local forest structure to the projection of forest development (Burton 1993; Pretzsch 2009; Weiskittel et al. 2011; Burkhart and Tomé 2012). Clutter et al. (1983) described the use of these indices as attempts to refine average stand density measures so that the varying degrees of crowding experienced by individual trees in a stand can be incorporated into the procedure of projecting individual tree growth. Burton (1993) saw competition indices as decision-support tools for forest management, specifically for naturally and artificially regenerated seedlings and saplings and their protection from vegetation other than trees, a problem which he criticised to be much neglected. He argued that competition should be viewed as one of many constraints rather than a determinant of tree performance. Burton (1993) also pointed out that the variation in growth response is often so great that a competition index has little predictive power. Initial tree size and environmental factors in his view play a much larger role.

With only few notable exceptions, to date most applications in forest science concern competition rather than interaction in general. Using the terminology of general plant science, all of them are intensity indices measured and take the "plant's eye view" (Pommerening and Sánchez Meador 2018).

Measures of competition can be used in growth estimations in two different ways, 1. in *direct estimations* and 2. as part of the so-called *potential-modifier approach*, see Sect. 5.2.5.

In both concepts, measures of competition are used as independent variables (regressors, explanatory variable) along with a number of other variables such as for example site factors. Additionally in some models the change in competition index over time is included as a separate independent variable. In the modifier function the competition index is usually incorporated in the exponent of an exponential function and the potential is derived from trees that have faced no or hardly any competition, e.g. open-grown trees or predominant forest trees. For further details see Pretzsch (2009).

---

[3]A response variable can be best defined as the property of a system in a structure/property relationship as described in the introduction. Response variables correspond with *dependent variable* and *regressand* in regression terminology.

The components of competition indices, i.e. the definition of the local neighbourhood and the construction of the mark, are usually optimised through correlation and regression analyses. The optimisation is facilitated by a clearly defined response or performance variable which in forest ecology and management most frequently is tree growth but Weigelt and Jolliffe (2003) also referred to other response variables in the general plant and vegetation science, e.g. reproduction and physiological performance.

With measures of competition in forest science there is usually little interest in summary characteristics, e.g. a mean competition index at forest stand level or a competition density distribution. Weigelt and Jolliffe (2003), however, also reported the use of competition summary characteristics in the general plant and vegetation science literature. Theoretically competition NNSS can be used in the same way as structural NNSS. Despite obvious similarities to measures of structure, the main focus of measures of competition is on the individual marks only, i.e. the index value of each individual tree in the observation window.

In the context of individual-based ecology, non-spatial measures of interaction/-competition are not considered, as they are not well suited to uncover interaction processes. In individual-based ecology, the definition of local neighbourhood is crucially important. The nearest neighbours of a given tree are those, that are likely to interact with this tree. Particularly important are size ratios and size differences between a subject tree and its nearest neighbours.

There is growing evidence that size matters more in studies of interaction and competition than species differences (Vogt et al. 2010; Kunstler et al. 2016) supporting the assumption that competition within species is generally stronger than between species. However, some authors have included species-specific traits such as light transmission factors, wood density or specific leaf area (Pretzsch et al. 2002; Canham et al. 2004) in the calculation of competition load to account for different light demands or shading (Pommerening and Sánchez Meador 2018).

Some modellers also used directional information in the construction of competition indices, since it is plausible that there are differences in the competitive effect between evenly distributed and clustered competitors (Gadow et al. 1998; Pretzsch et al. 2002; Miina and Pukkala 2002).

Pretzsch (2009), Weiskittel et al. (2011) and Burkhart and Tomé (2012) offer a good overview of competition indices.

Measures of Structure

Spatial measures of structure have been developed for mainly two purposes, 1. for the quantitative description of the spatial arrangement of trees and their attributes and 2. for providing spatial measures of biodiversity. There are many papers with overviews and example applications (see Neumann and Starlinger 2001; Aguirre et al. 2003; Pommerening 2002; McElhinny et al. 2005; Pommerening 2006; Szmyt

2014). As with competition/interaction measures, non-spatial measures of structure are not considered here, because they only poorly describe tree interactions.

For analysing the variability of spatial aspects of plant populations the first summary characteristics were proposed in the 1950 and 1960s, e.g. the aggregation index of Clark and Evans (1954) and Pielou's coefficient of segregation (Pielou 1977). These and similar early approaches reflected the state of the computer and mensuration technology of the time and expressed plant structure using a single number. Krebs (1999) and Dale and Fortin (2014) give a good overview. Later the advantages of estimating histograms and functional summary characteristics were recognised and these provided more detailed information about stand structure (Aguirre et al. 2003; Pommerening 2006).

More recently a good quantitative description of spatial forest structure has also been recognised as the key to the ability of simulating spatial patterns based on non-parametric modelling methods (Lewandowski and Gadow 1997; Pommerening 2006; Pommerening and Stoyan 2008; Lilleleht et al. 2014), see Sect. 5.1.2.

Since the sustainability concept has been extended beyond the traditional concept of simple timber sustainability (Pommerening and Murphy 2004) woodland managers are increasingly required to consider and improve biodiversity, conservation and habitat functions within the forest. There is an urgent need for practical, meaningful and quantitative criteria and measures of these functions. Because of their correlation with habitat functions and population dynamics of endangered mammal and bird species, structural indices have been proposed as surrogates for more direct measures of biodiversity (Pommerening 2002). To this end Gadow (1999) and Pommerening (2002) subdivided α-diversity into *location diversity*, *species diversity* and the *size diversity*, see Fig. 1.3 in Sect. 1.3. At a small scale, the diversity of tree locations reflects the pattern of tree locations: Are they regular, clumped (clustered), random or some combination of these? Species diversity is concerned with the spatial arrangement of species while size diversity involves the spatial arrangement of, for example, diameters or heights (Pommerening 2006). The use of structural indices is particularly effective in forest inventories with many small replicated observation windows (Pommerening and Stoyan 2008; Motz et al. 2010, see Sect. 1.4).

Defining a response or performance variable (see footnote 3 on "Nearest Neighbour Summary Statistics") is not as straightforward as with measures of competition, since the purpose of these measures is fundamentally different. Possibilities include the abundance of an endangered animal species, tree (population) growth and the degree to which allometric models can be improved. Especially in the first case, data are often difficult to gather. The difficulties in data acquisition and the absence of clearly defined response/performance variables explain why there is hardly any study concerned with this problem.

Through simulation Pretzsch (1995) for example investigated the relationship between the diversity of tree locations and absolute stand basal area growth rates. Using the aggregation index of Clark and Evans (1954) he could show that maximum stand basal area growth rate was achieved with regularly distributed tree locations, that 95% of the maximum absolute growth rate (AGR) was realised when the same trees were randomly distributed and a minimum of 50% of maximum AGR in the case of strongly clustered tree locations. Bravo and Guerra (2002) found relationships between stand and tree based structural indices and diameter growth for maritime pine (*Pinus pinaster* AIT.) in Spain and Davies and Pommerening (2008) have used measures of spatial structure for improving allometric models in Wales. The authors could show that spatial indices can significantly improve crown models for Sitka spruce (*Picea sitchensis* (BONG.) CARR.) and birch (*Betula* spp.) especially in forests with poor thinning history.

In materials science, *reconstruction* (Torquato 2002, p. 294) is used as a way of evaluating summary statistics: The extent to which the observed realisation of forest structure can be reconstructed with a given summary characteristic reveals the level of information embodied in it. Pommerening (2006) has independently developed the same idea when evaluating structural indices by reversing forest structural analysis, see Sect. 5.1.2.

In contrast to measures of competition, with measures of structure there is usually little interest in individual marks but rather in summary characteristics, e.g. a mean structural index at forest stand level or a probabilty density distribution.

Location Diversity (Point Patterns without Marks)

There are three different possibilities of expressing location diversity with NNSS, using 1. distances, 2. angles and 3. directions. For each of these options examples are given in this section. All of these indices assume that the stationarity assumption holds, i.e. that the underlying, unknown point process model is stationary. In the case of inhomogeneity, NNSS typically indicate clustering (Baddeley et al. 2016).

A bench mark location-diversity index is the *aggregation index R'* by Clark and Evans (1954). This index compares the mean of observed distances, $\bar{r}$, between any point of the point pattern and its first nearest neighbour with the mean distance in a Poisson point process (complete spatial randomness), $\mathbf{E}r$. The mean of observed distances depends on the point density of a given pattern.

$$R' = \frac{\bar{r}}{\mathbf{E}r} \quad \text{with} \quad \mathbf{E}r = \frac{1}{2 \cdot \sqrt{\frac{N}{A}}} \quad \text{and} \quad R' \in [0, 2.1491] \tag{4.4}$$

N and A are the number of points in the observation window and its area, respectively. $R' > 1$ indicates a tendency towards a regular point pattern (mean of observed distances > mean Poisson distance) as caused by inhibition, whilst $R' < 1$ highlights a trend towards clustering (mean of observed distances < mean Poisson distance) caused by mutual attraction. When mean observed distance and mean Poisson distance are roughly the same, $R' \approx 1$. It is possible to measure the individual distances r_i in-situ in the field, i.e. mapping is not absolutely required.

The aggregation index R' by Clark and Evans (1954) is comparatively straightforward to code. The spatstat package offers functions clarkevans() and

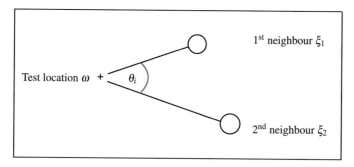

Fig. 4.14 Illustration of the principle of the "mean of angles" index θ_i by Assunção (1994)

`clarkevans.test()` to perform the calculations described in Eq. (4.4). How to use them is explained in the following listing. In line 1, the `spatstat` point process object `myDataP` is passed on to the function `clarkevans()`. As a result we obtain three values, one where no edge correction is performed and two were calculated using edge correction (see Sect. 4.4.8).

```
1  > clarkevans(myDataP)
2  naive Donnelly cdf
3  1.507010 1.469649 1.477755
4  > clarkevans.test(myDataP, correction = "cdf")
5
6  Clark-Evans test
7  CDF correction
8  Monte Carlo test based on 999 simulations of CSR with fixed n
9
10 data: myDataP
11 R = 1.4778, p-value = 0.002
```

The *means of angles index* by Assunção (1994, see Fig. 4.14), is an example of a location NNSS using angles. The means of angles index is test-location related: ξ_1 and ξ_2 are the locations of the trees closest to test location ω. The constructed mark θ_i is defined as the smallest of two possible angles formed by the points $\xi_1 \omega \xi_2$ so that $\theta_i < 180°$.

The l test locations can, for example, be sample point locations in forest inventory. For fully mapped plant patterns constructing a lattice and measuring θ_i at the grid points is a good option. It is also possible to use random test-point locations, however, the variance of θ_i is usually smaller when a lattice is used. The arithmetic mean of all θ_i is defined as

$$\overline{\theta} = \frac{1}{l} \sum_{i=1}^{l} \theta_i; \qquad \overline{\theta} \in [0, \pi] \tag{4.5}$$

For random point patterns $\overline{\theta} \approx 90°$. $\overline{\theta} < 90°$ indicates clustered point patterns and $\overline{\theta} > 90°$ is typical of regular point patterns. Similar to the aggregation index by Clark and Evans (1954) it is possible to divide $\overline{\theta}$ by the expected value of 90°, which reflects complete spatial randomness.

The listing below shows how $\overline{\theta}$ can be calculated using the spatstat and LearnGeom packages. After loading the data related to a fully mapped research plot (not shown) and after conversion to a spatstat point process object, a lattice needs to be defined. The last two numbers in function gridcentres() are crucial for this definition. We used a step width of 0.25 m (line 2). Afterwards the grid centre coordinates need to be converted to another spatstat point process object (line 3). In line 4, the spatstat function nncross() is used to find the two nearest tree neighbours for each grid centre. Here what = "which" specifies that we are interested in the nearest neighbour indices. In the following for loop (lines 6–15) we calculate all angles θ_i, where omega is the grid-centre point and xi1 and xi2 are the nearest tree neighbours.

```
1  > library(LearnGeom)
2  > A <- gridcentres(xwindow, 200, 100)
3  > myGridP <- ppp(A$x, A$y, window = xwindow)
4  > XY <- nncross(myGridP, myDataP, what = "which", k = 1 : 2)
5  > XY$angle <- NA
6  > for (i in 1 : length(XY$which.1)) {
7  + omega.x <- A$x[i] # Grid centre point
8  + omega.y <- A$y[i]
9  + xi1.x <- myData$x[XY$which.1[i]]
10 + xi1.y <- myData$y[XY$which.1[i]]
11 + xi2.x <- myData$x[XY$which.2[i]]
12 + xi2.y <- myData$y[XY$which.2[i]]
13 + XY$angle[i] <- Angle(c(xi1.x, xi1.y), c(omega.x, omega.y),
14 + c(xi2.x, xi2.y))
15 + }
16 > mean(XY$angle, na.rm = T)
```

An alternative to Assunção's means of angles index is the *uniform angle index* or contagion (Aguirre et al. 2003). This measure considers the angles subtended by adjacent neighbours at the reference tree. An indicator function assigns a value of 1 to all situations where an angle is smaller than the reference angle $\frac{360°}{k+1}$ representing regular patterns. The use of the indicator function, however, turns a continuous variable (angle) into a categorical leading to a loss of information, which is counterbalanced by the benefit of an easy in-situ application in the field, where no exact angle measurements are required. The uniform angle index can be computed both as test-location and point-related characteristic.

The *mean directional index* (Corral-Rivas 2006) is an example of a continuous NNSS using directions instead of distances or angles. The constructed mark R_i is defined as the length of sum of unit vectors $\overrightarrow{e_{ij}}$ pointing away from reference tree i to neighbours j (see Fig. 4.15):

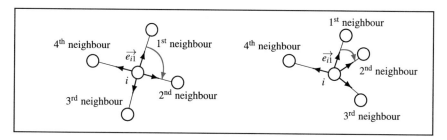

Fig. 4.15 Two different point configurations illustrating the principle of the mean directional index (Corral-Rivas 2006) applied as a point-related characteristic. The unit vectors $\vec{e}_{i1}$ are indicated in bold black; i is the typical or reference point; α_{ij} are the angles between the lines connecting i and neighbour 1 and i and neighbour j, respectively

$$R_i = \parallel \vec{e}_{i1} + \cdots + \vec{e}_{ik} \parallel = \sqrt{\left(\sum_{j=1}^{k} \cos\alpha_{ij}\right)^2 + \left(\sum_{j=1}^{k} \sin\alpha_{ij}\right)^2} \; ; \quad R_i \in [0, k]$$

(4.6)

If the neighbouring trees of tree i are located in a perfect lattice square, $R_i = 0$. The more clustered the pattern of neighbours is the larger the R_i value.

In Eq. (4.6), α_{ij} are the angles measured clockwise between a line connecting the typical point i and a nearest neighbour j and a reference bearing (e.g. due north or a line between the typical point i and the first nearest neighbour). The number of nearest neighbours is again denoted by k, i.e. in Fig. 4.15 $k = 4$. Note that the numbering of neighbours follows clockwise direction and is not related to neighbour distance. The mean directional index can be computed both as test-location and point-related characteristic and R_i can also be combined with a competition/interaction index to provide additional directional information. Dale and Fortin (2014, p. 333f.) suggested the mean directional index for the analysis of the directions of animal movements.

When the line between tree i and the first nearest neighbour is used as reference bearing, only $k - 1$ angle measurements are necessary because $\alpha_{i1} = 0°$ and $\cos\alpha_{i1} = 1$ and $\sin\alpha_{i1} = 0$. The angles of the left example in Fig. 4.15 are $\alpha_{i1} = 0$, $\alpha_{i2} = 86°$, $\alpha_{i3} = 176°$, $\alpha_{i4} = 276°$. This results in

$$R_i = \sqrt{(1 + 0.07 - 1 + 0.10)^2 + (0 + 1 + 0.07 - 0.99)^2} = \sqrt{0.17^2 + 0.08^2} = 0.19.$$

In the left example of Fig. 4.15, the four vectors more or less cancel each other out. Therefore the value of R_i is near 0 indicating a regular arrangement of points around the typical point i.

The angles of the right example in Fig. 4.15 are $\alpha_{i1} = 0$, $\alpha_{i2} = 39°$, $\alpha_{i3} = 110°$, $\alpha_{i4} = 266°$. This leads to

$$R_i = \sqrt{(1 + 0.78 - 0.34 - 0.07)^2 + (0 + 0.63 + 0.94 - 1)^2} = \sqrt{1.37^2 + 0.57^2} = 1.48.$$

In the right example of Fig. 4.15, vectors 3 and 4 almost cancel each other out while vector 1 and 2 point to similar directions. Therefore the value of R_i is much larger than in the previous example indicating a greater tendency towards clustering.

A naïve estimator of the mean directional index as a population characteristic is the arithmetic mean, i.e.

$$\overline{R} = \frac{1}{N} \sum_{i=1}^{N} R_i. \tag{4.7}$$

N is the number of points in the observation window. However, it is recommended to use the more sophisticated NN1 estimator (see Sect. 4.4.8), which takes edge effects into account. $\overline{R}$ compared with expected R_i under the conditions of a Poisson process, $\mathrm{E}R$, helps to interpret the point pattern. For $k = 4$ neighbours $\mathrm{E}R = 1.799$. However, the mean directional index can be applied to any number of neighbours.[4] Values of $\overline{R}$ larger than $\mathrm{E}R$ indicate clustered point patterns while values of $\overline{R}$ smaller than $\mathrm{E}R$ indicate regular point patterns.

The following listing gives the function `calcMDI()` which can calculate the mean directional index without edge correction. The data frame `myData` needs to include a matrix with the indices of the k nearest neighbours for each tree i. The first `for` loop includes all trees i and the second all neighbour trees j.

```
1   > calcMDI <- function(myData, k) {
2   + for (i in 1 : length(myData$x)) {
3   + ex <- 0
4   + ey <- 0
5   + for (j in 1 : k) {
6   + xx2 <- getX(myData$neighbour[i, j], myData)
7   + yy2 <- getY(myData$neighbour[i, j], myData)
8   + exx <- myData$x[i] - xx2
9   + eyy <- myData$y[i] - yy2
10  + dist <- myData$distance[i, j]
11  + ex <- ex + exx / dist
12  + ey <- ey + eyy / dist
13  + }
14  + myData$mdi[i] <- (ex ^ 2 + ey ^ 2) ^ 0.5
15  + }
16  + return(myData)
17  + }
```

For illustrating potential information gained from the application of the means of angles index and the mean directional index the data of an old mixed oak-beech forest and a middle-aged pure Sitka spruce plantation are used, see Fig. 4.16.

The analysis of the Manderscheid woodland produces $R' = 1.03, \overline{\theta} = 91.4°$ and $\overline{R} = 1.70$. For Clocaenog we obtain $R' = 1.48, \overline{\theta} = 119.8°$ and $\overline{R} = 1.13$. This confirms the visual impression from Fig. 4.16 of near random tree locations in Manderscheid and regular ones in Clocaenog. More detailed information we obtain from the density distributions in Fig. 4.17. For the means of angles index we can see an almost uniform distribution for Manderscheid, i.e. in this forest stand all angles between 0 and 180° occur with almost equal frequencies. By contrast, the Clocaenog data show a clear mode at larger distances. A similar impression we obtain from the density

---

[4]The expected values $\mathrm{E}R$ for $k = 3, \ldots, 6$ are 1.575, 1.799, 2.007 and 2.193 and can be approximated by $0.5\sqrt{k \cdot \pi}$ (Illian et al. 2008, p. 197).

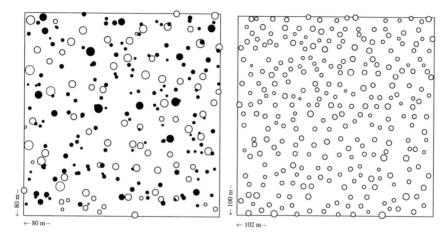

Fig. 4.16 Left: Map of a mixed sessile oak (*Quercus petraea* MATT., 81 trees, open circles)—European beech (*Fagus sylvatica* L., 163 trees, filled circles) forest stand at Manderscheid (Rhineland-Palatinate, Germany) in 1995, see Pommerening (2002) and Illian et al. (2008). Right: Map of a pure Sitka spruce (*Pinus sitchensis* (BONG.) CARR., 287 trees) plantation forest stand at Cefn Du (Clocaenog Forest, plot 1, North Wales, UK) in 2002. The radii of the disks denoting the tree locations are proportional to stem diameters

distributions of the mean directional index. For Manderscheid the mode of this distribution is further right than for Clocaenog indicating more regularity in the latter data.

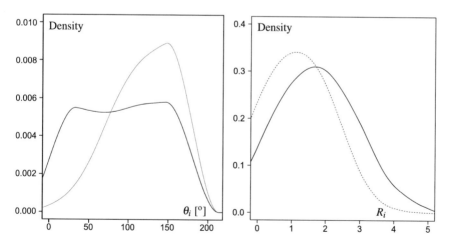

Fig. 4.17 Density distributions of θ_i (means of angles index, left) and of R_i (mean directional index, right) applied to the Manderscheid (solid lines) and the Clocaenog (dotted lines) forest stands. In both cases the Epanechnikov kernel (Eq. 4.28) was used to estimate the probability density functions with a bandwidth of 15° and 0.9, respectively

As with all such snapshot analyses (where only one point pattern in time is studied), the results often point to the legacy of past processes. In both cases human forest management in combination with natural processes have caused the current point pattern of tree locations. At Manderscheid, oak trees were managed to become regularly spaced so that they would not compete with each other. Beech trees partly colonised the stand and partly were planted. This species was frequently cut back to prevent intense competition with oak. The result was a near random pattern of tree locations. At Clocaenog (plot 1) there is only one species that was planted in a regular plantation fashion and thinned 3–5 times before mapping so that every tree was released from competition by others. This enforced regularity. Given the density at the spatial pattern at Clocaenog (plot 1), current tree interactions in this forest stand are low, although the test for the aggregation index of Clark and Evans (1954) was significant.

Interestingly the same test does not give a significant deviation from the CSR null hypothesis for Manderscheid, although local woodland managers based on their experience would argue that interactions between oak and beech were intense.

A significant test result does not necessarily indicate strong tree interactions and a lack of significance does not necessarily mean an absence of interactions (Rajala et al. 2018). This highlights that background information and experience are crucial in selecting meaningful summary characteristics and making correct interpretations. Still the point pattern information here has contributed interesting information on the past of these two forest stands. More information can be gained when considering qualitative and quantitative marks. Corral-Rivas (2006) and Illian et al. (2008) found evidence that distance-related measures perform best in statistical tests followed by directional indices.

Species Diversity (Point Patterns Marked with Qualitative Marks)

The most common qualitative mark in forest ecology and management is species. But there are many other options such as provenance (within the same species) or infections. In contrast to quantitative marks such as tree size, the mark variable is not on a continuous scale and therefore subsets the point pattern into groups of different types. These groups can for example be thought of as different species populations and there is a particular interest in studying interactions *within* and *between* such populations. As described in Sect. 4.4.5, this is similar to the concept of conspecific and heterospecfic interactions in ecology.

An early index quantifying species diversity was the coefficient of segregation by Pielou (1977). This index assumes a bivariate spatial species pattern and divides the observed number of heterospecific pairs by the expected number of heterospecific pairs. This ratio is then subtracted from 1 (Illian et al. 2008, p. 314). An index value of 0 points to independent marks, while a value of 1 describes a situation where the typical point and its nearest neighbour always have the same mark. The index value is negative with a minimum of -1, if the species of all pairs are different.

Gadow (1993) and Aguirre et al. (2003) extended Pielou's coefficient of segregation to general multivariate species patterns involving k neighbours. The mingling index is defined as the mean heterospecific fraction of plants among the k nearest neighbours of a given plant i (Eq. 4.8). In the analysis, every plant within a given research plot acts once as plant i (typical point).

$$M_i = \frac{1}{k} \sum_{j=1}^{k} \mathbf{1}(m_i \neq m_j); \qquad M_i \in [0, 1] \qquad (4.8)$$

Here m_i and m_j denote the marks of point i and j as in Table 4.1. The marks in Eq. (4.8) have so far mostly been applied to species, but they are certainly not limited to this variable. The general meaning of indicator function $\mathbf{1}(\ )$ was explained in Table 4.1: The value returned by the function is 1, if the condition inside the round brackets is fulfilled, otherwise it is 0. Naturally it is also possible to study the complementary case $\mathbf{1}(m_i = m_j)$ (Baddeley et al. 2016, p. 645). The specific construction method of mark comparison (Table 4.1) used here leads to a binary data problem, where each comparison can have outcome 0 or 1. Due to this discrete nature of outcomes for a given k there are only $k + 1$ possible values that M_i can take. In the theoretically possible outcomes $0/k$, $1/k$, ..., k/k of M_i (see Fig. 4.18 for an example), the number in the numerator denotes the number of neighbours with a

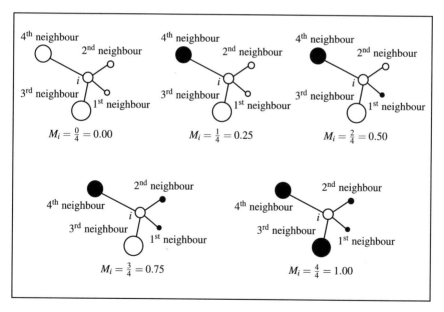

Fig. 4.18 Principle of the species mingling index (Gadow 1993) with $k = 4$ nearest neighbours and $k + 1 = 5$ possible discrete outcomes. The neighbours are numbered according to increasing distance from the reference plant i, but this ordering is not important

mark type different from that of tree i. M_i can be determined in-situ in the field
and the $k + 1$ different outcomes can serve as a basis for a mark distribution, i.e. in
a simple bar chart, the frequencies of trees with any of the $k + 1$ M_i values can be
summarised in absolute or relative terms. As for the mean directional index, again the
arithmetic mean $\overline{M}$ (Eq. 4.9) can serve as a naïve estimator of population mingling.
However, it is again recommended to use an estimator that takes edge effects into
account, see Sect. 4.4.8. $\overline{M}$ can also be calculated from the proportion of trees in
each class of the mingling mark distribution (Lewandowski and Pommerening 1997;
Pommerening and Stoyan 2006), i.e.

$$\overline{M} = \frac{1}{N} \sum_{i=1}^{N} M_i = \sum_{i=0}^{k} \frac{i}{k} b_i, \qquad (4.9)$$

where $b_0, \ldots, b_k$ are the proportions in the $k + 1$ classes of the mingling mark distribution. In mixed forest stands, it is interesting to calculate mark distribution and $\overline{M}$
separately for all or some species a of particular interest, e.g. for the most abundant
or for rare, protected species. This often is even more informative than the characteristics for the whole forest stand and can be achieved by using only those M_i in the
calculation where the species of tree i matches the species of interest.

According to Lewandowski and Pommerening (1997) expected mingling at population level (implying independent species marks), EM, is independent of the number
of neighbours, k, and can be calculated as

$$EM = \sum_{i=1}^{s} \frac{N_i(N - N_i)}{N(N - 1)}, \qquad (4.10)$$

where s is the number of species (or qualitative marks), N is the total number of trees
in the observation window and N_i is the number of trees of species i. EM describes
the mean number of k neighbours with a type of species different from the type or
species of reference tree i when the species or type marks are randomly dispersed.
The formula of EM suggests that the mingling concept highly depends on species
richness in relation to the total number of plants.

In analogy to Pielou's segregation index, $\overline{M}$ and EM can be combined in an index
Ψ expressing the relationship between observed species mingling and completely
random species mingling according to

$$\Psi = 1 - \frac{\overline{M}}{EM}, \qquad (4.11)$$

which Pommerening and Uria-Diez (2017) referred to as *species segregation index*.
Consequently, $\Psi = 0$, if the species are independently dispersed. If the nearest neighbours and a given tree always share the same species, $\Psi = 1$ (attraction of the same
species). If all neighbours always have a species different from that of a tree under
study, Ψ is negative (attraction of different species) with a minimum of -1. $\overline{M}$ and

Ψ provide different information, Ψ, for example, is less dependent on the number of individuals per species. The species segregation index includes and extends the original Pielou index.

In the case of the aforementioned type-specific analysis, expected mingling of type or species a is defined as

$$EM_a = \frac{N - N_a}{N - 1}, \qquad (4.12)$$

where N_a is in the number of points of type a or number of trees of species a (Lewandowski and Pommerening 1997). EM and EM_a relate through the *law of total probability*:

$$EM = \sum_{a=1}^{s} p_a \cdot EM_a, \qquad (4.13)$$

where $p_a = N_a/N$. Lewandowski and Pommerening (1997) also described expected values for the classes of the mingling mark distribution. Based on EM_a, a type or species specific species segregation index Ψ_a can be constructed in analogy to Eq. 4.11.

In the listing below, the indices of the four nearest neighbours are identified by the `spatstat` function `nnwhich()`. The individual-tree indices M_i (Eq. 4.8) are calculated in line 3 using function `calcMingling()` that we will introduce in a separate listing below. Mean mingling is computed in line 4. Expected mingling is calculated in line 6 using function `calcExpectedMinglingAllSpecies()` that follows Eq. (4.10). Ψ (Eq. 4.11) is then computed in line 8.

```
1  > neighbours <- nnwhich(myDataP, k = 1 : 4)
2  > k <- 4
3  > mi <- calcMingling(myData$species, neighbours, k)
4  > (mm <- mean(mi))
5  [1] 0.439549
6  > (em <- calcExpectedMinglingAllSpecies(myData$species))
7  [1] 0.445355
8  > (m.s <- 1 - mm / em)
```

The key function `calcMingling()` is listed below. It uses a `type` vector (species), the `neighbour` matrix and the number of nearest neighbours `k` as arguments.

```
> calcMingling <- function(mark, neighbours, k) {
+ mingling <- NA
+ for (i in 1 : length(mark)) {
+ msum <- 0
+ for (j in 1 : k) {
+ if(mark[i] != mark[neighbours[i, j]])
+ msum <- msum + 1
+ }
+ mingling[i] <- msum / k
+ }
+ return(mingling)
+ }
```

Table 4.2 Values of $\overline{M}^{E}$, *EM* and Ψ^{E} and $\overline{M}^{V}$, Ψ^{V}, respectively, for the mixed-species Manderscheid stand (see Fig. 4.16, left) separately for the two species and the total stand. 'E' denotes simple Euclidean neighbourhood whilst 'V' indicates Voronoi neighbourhoods, see Sect. 4.4.5

	$\overline{M}^{E}$	$\overline{M}^{V}$	*EM*	Ψ^{E}	Ψ^{V}
Oak	0.70	0.65	0.67	−0.05	0.03
Beech	0.31	0.32	0.33	0.08	0.03
Total	0.44	0.43	0.45	0.01	0.03

For calculating type or species specific mingling characteristics, the data need to be subset:

```
> mi1 <- mi[myData$species == 1] # oak
> (mm1 <- mean(mi1))
[1] 0.703704
> (em1 <- calcExpectedMinglingOneSpecies(myData$species, 1))
[1] 0.670782
> (m.s1 <- 1 - mm1 / em1)
[1] -0.0490798
```

Here function `calcExpectedMinglingOneSpecies()` is an implementation of Eq. (4.12). Using simple Euclidean neighbourhood, the population values of $\overline{M}^{E}$, *EM* and Ψ^{E} for the Manderscheid forest stand (line "Total" in Table 4.2) convey the impression of average mingling and nearly independent species marks. The situation is quite different when analysing the species populations separately: Oak has a very high mean mingling whilst that of beech is quite low. Still both observed mingling values are close to the expectation for independent marks. However, Ψ^{E} gives a weak signal suggesting that oak attracts beech whilst beech is weakly segregated. Testing as described in Sect. 4.4.9 can refine these results.

A slightly different picture is conveyed when using Voronoi neighbours for the mingling estimation. For oak $\overline{M}^{V}$ is smaller than $\overline{M}^{E}$, whilst for beech $\overline{M}^{V}$ is slightly larger than $\overline{M}^{E}$ eventually resulting in an $\overline{M}^{V}$ for all trees together (line "Total" in Table 4.2) that is slightly smaller than that estimated from Euclidean neighbours.

The differences in the mingling values between the two neighbourhoods is only slight because the overall point pattern is close to a situation of independent species marks. However, oak on average occupies much larger Voronoi territories than beech (0.3 ha as opposed to 0.008 ha, see Fig. 4.11) so that Voronoi neighbours of oak may include more oak neighbours than in the case of the simple Euclidean neighbourhood, hence the corresponding mean mingling value is smaller. By contrast, the Voronoi neighbours of beech include potentially more oak than the Euclidean neighbours. Naturally the number of Voronoi neighbours varied from tree to tree and the average number of Voronoi neighbours for oak was 5.9 and 5.8 for beech, respectively. Interestingly the values of Ψ^{V} are the same for both species and the stand as a whole suggesting a slight attraction of conspecific trees.

Finally, the aforementioned mingling mark distribution offers the opportunity to study the mingling behaviour in greater detail. In Fig. 4.19, we can see that the

Fig. 4.19 Mingling mark
distributions of oak (white)
and beech (black) at
Manderscheid (see Fig. 4.16,
left) considering $k = 4$
neighbours

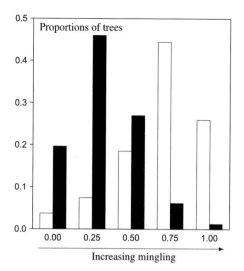

majority of oak trees are surrounded by three or four beech neighbours, whilst most
beech trees only have one or two oak neighbours. This suggests that beech occurs in
conspecific clusters whilst oak is individually mixed with beech. Apparently the use
of additional species marks puts the information on point patterns into perspective
and helps to better understand structure and interactions of a forest stand under study.

The number of nearest neighbours, k, can take any number that is justified by the
ecological context of a given study and Pommerening (2006) has demonstrated that
k depends on the properties of the pattern under study and can be optimised for a
given plant pattern. However, the problem remains that optimal k cannot be easily
determined ad hoc for a given population or forest stand. Pommerening et al. (2019)
have therefore suggested calculating Ψ for multiple k and to combine the values to
form a scale-dependent function $\Psi(r)$, where r is distance between trees:

$$\Psi'(r) = \begin{cases} \Psi(k) & \text{for } r = \bar{r}_k, \ k = 1, 2, 3, \ldots, \\ \Psi(k) + \frac{\Psi(k+1)-\Psi(k)}{\bar{r}_{k+1}-\bar{r}_k}(r - \bar{r}_k) & \text{for } \bar{r}_k < r < \bar{r}_{k+1}, \ k = 1, 2, 3, \ldots \end{cases}$$

(4.14)

The authors termed $\Psi'(r)$ the *species segregation function*. $\bar{r}_k$ is the population mean
distance $\bar{r}_k = \frac{1}{N} \sum_i^N r_{ik}$ between any individual i and its kth nearest neighbour.
Relating $\Psi(k)$ to $\bar{r}_k$ provides additional information on the scale of species segrega-
tion. At the population mean distances $\bar{r}_k$ the function has the value $\Psi(k) = 1 - \frac{\overline{M(k)}}{\text{EM}}$
and between the mean distances linear interpolation is performed. Linear interpola-
tion implies that the $\Psi(k)$ values calculated at the corresponding $\bar{r}_k$ are connected
by straight lines. As a consequence the value of $\Psi'(r)$ for a distance r between $\bar{r}_k$
and $\bar{r}_{k+1}$ is taken to be a weighted average of $\Psi(k)$ and $\Psi(k + 1)$.

With increasing r, $\Psi'(r) \to 0$ denoting mark independence. The shape of $\Psi'(r)$
whilst gradually approaching zero is a good characteristic of species mingling in a

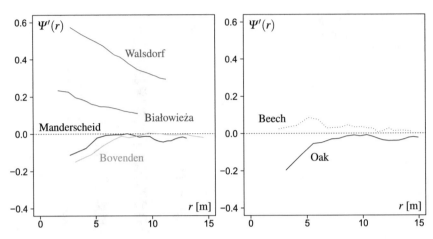

Fig. 4.20 The species segregation function for four forest stands (left) and for two species of the Manderscheid stand (right) with $k = 1, \ldots, 20$ neighbours

forest stand. The authors particularly considered $\Psi(1)$, average slope and departure from linearity as important features of the species segregation curve providing additional information on species mingling in a forest ecosystem. $\Psi(1)$ is an expression of maximum species segregation, while average slope is a measure of how rapidly the species or segregation effect decays with distance. Since nonlinear curves often indicate a fast decline of the species segregation effect, deviation from linearity is another measure of decay.

To give examples, Fig. 4.20 (left) shows the species segregation function for four mixed-species forest stands from Germany and Poland. In Walsdorf there is high species segregation at low distances with a rapid decline. By contrast Białowieża shows a much lower initial species segregation with a decline that is more gradual than in Walsdorf.

The curves of $\Psi'(r)$ for Manderscheid and Bovenden are similar: There is an aggregation of species at short distances, a bit more at Bovenden than at Manderscheid, followed by a rapid nonlinear decline of this effect and species independence at about 5 m at Manderscheid and 7 m at Bovenden.

The same species segregation function can also be calculated for the two species at Manderscheid (see also Fig. 4.16, left). Although both beech and oak are not far from species independence, we can clearly see a confirmation for what we concluded from Table 4.2: Particularly at small distances, the oak curve indicates species aggregation (followed by a nonlinear decline) while beech tends towards (mild) species segregation (Fig. 4.20, right).

Based on the Janzen-Connell, herd-immunity and size-inequality hypotheses explained in Chap. 2, Pommerening and Uria-Diez (2017) have put forward the *mingling-size hypothesis*, which suggests that in many forest ecosystems there is a significant tendency for large trees to be surrounded by other species. For studying this new hypothesis, the authors used the mingling concept as outlined in this chapter.

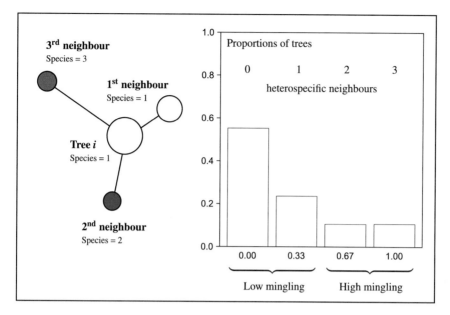

Fig. 4.21 Left: Principle and example of the structural unit of four trees used to assign a mingling index to a tree i with $M_i = 0.67$ (two heterospecific neighbours corresponding to "high mingling"). The colours represent different hypothetical species. Right: Empirical mingling distribution using $k = 3$ neighbour trees and a hypothetical data set. The labels indicate the definition of "low" and "high" mingling

In order to link species mingling with size, the authors applied logistic regression and the mingling concept had to be adapted to satisfy the requirements of this technique. For this purpose, $k = 3$ nearest neighbours were selected leading to $k + 1 = 4$ possible discrete mingling classes. The chosen mingling mark distribution suggests that the situation of 0 or 1 neighbour with a species different from that of tree i can be referred to as *low mingling*, because in this case there is either no species mingling at all or only very weak mingling. Consequently the situation that there are two or three heterospecific neighbours qualifies for "high mingling", for there is either maximum or near maximum species mingling in this situation (see Fig. 4.21).

Although this is a simplification, Pommerening and Uria-Diez (2017) could show that the proportion of high mingling is always very close to $\overline{M}$ (with $k = 3$ neighbours). The binary classification of low and high mingling allowed the use of the simple logistic regression function

$$P_m = \frac{e^{\beta_0 + \beta_1 x}}{1 + e^{\beta_0 + \beta_1 x}}, \tag{4.15}$$

where P_m is the probability of high mingling and x is an arbitrary explanatory variable. β_0 and β_1 are regression coefficients similar to the intercept and slope parameters of simple linear regression (Dalgaard 2008). Large slope values indicate a stronger

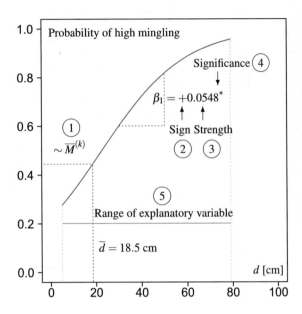

Fig. 4.22 Illustration of the information provided by the logistic regression curve after Pommerening and Uria-Diez (2017)

dependence of the probability of high mingling on the explanatory variable than small slope values. Given the objective of their paper the authors primarily used stem diameter, d, and independently stem diameter differentiation T (Eq. 4.16) for x. The logistic function P_m offers a number of useful and interpretable details (Fig. 4.22).

Drawing a vertical line from the mean stem diameter, $\overline{d}$ to the curve and a horizontal line from the point on the curve to the ordinate gives a good estimate of mean mingling, $\overline{M}$. This determines the relative location of the curve in the graph (Fig. 4.22, ①). The sign provides information on the general trend between the two variables under consideration: If positive the probability of high mingling increases with increasing stem diameter, d, otherwise it decreases (Fig. 4.22, ②). The value of the slope parameter, β_1, offers information on the strength of the relationship between the probability of high mingling and stem diameter (Fig. 4.22, ③). The larger the value of β_1 the stronger the relationship. In addition, the significance of β_1 is tested using the generalised likelihood ratio test (Fig. 4.22, ④). Finally, the extent of the logistic regression curve gives the range of the explanatory variable, d (Fig. 4.22, ⑤).

The logistic function of Eq. 4.15 is therefore a useful characteristic to link mingling with other structural measures and with size characteristics of trees. This method is also a good alternative to bivariate mark distributions studying the relationship between two NNSS distribution. Naturally such an analysis can also be done separately for particular species populations. The logistic-regression approach can also be applied to size dominance and uniform angle index discussed in the next section.

The authors found evidence that large trees and trees growing at low densities often have indeed a tendency towards high species mingling and this trend appeared to be largely independent of climate and the number of species involved. This lent strong support to the idea that human management and natural disturbances as well as Janzen-Connell and herd immunity effects influence spatial species mingling patterns in the way the mingling-size hypothesis suggested.

However, the authors' hypothesis did not universally apply, because there were also notable deviations from this expectation which require further study in the future.

Size Diversity (Point Patterns Marked with Quantitative Marks)

Quantitative marks are continuous variables that typically can be used in a more flexible way than qualitative marks. With trees size variables that relate to heights, lengths, diameter, volume and biomass but also leaf-area index and growth rates are such quantitative marks, hence the term *size diversity* in the literature related to forest structure.

Gadow (1993) suggested size differentiation, which follows the size-ratio principle of Table 4.1. This NNSS is defined as the mean of the ratio of smaller-sized and larger-sized marks of the k nearest neighbours subtracted from one:

$$T_i = 1 - \frac{1}{k} \sum_{j=1}^{k} \frac{\min(m_i, m_j)}{\max(m_i, m_j)}; \qquad T_i \in [0, 1] \qquad (4.16)$$

The value T_i increases with increasing average size difference between neighbouring trees. $T_i = 0$ implies that neighbouring trees have equal size (Pommerening 2002). For size differentiation to work all marks should ideally be larger than zero. Mean size differentiation and a density distribution can be estimated in analogy to the previously discussed NNSS. An interpretation guide is offered in Table 4.3 (Pommerening 2002). The table has also served as the basis of an empirical mark distribution, but since a continuous mark is considered, a kernel function is recommended for describing this mark distribution.

Table 4.3 Interpretation of values of the size differentiation index, Eq. 4.16

T_i interval	Qualitative descriptor	Interpretation
[0.0, 0.3)	Weak	Smaller plant has at least 70% of the neighbour plant's size
[0.3, 0.5)	Moderate	Smaller plant has 50–70% of the neighbour plant's size
[0.5, 0.7)	Strong	Smaller plant has 30–50% of the neighbour plant's size
[0.7, 1.0)	Very strong	Smaller plant has less than 30% of the neighbour plant's size

The following listing shows the key functions used for calculating T_i. The first function xdiff() is an auxiliary function ensuring that all size marks are greater than zero. Then the two marks are correctly assigned to numerator and denominator according to Eq. (4.16).

```
1   > xdiff <- function(m1, m2) {
2   + stopifnot(all(m1 > 0))
3   + stopifnot(all(m2 > 0))
4   + m <- m1 / m2
5   + if(m > 1)
6   + m <- 1 / m
7   + return(m)
8   + }
9
10  > calcDiff <- function(mark, neighbours, k) {
11  + tm <- NA
12  + for (i in 1 : length(mark)) {
13  + tsum <- 0
14  + for (j in 1 : k) {
15  + tsum <- tsum + xdiff(mark[i], mark[neighbours[i, j]])
16  + }
17  + tm[i] <- 1 - tsum / k
18  + }
19  + return(tm)
20  + }
```

calcDiff() calculates T_i based on the neighbours matrix obtained from the spatstat function nnwhich().

Using the mark construction principles of Table 4.1 it is, of course, also possible to define an alternative size differentiation NNSS, for example based on the mark difference principle of the mark variogram:

$$T_i' = \frac{1}{2k\sigma_m^2} \sum_{j=1}^{k} (m_i - m_j)^2; \qquad T_i' \in [0, 1] \qquad (4.17)$$

where σ_m^2 is the mark variance (Pommerening et al. 2011). This definition has the benefit that it does not require all marks to be larger than zero.

Expected size differentiation is not as straightforward as expected mark mingling. The marks need to be sorted in ascending order, i.e. $m_1 \leq m_2 \leq \cdots \leq m_N$. Based on this the cumulative measure D_i is defined as

$$D_i = \begin{cases} 0 & \text{for } i = 1, \\ m_1 + \ldots + m_i & \text{for } i = 2, \ldots, N. \end{cases} \qquad (4.18)$$

Expected size differentiation across species, $\mathbf{E}T$, can now be calculated as

$$\mathbf{E}T = 1 - \frac{2}{N(N-1)} \sum_{i=1}^{N} \frac{D_i}{m_i}. \qquad (4.19)$$

The R code required for computing Eq. (4.19) can look like this:

```
> calcExpectedDiffAllSpecies <- function(mark) {
+ r <- NA
+ r[1] <- 0
+ mark <- sort(mark)
+ for (i in 2 : length(mark))
+ r[i] <- r[i - 1] + mark[i - 1]
+ ET <- 0
+ for (i in 1 : length(mark))
+ ET <- ET + 2 * r[i] / mark[i]
+ ET <- 1 - 1 / ((length(mark) - 1) * length(mark)) * ET
+ return(ET)
+ }
```

In analogy to Ψ (Eq. 4.11) it is now possible to define the size segregation index, Υ (Pommerening and Uria-Diez 2017):

$$\Upsilon = 1 - \frac{\overline{T}}{\overline{ET}} \tag{4.20}$$

Consequently, $\Upsilon = 0$, if the size marks are independently dispersed without any spatial correlation. If the sizes of the nearest neighbours and a typical tree are always of similar size, $\Upsilon \approx 1$ (attraction or aggregation of similar sizes = segregation of sizes). If all neighbours always have size marks quite different from that of the reference tree, Υ is negative and tends towards -1 in the extreme case (attraction or aggregation of different sizes; aggregation in the classical sense). In the same way as for Ψ it is now also possible to consider Υ for different k and to define a function $\Upsilon'(r)$ in analogy to Eq. (4.14).

Size differentiation applied to the stem diameters of Clocaenog and Manderscheid forest stands reveals important differences (Fig. 4.23). In the plantation stand at Clocaenog there is a markedly lower spatial size differentiation than at the oak-beech forest. The density distribution shows this particularly clearly. $\overline{T} = 0.17$ and $\Upsilon = -0.006$ at Clocaenog, i.e. there is a very low diameter differentiation and the stem diameters are as good as spatially uncorrelated. At Manderscheid, $\overline{T} = 0.37$ and $\Upsilon = -0.05$, i.e. stem diameter differentiation is moderate here and there is a weak attraction of trees of different sizes. Again refined results can be obtained through testing (see Sect. 4.4.9).

Hui et al. (1998) and Aguirre et al. (2003) have proposed an index using the construction principle of mark comparison (Table 4.1) in analogy to the aforementioned mingling index. This method turns the continuous mark into a binary problem, see Fig. 4.24 and Eq. 4.21, but also is more focussed on size dominance than on diversity.

$$U_i = \frac{1}{k} \sum_{j=1}^{k} \mathbf{1}(m_i > m_j); \qquad U_i \in [0, 1] \tag{4.21}$$

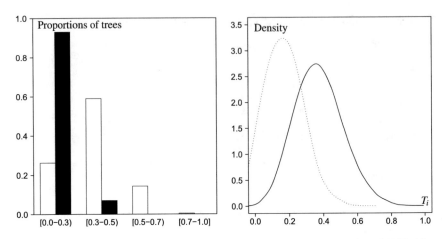

Fig. 4.23 Left: Size differentiation mark distribution according to Eq. (4.16) and Table 4.3 at Clocaenog (black) and Manderscheid (white) with $k = 4$ neighbours and stem diameter as mark. Right: The corresponding density functions based on the Epanechnikov kernel (Eq. 4.28) and a bandwidth of $h = 0.09$. Clocaenog—dotted line, Manderscheid—solid line

The indicator variable turns 1 if the size mark of tree i exceeds that of neighbouring tree j, otherwise 0. Hui et al. (1998) originally proposed the complementary case $\mathbf{1}(m_i < m_j)$. Like with the mingling NNSS, there are $k + 1$ possible discrete outcomes (Fig. 4.24) which can serve as the basis of a mark distribution.

The basic code for the calculation of the dominance index U_i is not surprisingly very similar to that for the mingling index M_i, since both indices share the same mark construction principle. The `mark` argument contains the size variable used for the mark definition and `neighbours` is the matrix with the indices of the k nearest neighbours of each tree.

```
1  > calcDominance <- function(mark, neighbours, k) {
2  + dm <- NA
3  + for (i in 1 : length(mark)) {
4  + dsum <- 0
5  + for (j in 1 : k) {
6  + if(mark[i] > mark[neighbours[i, j]])
7  + dsum <- dsum + 1
8  + }
9  + dm[i] <- dsum / k
10 + }
11 + return(dm)
12 +}
```

Gadow and Hui (2002) proposed using the $k + 1$ possible discrete outcomes of the dominance mark distribution as spatial variants of *relative crown classes* (Table 4.4). "Relative" in this context means that trees are not classified according to global canopy layers as in Kraft's crown classes (see Sect. 3.6.1) but rather classified individually in the context of their nearest neighbours.

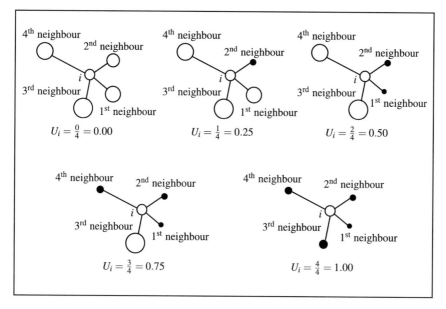

Fig. 4.24 Principle of the size dominance index (Hui et al. 1998; Aguirre et al. 2003) with $k = 4$ nearest neighbours and $k + 1 = 5$ possible discrete outcomes. The neighbours are numbered with increasing distance from the reference plant i, but this ordering is not important

Also for size dominance it is possible to estimate a population mean, which for very large observation windows with many points can be the arithmetic mean $\overline{U}$, but for sparser data edge effects have to be taken into account, see Sect. 4.4.8.

Coming back to our Manderscheid example, Fig. 4.25 shows the dominance mark distributions for the two species in this woodland. Here the species-specific distributions were calculated in such a way that the typical tree was of one specific species and the nearest neighbours were selected purely by Euclidean distance regardless of species.

We can clearly see that oak in the structural context of the four nearest neighbours mostly is a dominant species. This is contrasted by beech, where the majority of individuals is dominated by their neighbours. This is a reflection of the forest management practice at Manderscheid, where good-quality oak was favoured in thinnings at the expense of beech the prime function of which was to prevent epicormic growth at oak stems. $\overline{U}$ of oak was 0.80 whilst that of beech was 0.37.

In 2004, the CCF Sitka spruce (*Picea sitchensis* (BONG.) CARR.) trial area in Clocaenog Forest (Cefn Du, North Wales, UK) was thinned. Prior to this the Tyfiant Coed project team at Bangor University marked frame trees and trees for thinning, see Sect. 3.6.1. Plot 4 was part of a uniform shelterwood system (see Sect. 3.7) and because of exposure and altitude it was important to recruit frame trees (see Sect. 3.6.1) from dominant, windfirm canopy trees. Potential competitors were to be selected in the

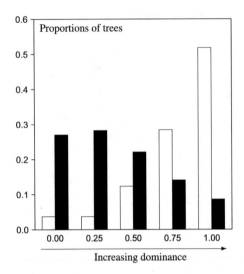

Fig. 4.25 Dominance mark distributions of oak (white) and beech (black) at Manderscheid (see Fig. 4.16, left) considering $k = 4$ neighbours and stem diameter as mark

spirit of a thinning from below, which is common practice in wind-exposed mature spruce forests (Kramer 1988).

After the marking was carried out by a silvicultural specialist, the dominance mark distribution was computed using stem diameter as mark (Fig. 4.26). The results showed very clearly that the appointed frame trees were indeed the most dominant trees of the plot whilst the trees marked for thinning were dominated. The indifferent matrix trees occurred almost uniformly in all five classes but were more frequent in the lower, first three dominance classes. Like in the previous example the neighbours of frame, matrix and trees to be thinned, categories that play the role of "species" or type here, where identified purely by Euclidean distance regardless of species.

Table 4.4 Interpretation of values of the size dominance index, Eq. 4.21 from the perspective of reference plant i with $k = 4$ neighbours (modified from Gadow and Hui 2002)

U_i	Qualitative descriptor	Interpretation
0.00	All four neighbours larger than reference plant	Very suppressed
0.25	Three of four neighbours larger than reference plant	Moderately suppressed
0.50	Two of four neighbours larger than reference plant	Co-dominant
0.75	One of four neighbours larger than reference plant	Dominant
1.00	All neighbours smaller than reference plant	Strongly dominant

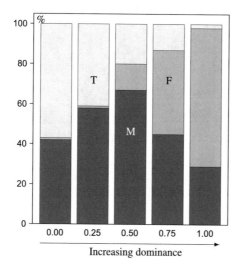

Fig. 4.26 Dominance mark distribution for frame trees (F), trees selected for thinning (T) and for indifferent matrix trees (M) at Clocaenog Forest (Cefn Du, plot 4) in 2004

An interesting and intuitively appealing variant of the size dominance characteristic was suggested by Hu and Hui (2015). As with mingling and size dominance this NNSS is also based on the construction principle of mark comparison, however, here the indicator function takes the value of 1, if the crowns of the pair of trees considered overlap, otherwise the value is 0. The authors referred to this measure as the *crowding index*, see Fig. 4.28. Larger values of C_i are associated with increased competition in the vicinity of reference tree i. At stand level, $\overline{C}$ can be interpreted as a measure of crown coverage and gap structure. The crowding index C_i is straightforward to sample in-situ in the field.

Calculations of marks in the office require several decisions to be made, particularly on how tree crowns, perhaps based on several crown radii measurements in the field, are to be modelled for the NNSS calculation, e.g. as polygons or as circular projection areas using the quadratic mean crown radius (Davies and Pommerening 2008). The latter case of circular projection areas is easy to apply and an equation of C_i could in that case look like this (see also Fig. 5.10):

$$C_i = \frac{1}{k}\sum_{j=1}^{k}\mathbf{1}(m_i + m_j > r_{i,j}); \qquad C_i \in [0, 1] \qquad (4.22)$$

Here m_i is the mean quadratic crown radius of tree i, whilst m_j is the mean quadratic crown radius of tree j. The distance between the stem centre locations of two trees

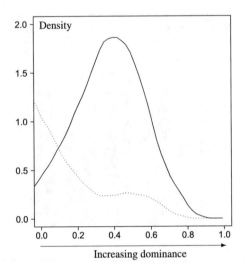

Fig. 4.27 Density function of size dominance U_i' (Albert 1999) based on stem diameter, the Epanechnikov kernel (Eq. 4.28) and a bandwidth of $h = 0.09$ for Manderscheid. Beech—dotted line, oak—solid line

is denoted as $r_{i,j}$. Crowns do not overlap if $m_i + m_j < r_{i,j}$. If crown radii measurements are not available for all trees, it is possible to model the mean quadratic crown radius in dependency on stem diameter, e.g. using the Michaelis-Menten equation

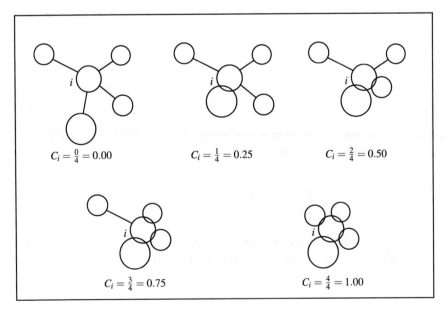

Fig. 4.28 Principle of the crowding index (Hu and Hui 2015) with $k = 4$ nearest neighbours and $k + 1 = 5$ possible discrete outcomes. i is the reference or typical plant

Table 4.5 Interpretation of values the size dominance index U_i' by Albert (1999), Eq. 4.23

U_i' interval	Interpretation for plant i
$[-1.0, -0.6)$	Very suppressed
$[-0.6, -0.2)$	Suppressed
$[-0.2, +0.2)$	Indifferent
$[+0.2, +0.6)$	Co-dominant
$[+0.6, +1.0)$	Dominant

(Pommerening and Maleki 2014). The crowding NNSS should also be straightforward to apply to remote sensing data in an automated way. Here possibly no crown-radius model is required, as it is clear from the pixel clouds whether tree crowns touch or not. In a practical context, Euclidean distances do not need to be considered but the k nearest neighbours are defined by the proximity of their crowns to that of the typical tree.

Albert (1999, p. 51ff.) suggested an intriguing combination of size differentiation and size dominance NNSS:

$$U_i' = \frac{1}{k} \left(\sum_{j=1}^{k} \mathbf{1}(m_i > m_j) \left(1 - \frac{m_j}{m_i} \right) - \sum_{j=1}^{k} \mathbf{1}(m_i < m_j) \left(1 - \frac{m_i}{m_j} \right) \right) \quad (4.23)$$

This NNSS is based on the mark difference construction principle of Table 4.1 similar to the competition index by Tomé and Burkhart (1989), i.e. size differentiation where neighbours are large than tree i are subtracted from size differentiation with smaller neighbours.

In the context of competition and facilitation, the sum indicating dominant size differentiation is reduced by size differentiation where tree i is not dominant. Like in Tomé and Burkhart (1989) this NNSS includes a compensation effect. Equation 4.23 leads to continuous values of U_i' between -1 and 1. The larger U_i' the more dominant is tree i. Negative values of U_i' indicate suppression by neighbouring trees. With values of $U_i' \approx 0$ either the neighbouring trees are of similar size as tree i or the differentiation values of smaller and larger neighbours even out. Values of $U_i' = 0$ are expected with mark independence. Albert (1999) also suggested the interpretation guide given in Table 4.5.

In analogy to size differentiation U_i' can be coded as in the listing below. Equation (4.23) is implemented in line 4, where automatic type coercion from boolean to integer is used (see Appendix C, Sect. C.1). Lines 9–19 follow the template of the coding for size differentiation.

```
1  > xdiff <- function(m1, m2) {
2  + stopifnot(all(m1 > 0))
3  + stopifnot(all(m2 > 0))
4  + m <- (m1 > m2) * (1 - m2 / m1) - ((m1 < m2) * (1 - m1 /
5  + m2))
6  + return(m)
7  + }
8  >
9  > calcDD <- function(mark, neighbours, k) {
10 + dd <- NA
11 + for (i in 1 : length(mark)) {
12 + ddsum <- 0
13 + for (j in 1 : k) {
14 + ddsum <- ddsum + xdiff(mark[i], mark[neighbours[i, j]])
15 + }
16 + dd[i] <- ddsum / k
17 + }
18 + return(dd)
19 + }
```

Applied to the Manderscheid woodland (see Fig. 4.16) we see clear differences in the two species: The nurse species beech has one mode around 0, indicating indifference, and another, weaker one around 0.6 suggesting co-dominance. Obviously the majority of beech trees do not "threaten" oak, however, there are a few that come close to being a threat. By contrast oak has only one mode around 0.4 suggesting co-dominance. For beech $\overline{U}' = -0.13$ whilst for oak $\overline{U}' = 0.32$. For the whole forest stand (trees of both species pooled) $\overline{U}' = 0.02$, i.e. near the expectation for mark independence (Fig. 4.27).

Care has to be taken when analysing point patterns with more than one qualitative type (species) in addition to quantitative marks. Here often the question arises how best to compute species or type specific variants of NNSS for quantitative marks, e.g. species specific size differentiation or dominance.

Initially this was decided by typical or reference point, i.e. the individual-tree index was calculated for all points and then a subset for the points of a specific type or species was used for the NNSS calculation regardless of the species of the k nearest neighbours. The work by Goreaud and Pélissier (2003) and Wiegand and Moloney (2014), however, lends support to the view that in certain situations NNSS should be calculated more strictly for *within* and *between* type point patterns (see also Sect. 4.4.5). This implies that for within-type analyses typical points and neighbours should be of one species or type and this can be achieved by subsetting a composite pattern for one species and analysing the subset. This is probably the best way of defining species-specific NNSS for quantitative marks. However, it is also possible to study between-type interactions where the typical point is of one particular species and the k nearest neighbours of another. This can be achieved by using the spatstat function nncross(), which can be employed to identify the nearest neighbours of a species other than that of typical tree i. In the end it depends on the research question which definition of species-specific NNSS is applied and there are also many problems where it is appropriate that the typical tree is of one specific species and the nearest neighbours are selected purely by Euclidean distance regardless of species.

4.4.7.2   Second-Order Summary Characteristics

Second-order summary characteristics were initially developed within the theoretical framework of mathematical statistics (Baddeley et al. 2016; Illian et al. 2008; Møller and Waagepetersen 2007; Ripley 1976) and then applied in various fields of natural sciences including forest ecology (Dale and Fortin 2014; Wiegand and Moloney 2014) and management. They are functional summary characteristics describing variability and correlations in marked and non-marked point processes by considering pairs of points.

Functional second-order characteristics depend on a distance variable r and quantify structural properties of a point process (or pattern) depending on the probability that two points occupy locations r distance away from each other. This allows them to be related to various ecological scales and also, to a certain degree, to account for long-range point interactions (Pommerening 2002). Second-order characteristics are considered less ambiguous and more precise than NNSS, i.e. their use is recommended provided the data are of sufficient quality and quantity (see Sect. 4.4.7). Several examples are given in this section but more can be found in the literature provided.

Location Diversity (Point Patterns without Marks)

Traditionally the most popular second-order characteristic has been Ripley's K-function (Ripley 1976). $\lambda K(r)$ denotes the mean number of points in a disc $b(\xi_i, r)$ of radius r centred at the typical point ξ_i (which is not counted) where λ is the intensity (point density), see Fig. 4.29. This function has a cumulative nature.

Besag (1977) suggested transforming the K-function by dividing it by π and by taking the square root of the quotient, which yields the L-function with both statistical and graphical advantages over the K-function:

$$L(r) = \sqrt{\frac{K(r)}{\pi}} \tag{4.24}$$

Like other cumulative characteristics the L-function is often used for testing the CSR hypothesis (see Sect. 4.4.9), e.g. in Ripley's L-test (Stoyan and Stoyan 1994). In the case of a Poisson process, $L(r) = r$. For clustered point processes, $L(r) > r$ and regular point processes exhibit L-functions with $L(r) < r$ (see Fig. 4.30, left, for an illustrated example). Instead of the classical definition often another transformation, $L(r) - r$, is used in the literature frequently under the same name, which results

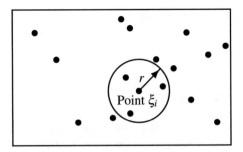

Fig. 4.29 The principle of the construction of Ripley's K function

in horizontal graphs and $L(r) = 0$ in the Poisson case (see Fig. 4.30, right). Whilst clustered patterns can have a minimum distance between points close to zero, regular patterns usually have a larger minimum distance, r_0, which is also referred to as *hard-core distance*.

Despite its graphical and statistical advantages the classical $L(r)$ function is not easy to interpret, since observed curves often do not differ much from the 45° line indicating CSR. Also the cumulative nature of the graphs often renders interpretations difficult. In that case the horizontal graph of $L(r) - r$ is easier to interpret, see Fig. 4.30 (right).

However, for the detailed analysis of interactions functions of the nature of derivations are preferred. One of these is the *pair correlation function* $g(r)$, which is related to the first derivative of the K-function (Eq. 4.25) (Illian et al. 2008),

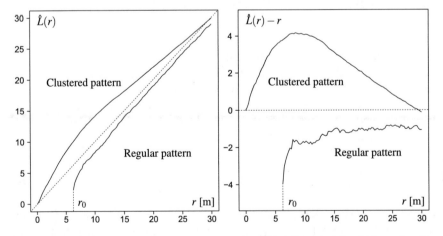

Fig. 4.30 Different shapes of Besag's L-function (Eq. 4.24, left) and of the $L(r) - r$ function (right) estimated from simulated point process models along with their interpretation. The dashed reference lines indicate CSR (Poisson process) and r_0 is the hard-core distance. For maps of the corresponding patterns see Fig. 4.7

$$g(r) = \frac{K'(r)}{2\pi r}. \tag{4.25}$$

For a heuristic interpretation of the pair correlation function $g(r)$ consider the probability P that two points of the point process occur at two locations with distance r between them. The probability that there is a point of the point process in a circle of an infinitesimally small area dF is λdF, where the intensity λ is a constant due to the stationarity assumption. Also due to isotropy, directions do not play a role (see Sect. 4.4.3). Therefore the probability $P(r)$ depends on distance r between the two points only. Then we have

$$dF \bigcirc\!\!\longleftarrow\!\! r \!\longrightarrow\!\! \bigcirc dF \qquad P(r) = \lambda dF\, \lambda dF\, g(r).$$

In this approach, the pair correlation function $g(r)$ acts as a correction factor. For a Poisson process and for large distances the points are stochastically independent and as a result $g(r) = 1$. In the case of cluster processes $g(r) > 1$. This can be interpreted as an attraction among points. For regular patterns $g(r) < 1$ indicating inhibition between points (see Fig. 4.31).

For cases other than a Poisson process, it is interesting to consider specific characteristic distances such as those given as $r_0, \ldots, r_3$ in Fig. 4.31 (Illian et al. 2008, p. 239ff.). r_0 is the aforementioned minimum interpoint or hard-core distance, where as r_1 is the distance at which the first maximum of $g(r)$ occurs, i.e. the range of most frequent short distances between the typical point and its nearest neighbour. This is often but not always followed by a minimum at r_2 indicating regions in the pattern with a small number of points beyond the nearest neighbours. Further sequences of local minima and maxima can follow, which are typically smaller in extent than those at r_1 and r_2. Eventually the correlation range, r_{corr}, is reached, perhaps at r_3 in Fig. 4.31. After that point there are only random fluctuations around 1. Sometimes this limit may differ from 1 due to statistical fluctuations and spatial inhomogeneity. r_{corr} marks an important point because statistical interactions cease beyond this distance. Distances $r_0, \ldots, r_3$ are particularly important for regular and clustered patterns.

Degenhardt (1999) argued that r_0 and r_{corr} are closely related to point density λ and can be estimated as $r_0 = a\sqrt{\frac{1}{\lambda}}$ and $r_{\text{corr}} = b\sqrt{\frac{1}{\lambda}}$, where $a \approx 0.1$ and b between 1.2 and 1.5 (Illian et al. 2008, p. 159f.).

For the estimation of density functions such as the pair correlation function non-parametric kernel estimator methods are commonly used Diggle 2014; Illian et al. 2008, which are not based on model assumptions. An unknown probability density function $f(x)$ can be estimated from a sample $x_1, \ldots, x_n$ by using a symmetric kernel function $k(x)$:

$$\hat{f}(x) = \frac{1}{n} \sum_{i=1}^{n} k(x - x_i), \tag{4.26}$$

Fig. 4.31 Estimated pair
correlation functions $\hat{g}(r)$
corresponding to the
$\hat{L}$-functions in Fig. 4.30

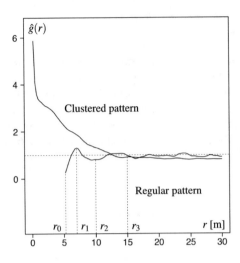

where $\hat{f}(x)$ is an estimator for $f(x)$, n is the sample size and x are discrete values
throughout the sample range for which values of $f(x)$ are estimated, e.g. discrete
distance values $0 = 0, 0.25, 0.5, 0.75, \ldots$. There are many possible kernel functions
to choose from and most frequently used are the *box kernel*

$$k(x) = \begin{cases} \frac{1}{2h} & \text{for } -h \leq x \leq h, \\ 0 & \text{otherwise} \end{cases} \tag{4.27}$$

and the *Epanechnikov kernel*

$$k(x) = \begin{cases} \frac{3}{4h}\left(1 - \frac{x^2}{h^2}\right) & \text{for } -h \leq x \leq h, \\ 0 & \text{otherwise,} \end{cases} \tag{4.28}$$

where h is referred to as bandwidth and acts as a smoothing parameter. When the
discrete test value considered is x and the bandwidth is h, the idea of kernel estimators consists in taking all sample values $x_1, \ldots, x_m$ between $x - h$ and $x + h$ and
giving them weights which decrease with increasing deviation from x. In the case
of second-order and related functions, x corresponds with the interpoint distance r
(see Fig. 4.32).

The bandwidth h balances the trade-off between bias and variance of the estimator. Large values of h result in smooth curves of estimated density functions, small
h can potentially carry forward much statistical noise. The choice of h has, therefore, a major impact on the resulting probability density function but the choice of
kernel function is generally held to be of secondary importance (Diggle et al. 2014).
Identifying a suitable h is a task similar to the choice of suitable class widths for
histograms. Illian et al. (2008) emphasized that selecting h should be the result of an
iterative process where several values are tried and the results compared. The authors

Fig. 4.32 The principle of
using kernel functions in the
estimation of the pair
correlation and similar
probability density functions

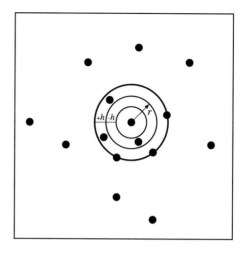

recommended $h \approx 0.1/\sqrt{\lambda}$ as a starting point, where λ is again point density. For identifying general trends, larger values of $h = 2$ m are often good starting points for tree data. However, since h also influences the locations of $r_0, \ldots, r_3$ in Fig. 4.31, for an accurate determination of these distances it is recommended to use low values of h here and to compare the results for these distances with those discernible from the L functions. Often one third to half of the diagonal of the observation window is recommended as the maximum value of r to be included in the analysis (Illian et al. 2008, p. 96), but this also depends on research objectives.

Illian et al. (2008, p. 232) gave the estimator of the pair correlation function as

$$\hat{g}(r) = \sum_{\xi_i, \xi_j \in W}^{\neq} \frac{k_h(\|\xi_i - \xi_j\| - r)}{2\pi r A(W_{\xi_i} \cap W_{\xi_j})}. \tag{4.29}$$

Here ξ_i and ξ_j are arbitrary points of the point pattern in the observation window W. k_h is a suitable kernel function, e.g. the Epanechnikov kernel (Eq. 4.28), $A(W_{\xi_i} \cap W_{\xi_j})$ is the area of intersection of W_{ξ_i} and W_{ξ_j}, see Illian et al. (2008, p. 481f. and p. 188), relating to the translation edge correction (Ohser and Stoyan 1981), see Sect. 4.4.8.

In line 1 of the following code listing, the discrete values of r are defined for which the pair correlation function is estimated. In lines 2 and 3, the spatstat pcf() function is used for estimating the pair correlation function. correction = "translate" relates to the translation edge correction (see Sect. 4.4.8), kernel = "epanechnikov" defines the kernel function as previously discussed and bw = 0.8 provides the bandwidth information. The code in line 4 is a manual check of the hard-core distance. After calculating the function the graph can be plotted as indicated in line 7.

```
1  > myR <- seq(0, 30, 0.25)
2  > myPcf <- pcf(myDataP, r = myR, correction = "translate",
```

Fig. 4.33 Estimated pair
correlation functions $\hat{g}(r)$ for
Clocaenog (see Fig. 4.16,
solid curve) and Pen yr Allt
Ganol (dashed curve) from
North Wales using the
Epanechnikov kernel
(Eq. 4.28) and a bandwidth
of 0.8 m

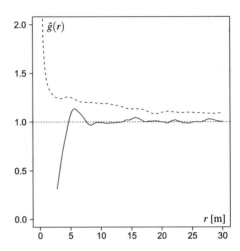

```
3   + kernel = "epanechnikov", bw = 0.8)
4   > hardcore <- min(nndist(myDataP, k = 1))
5   >
6   > par(mar = c(2, 3, 0.5, 0.5))
7   > plot(myPcf$r, myPcf$trans, ... )
```

We applied the above code to the data from Clocaenog (see Fig. 4.16, right) and Pen yr Allt Ganol (Pommerening and Uria-Diez 2017) by ignoring the species marks in the latter case, see Fig. 4.33. From the $\hat{g}(r)$ curves it is obvious that Clocaenog has a very regular pattern of tree locations with a hard-core distance of 2.5 m, whilst at Pen yr Allt Ganol there is a heavy clustering of tree locations due to an ongoing patchy regeneration process.

In the Clocaenog graph we can also recognise a first maximum at $r_1 \approx 5$ m followed by a weak minimum at $r_2 \approx 9$ m. The correlation range is owed to past interactions and probably is about 10–11 m (Fig. 4.33). It is recommended to show graphs of $\hat{g}(r)$ only for distances $r \geq r_0$, i.e. for the range of distances that occur in the actual data in order to avoid statistical artefacts and misinterpretations.

LeMay et al. (2009) studied the spatio-temporal structure of a multi-storied, multi-aged interior natural Douglas fir (*Pseudotsuga menziesii* var *glauca* (MIRB.) FRANCO) forest in British Columbia (Canada). While applying the pair correlation function to the data from six research plots the authors noticed that in the same forest there was more variation in space (between the plots) than there was in time within the same plots (Fig. 4.34). This suggests that changes in space are often greater in natural forests than they are in time. In plot 1, tree locations were closer to a complete random dispersion with flat maximum between 2 and 4 m. By contrast, a clustered tree dispersion was found in plot 2 with a cluster radius of approximately 3 m. That difference can often be greater in space than in time also needs to be considered in experimental design, where replications play an important role (Montgomery 2013).

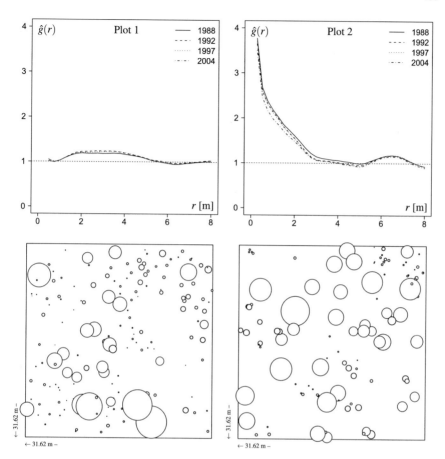

Fig. 4.34 Top: The pair correlation function $\hat{g}(r)$ estimated for plots 1 and 2 of the Alex Fraser Research Forest (BC, Canada) with bandwidth $h = 0.5$ m and the Epanechnikov kernel (Eq. 4.28) in a mostly pure stand of interior Douglas fir (*Pseudotsuga menziesii* var *glauca* (MIRB.) FRANCO). Bottom: The corresponding plot maps in 2004

Illian et al. (2008), Baddeley et al. (2016) and Bagchi and Illian (2015) described methods of pooling data and treating replications.

Gavrikov et al. (1993) studied the differences in stem-centre and crown-centre coordinates of a Scots pine (*Pinus sylvestris* L.) stand in the Irkutsk region of Siberia in Russia. The stand originated from a large-scale fire disturbance followed by a rapid colonisation by Scots pine seedlings leading to a mono-specific even-aged stand. At the time of measurement the trees in the plot were 90 years old. By that time the Scots pine stand had undergone a heavy self-thinning process.

The pair correlation function was estimated twice, 1. by using the stem-centre locations and 2. based on the crown-tip locations of the 484 pine trees (Fig. 4.35). Although the differences in coordinates seem small on first sight, it turned out that

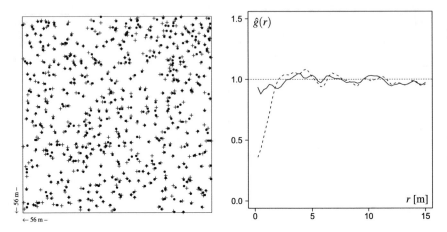

Fig. 4.35 Left: Two sets of locations of Siberian Scots pine (*Pinus sylvestris* L.) trees, i.e. stem-centre coordinates (filled circles) and crown-centre locations (crosses). Right: The corresponding estimated pair correlation functions $\hat{g}(r)$ based on stem-centre coordinates (solid curve) and on crown-centre locations (dashed curve). The Epanechnikov kernel (Eq. 4.28) and a bandwidth of $h = 0.25$ m were used

the curves of $\hat{g}(r)$ were quite different for the two location definitions: Whilst the pair correlation function for the stem centre-locations seemed to suggest a largely random pattern, $\hat{g}(r)$ of the crown-tip coordinates indicated a much more regular pattern and a small hard-core distance had formed. This illustrates that stem-centre tree locations, particularly of light demanding trees and with trees that do not naturally tend to develop a straight stem axis, are not necessarily the best definition of tree locations, because these locations are very conservative. However, since trees can avoid shading and obstruction by moving their crowns and/or their crown locations are moved by environmental factors, it is important to include such signals in the analysis and to consider them in the experimental design. The phenomenon of shifting tree crowns is also known as *crown plasticity* and has been studied in a number of research papers (Uria-Diez and Pommerening 2017; Vovides et al. 2018).

Other important related characteristics describing point patterns include the nearest-neighbour distance distribution $d(r)$, the aforementioned spherical contact distribution function or empty-space function $h_S(r)$ and their combination, the J-function (Illian et al. 2008; Baddeley et al. 2016). The cumulative empty space function and nearest-neighbour distance distribution are also denoted as $F(r)$ and $G(r)$ (Diggle 2014; Baddeley et al. 2016).

Species Diversity (Point Patterns with Qualitative Marks)

As described in Sect. 4.4.5, in point process statistics qualitative marks are usually treated as indicating ecological and statistical populations of different types or species, i.e. a point pattern with points of several types. These populations are then analysed separately but also the relationships between them is studied. If only two types of points are considered, the point pattern is referred to as *bivariate*, otherwise it is *multivariate*. Quantitative marks can theoretically be reduced to qualitative marks by aggregating them to size classes, which usually is not recommended for the loss of information. Also species marks can be aggregated to broader trait groups, such as conifers and broadleaves or shade-tolerant and light-demanding species. However, it is also possible to go the other way and consider different provenances or genotypes of the same species as types.

In analogy to the K- and L-functions also multivariate or inter-type K_{ij}- and L_{ij}-functions have been defined (Lotwick and Silverman 1982). For example $\lambda_j K_{ij}$ is defined as the mean number of points of type j in a disc of radius r centred at the typical point of type i. However, greater importance for interaction research has a derived measure, the *partial pair* or *cross-pair correlation function* $g_{ij}(r)$, which by analogy to $K_{ij}(r)$ can also be referred to as the intertype pair correlation function. It is a tool for investigating multivariate point patterns (Penttinen et al. 1992; Stoyan and Penttinen 2000; Illian et al. 2008) and its interpretation is similar to that of $g(r)$: Consider $P_{ij}(r)$ as the probability of finding a point of type i (e.g. i = species 1) in a circle with an infinitesimally small area dF and a point of type j (e.g. j = species 2) in another one of area dF, where the distance between the two circle centres is r. Then

$$\lambda_i dF \bullet\!\!\longleftarrow\!\!- r \longrightarrow\!\!\circ \lambda_j dF \quad P_{ij}(r) = \lambda_i dF \, \lambda_j dF \, g_{ij}(r).$$
$$i(j) \qquad\qquad\qquad j(i)$$

λ_i and λ_j is the intensity of the points of type i and of type j, respectively. The global behaviour of $g_{ij}(r)$ is the same as that of $g(r)$ and can also be interpreted in the same way (Illian et al. 2008).

In the code listing provided below, an implementation of estimating $g_{ij}(r)$ for the Manderscheid example (Fig. 4.16, left) is shown. It is important to assign factor levels as marks when defining the `ppp` object (line 2). After determining the evaluation distances using the `seq()` function in line 3 we calculate $\hat{g}_{11}(r)$ (oak-oak interations) using the `spatstat` function `pcfcross()` (lines 4–6). Here specifying the marks i and j is an additional task compared to function `pcf()`. The same applies to the relationships oak-beech (`myPcf12`) and beech-beech (`myPcf22`).

```
1  > myDataP <- ppp(myData$x, myData$y, window = xwindow,
2  + marks = factor(myData$species))
3  > myR <- seq(0, 10, 0.25)
4  > myPcf11 <- pcfcross(myDataP, i = 1, j = 1, r = myR,
5  + correction = "translate", kernel = "epanechnikov",
6  + bw = 0.5)
7  > myPcf12 <- pcfcross(myDataP, i = 1, j = 2, r = myR,
8  + correction = "translate", kernel = "epanechnikov",
9  + bw = 0.5)
10 > myPcf22 <- pcfcross(myDataP, i = 2, j = 2, r = myR,
11 + correction = "translate", kernel = "epanechnikov",
12 + bw = 0.5)
```

Fig. 4.36 Estimated partial
pair correlation functions
$\hat{g}_{ij}(r)$ for the mixed
oak-beech woodland at
Manderscheid
(Rhineland-Palatinate,
Germany, see Fig. 4.16)
using the Epanechnikov
kernel (Eq. 4.28) and a
bandwidth of 0.5 m

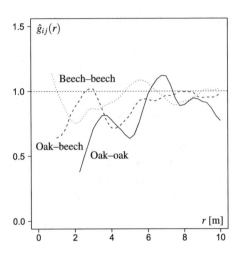

The corresponding minimum distances for oak-oak and beech-beech can be calculated by subsetting the data for each species and then by applying the function `min(nndist(myDataP1, k = 1))` in the case of oak-oak. The intertype minimum distance can be obtained from `min(nncross(myDataP1, myDataP2, k =
1, which = "dist"))`, where `myDataP1` represents the oak and `myDataP2` the
beech pattern.

The results reveal different types of interactions (Fig. 4.36). $\hat{g}_{11}(r)$ for the oak-oak
pattern reveals some regularity with a hard-core distance of approximately 2.0 m. We
also recognise the aforementioned short-range order with local maxima at $r = 3$ m
and $r = 7$ m. The beech pattern, by contrast, shows a cluster process at short distances.
There is an interesting local maximum at $r = 6$ m between two other local maxima
of $\hat{g}_{11}(r)$, which may indicate the distances between beech clusters and the spatial
arrangement of both species in this stand. The function $\hat{g}_{12}(r)$ remains below 1 for
almost the whole range of r. This suggests repulsion between the two species. The
range of correlation is around 8 m for beech-beech and oak-beech, but about 12 m
for oak-oak which reflects well the forest management type where the oak trees are
the frame trees and beech is a nurse species and by-product of oak management. The
oak trees form a regular hard-core pattern, whereas beech occur in clusters in weak
dependence on oak (Illian et al. 2008, p. 327f.).

At Coed y Brenin (plot 7) in North Wales a clearfelled site was replanted with
Douglas fir (*Pseudotsuga menziesii* (MIRB.) FRANCO) in 1985. However, many Douglas
fir saplings died soon after and broadleaved and other conifer species colonised
the site eventually resulting in ten different species when the plot was measured
in 2006. In this colonisation context, the partial pair correlation function can shed
light into the interactions between the 92 broadleaved and 287 conifer trees. The
broadleaved trees apparently formed clusters with a radius of approximately 2 m,
whereas the conifers showed some regularity with a hard-core distance of 44 cm
(compare with Fig. 4.37, left). This is plausible, since many conifers where planted

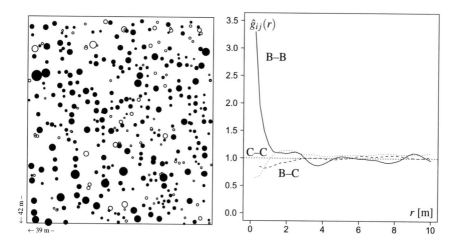

Fig. 4.37 Left: Mixed-species woodland at Coed y Brenin (plot 7) in North Wales (UK) in 2006. The ten species were grouped together as broadleaves (B, open circles) and conifers (C, closed circles). Right: The corresponding partial pair correlation functions $\hat{g}_{ij}(r)$. The Epanechnikov kernel and a bandwidth of $h = 0.5$ m were used

in a regular pattern and the broadleaves could only colonise space between these planting locations and where conifers had died. The relationship between broadleaves and conifers was characterised by repulsion, which however, was not too strong at this stage of woodland development. The correlation range of $\hat{g}_{BC}(r)$ and $\hat{g}_{CC}(r)$ in 2006 was approximately 10 m, whilst that of $\hat{g}_{BB}(r)$ reached further. Function $\hat{g}_{BB}(r)$ also shows a series of local maxima and minima reflecting the limited space available for colonisation.

The *mark connection function* $p_{ij}(r)$ is another important second-order characteristic used for the analysis of point patterns marked with qualitative marks. Consider a randomly selected pair of trees from a mixed-species forest with distance r between them. Then the species of both trees are random and the probability that one tree is of species i and the other of species j depends on distance. This probability is described by the mark connection function. It is related to the partial pair correlation function and the pair correlation function through $p_{ij}(r) = p_i p_j \cdot g_{ij}(r)/g(r)$ (Illian et al. 2008, p. 331). The measure can be interpreted as the probability P_{or} that two points at distance r have marks i and j given that these points are of the point pattern under study:

$$p_{ij}(r) = P_{or}\left(m(o) = i, m(\mathbf{r}) = j\right)$$

If $p_{ij}(r)$ is large for a given r then there is a tendency that at this distance preferably pairs of trees occur, where one tree is of species i and the other of species j. For very large distances it can be expected that there is no interaction between the two species any more. Then the values of the function $p_{ij}(r)$ are likely to be around the specific values

$$p_{ii}(r) = p_i^2 \qquad\qquad \text{for } r \to \infty,$$

$$p_{jj}(r) = p_j^2 \qquad\qquad \text{for } r \to \infty,$$

$$p_{ij}(r) = 2 \cdot p_i \cdot p_j \qquad\qquad \text{for } r \to \infty.$$

Here p_i (p_j) is the proportion of trees of species i (j) or their probability that a randomly selected tree is of species i (j). Factor 2 arises from the fact that any of the two trees can be of species i, whilst the other is of species j. When the two species are spatially (stochastically) independent from each other, $p_{ij}(r)$ is constant and equal to p_i^2 or $2 \cdot p_i \cdot p_j$. In tree interaction research, this behaviour of $p_{ij}(r)$ can be used to identify the range of mark correlation. This provides valuable information on the range up to which interaction between the species of a mixed forest stand can be expected. The sum of function values over all possible mark connection functions should sum up to one at any distance r.

In the R code listing shown below, an implementation of estimating $p_{ij}(r)$ for the Manderscheid example (Fig. 4.16) is given. Again, it is important to assign factor levels as marks when defining the ppp object (line 2). After determining the evaluation distances using the seq() function in line 3 we calculate $\hat{p}_{11}(r)$ (oak-oak interactions) using the spatstat function markconnect() (lines 4–6). The same applies to the relationships oak-beech (myP12) and beech-beech (myP22).

```
1  > myDataP <- ppp(myData$x, myData$y, window = xwindow,
2  + marks = factor(myData$species))
3  > myR <- seq(0, 10, 0.25)
4  > myP11 <- markconnect(myDataP, i = 1, j = 1, r = myR,
5  + correction = "translate", bw = 0.5)
6  > myP12 <- markconnect(myDataP, i = 1, j = 2, r = myR,
7  + correction = "translate", bw = 0.5)
8  > myP22 <- markconnect(myDataP, i = 2, j = 2, r = myR,
9  + correction = "translate", bw = 0.5)
```

We analysed the Manderscheid and Coed y Brenin woodlands with the mark connection function $p_{ij}(r)$ using our own estimation code rather than spatstat (Fig. 4.38, left). The function $\hat{p}_{11}(r)$ reflects inhibition among oak trees, i.e. oak trees appear to occur at a distance to each other, and $\hat{p}_{22}(r)$ mutual attraction among beech, i.e. these trees can be located quite close to each other. The range of mark correlation in both cases is around 8 m. The prominent local maxima of $\hat{p}_{12}(r)$ and $\hat{p}_{22}(r)$ at $r = 2$ m and $r = 5$ m reflect interactions between beech clusters and their oak neighbours, whilst the second local maximum may correspond to pairs of trees from neighbouring clusters (Illian et al. 2008, p. 334).

At Coed y Brenin (plot 7), there is moderate attraction among broadleaves up to 1 m and then rapidly turns to "inhibition", which marks the boundary of colonisation space that was available to these species (Fig. 4.38, right). There is clearly attraction among conifers and the alternating local maxima and minima may be a legacy of the planting design. Function $\hat{p}_{BC}(r)$ describing the interaction between broadleaves and conifers is halfway between $\hat{p}_{BB}(r)$ and $\hat{p}_{CC}(r)$ with moderate attraction at $r = 1$ m and stronger inhibition at $r = 1.8$ m. The range of mark correlation in the case of B-B is around 6 m, for B-C and C-C it is close to 10 m.

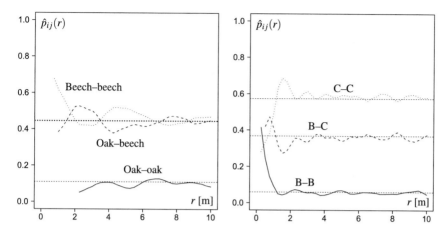

Fig. 4.38 Mark connection functions $\hat{p}_{ij}(r)$ for the mixed-species stands at Manderscheid (left) and Coed y Brenin (right, see also Figs. 4.16 and 4.37). The Epanechnikov kernel (Eq. 4.28) and bandwidths of $h = 1.0$ m and $h = 0.5$ m were used, respectively. The asymptotic values of the mark connection functions indicating stochastic independence are given by dotted straight horizontal lines

In another research plot at Coed y Brenin, a mixed birch-Sitka spruce woodland was thinned in June 2003 with the objective to release birch from dominating Sitka spruce (*Picea sitchensis* (BONG.) CARR.) neighbours to conserve the nature of a mixed birch-spruce woodland. At the time of thinning the forest stand was 34 years old and

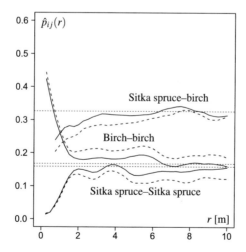

Fig. 4.39 Estimated mark connection functions $\hat{p}_{ij}(r)$ for the mixed birch-Sitka spruce woodland Coed y Brenin (plot 1) (North-Wales, UK) using the Epanechnikov kernel (Eq. 4.28) and a bandwidth of $h = 1.0$ m. The solid curves represent $\hat{p}_{ij}(r)$ before and the dashed ones $\hat{p}_{ij}(r)$ after thinning. The dotted straight horizontal lines show the asymptotic values of the mark connection functions before thinning. Modified from Mason et al. (2004)

birch (silver birch, *Betula pendula* ROTH, and downy birch, *Betula pubescens* EHRH.) suffered from spruce competition with signs of heavy decline. The crown thinning reduced total stand basal area from 42 m^2 to 31 m^2 (see Table 7.3). The results in terms of interaction within and between the two species are shown in Fig. 4.39.

On average the combination of Sitka spruce-birch is the most likely pairing. However, at distances around 1.0 m, there is a high probability of birch-birch combinations occurring. Within birch there is mutual attraction up to 2 m, whilst there is mutual inhibition up to that distance in Sitka spruce. As expected there is also inhibition between birch and Sitka spruce trees almost throughout the whole range of $r = 10$ m considered.

The thinning clearly reduced the probability of Sitka spruce-birch pairings and increased the probability of birch trees having other birch trees in their immediate vicinity. As a result of removing mostly Sitka spruce trees the probability of pairings within this species was also reduced. These results show that the thinning has successfully released birch trees from Sitka spruce competition by consolidating birch clusters and reducing mixed-species pairs at close proximity. However, as intended the general character of a mixed Sitka spruce-birch woodland has remained unchanged (Mason et al. 2004).

Partial pair correlation and mark connection functions are very useful in forest ecosystems with only few tree species. However, in highly diverse woodlands, their application is difficult. With only three tree species there are $\binom{4}{2} = 6$ partial pair correlation and mark connection functions to consider and many forests, for example in temperate China, have 30 or more species not to mention the situation in tropical forests. Even if one focuses only on the intertype functions and/or forms species groups, this remains a difficult task. To offer a solution Pommerening et al. (2011) and Hui and Pommerening (2014) introduced the *mark mingling function* $v(r)$. Strictly speaking the mark mingling function is a mark correlation function, but also shares similarities with the intertype mark connection function. The fundamental idea of $v(r)$ is to use the mingling test function $\mathbf{1}\left(m(\xi_i) \neq m(\xi_j)\right)$, i.e. assessing only, whether the species or types of a pair of points under consideration are different. This relates to the principle of the mingling NNSS discussed in Sect. 4.4.7.1 and to the mark comparison principle of Table 4.1.

In analogy to the estimator of the mark correlation function in Illian et al. (2008, p. 354f.) the estimator of the mark mingling function is defined as

$$\hat{v}(r) = \frac{1}{\mathbf{E}M} \sum_{\xi_i, \xi_j \in W}^{\neq} \frac{\mathbf{1}(m(\xi_i) \neq m(\xi_j)) \, k_h(\|\xi_i - \xi_j\| - r)}{2\pi r \, A(W_{\xi_i} \cap W_{\xi_j})}. \tag{4.30}$$

Here ξ_i and ξ_j are arbitrary points of the point pattern in the observation window W. k_h here is the Epanechnikov kernel function (Eq. 4.28) but other kernel functions can be used as well, $A(W_{\xi_i} \cap W_{\xi_j})$ is the area of intersection of W_{ξ_i} and W_{ξ_j}, see Illian et al. (2008, p. 481f. and p. 188), relating to the translation edge correction (Ohser and Stoyan 1981), see Sect. 4.4.8. Expected mingling, $\mathbf{E}M$ (Eq. 4.10), is used as a normalising term, see Illian et al. (2008, p. 346).

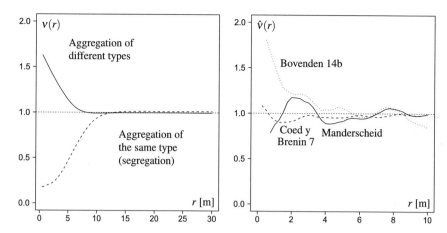

Fig. 4.40 Left: Schematic diagram of the mark mingling function $\nu(r)$. The straight horizontal line through 1 indicates spatially independent type marks. Right: Mark mingling function $\hat{\nu}(r)$ estimated for Manderscheid, Coed y Brenin (plot 7) and Bovenden 14b using the Epanechnikov kernel (Eq. 4.28) and a bandwidth $h = 0.5$ m

For $\nu(r) > 1$ we can conclude that there is an aggregation of different types or species, i.e. aggregation or attraction in the classical sense, whilst for $\nu(r) < 1$ we have within-type or within-species aggregation, traditionally termed segregation, (see Fig. 4.40, left). As with any second-order characteristic also for the mark mingling function we can determine the correlation or interaction range, which may differ from that found for other functions.

It is straightforward to implement the estimation of $\nu(r)$ in R using `spatstat`. Again, it is important to assign factor levels as marks when defining the `ppp` object (line 2). After determining the evaluation distances using the `seq()` function in line 3 we calculate $\hat{\nu}(r)$ using the `spatstat` function `markcorr()` (lines 4–6). In line 4, we recognise the aforementioned mingling test function $\mathbf{1}\left(m(\xi_i) \neq m(\xi_j)\right)$.

```
1  > myDataP <- ppp(myData$x, myData$y, window = xwindow, marks =
2  + factor(myData$Species))
3  > myR <- seq(0, 10, 0.25)
4  > myNu <- markcorr(myDataP, f = function(m1, m2) { m1 != m2 },
5  + r = myR, correction = "translate", kernel = "epanechnikov",
6  + bw = 0.5)
```

We used the mark mingling function for re-analysing the woodlands of Manderscheid, Coed y Brenin (plot 7, see Fig. 4.37) and additionally Bovenden 14b (Germany, see Pommerening and Uria-Diez 2017) and to compare their mingling patterns. The Manderscheid curve of $\hat{\nu}(r)$ is in fact very similar in shape to $\hat{p}_{12}(r)$ (oak-beech) in Fig. 4.38 (left), which is always the case in bivariate point patterns. Manderscheid $\hat{\nu}(r)$ starts with species segregation and has a local maximum at around 2 m indicating moderate species attraction and continues to show species segregation between $r = 4-7$ m followed by another maximum at 8 m. Coed y Brenin (plot 7) has ten species, i.e. the situation is more complex in this woodland. Still the dashed curve has a shape similar to the intertype B-C mark connection function in Fig. 4.38 (right). In contrast to Manderscheid, for Coed y Brenin 7 $\hat{v}(r)$ starts with species aggregation and then has a local minimum around 2 m indicating species segregation and retains this behaviour throughout the distance range. The remarkable woodland Bovenden 14b near Göttingen in Germany demonstrates a very different mingling pattern with strong species attraction up to $r = 6$ m. This was caused by specific diversity-oriented woodland management in a mixed ash-sycamore beech woodland with five different species. Naturally dominant beech (*Fagus sylvatica* L.) was continuously removed to favour individual trees of ash (*Fraxinus excelsior* L.) and sycamore (*Acer pseudoplatanus* L.).

Size Diversity (Point Patterns Marked with Quantitative Marks)

Quantitative marks, particularly size, size ratios, number or weight of fruits, isotopic nutrient uptake by plants and biomass as well as growth rates are of particular interest in the analysis of marked point patterns. In ecological-statistical analyses, summary functions from point process statistics yield valuable information on the correlations between the marks of point pairs in dependence on the interpoint distance r, about mutual inhibition or mutual stimulation and on the degree of mark similarity.

The analysis of marked point patterns is a multistep, iterative process. The map of plant locations and marks is first visually assessed and this may already result in working hypotheses or even in tentative ecological theories. The next logical step in the analysis is the estimation and interpretation of mark distributions. These can, for example, be simple empirical histograms of tree stem diameter or total height but also boxplots. It is important to learn about the shape of these mark distributions, e.g. how many modes they have and if they are skewed. Sometimes the structure of a mark distribution even suggests a transformation of marks before any second-order characteristics are applied. By interpreting this characteristic one learns important facts about mark structure and a trained ecologist can often link the shape of an observed mark distribution with certain ontogenetic stages in a population of organisms or with stand management (Ballani et al. 2019).

Stem diameter has for example traditionally been the most frequently used tree characteristics in forest ecology and management. This has much to do with the fact that stem diameters can be efficiently measured in terrestrial surveys and are therefore the most commonly available tree variable. Figure 4.41 visualises six common types of mark distributions for stem diameters.

Following the analysis and interpretation of mark distributions, Ballani et al. (2019) recommended constructing mark-mark scatterplots, see Fig. 4.42. The mark-mark scatterplot is obtained by plotting the quantitative marks of all point pairs with an inter-point distance r smaller than a suitable r_{max}. The mark pairs of these points are arranged in a mark-mark coordinate system, where the abscissa is related to the mark of the first point i and the ordinate to that of the second point j. For ecological

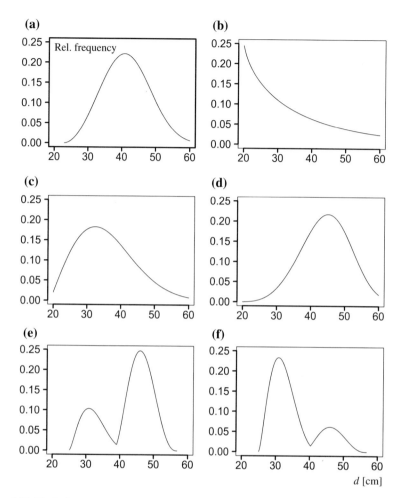

Fig. 4.41 Typical mark distributions of diameters at breast height (d) of **a** an even-aged pure species stand (plantation), **b** an uneven-aged selection or natural forest (negative exponential), **c** an even-aged pure species stand (right skewed due to a few exceptionally big trees), **d** an even-aged pure species stand (left skewed due to a few exceptionally small trees), **e** a two-storied mixed forest and **f** a young (regenerated) stand with a few standards/seed trees

applications intervals $[0, r_{max}]$ for suitable r_{max} are of main interest, since interactions of ecological importance mainly occur at short distances.

When plotting pairs of marks, it is not obvious which is the first and which the second data point. Therefore, in the scatterplot two points are assigned to each point pair, i.e. (i, j) and (j, i). The resulting graph is symmetric with respect to the line $m_i = m_j$.

The authors used grey tones to highlight point pairs at specific distance $r < r_{max}$. According to the inter-point distance of a point pair in the interval $[0, r_{max}]$, the points

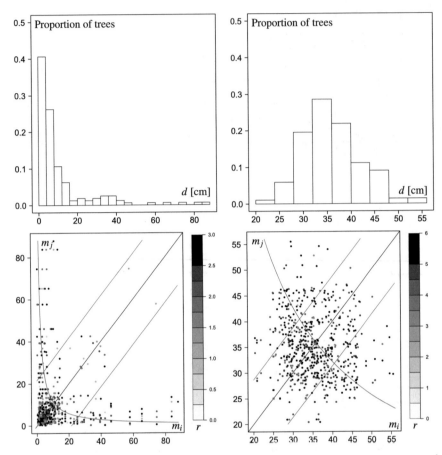

Fig. 4.42 Mark distributions and mark-mark scatterplots including the contour lines at $m_i m_j = \overline{m}^2$ (blue) and $0.5(m_i - m_j)^2 = \sigma_m^2$ (red) for plot 1 ($r_{\max} = 3$ m, left) from the Alex Fraser Research Forest in British Columbia (Canada) in 1988, see Fig. 4.34 and for Clocaenog Forest plot 1 (Wales, UK) in 2002 (right, $r_{\max} = 6$ m), see Fig. 4.16. d is stem diameter

are then plotted in the corresponding grey tone between white (= distance 0) and black (= distance $r_{\max}$), see Fig. 4.42.

The choice of the limiting distance $r_{\max}$ is crucial. Ballani et al. (2019) recommended values of $r_{\max}$ markedly smaller than the range of correlation. For this the authors have three reasons: 1. The ecologically most interesting interaction occurs at short distances corresponding to the distances to near neighbours, 2. the shape of the summary functions, which are aimed to be interpreted by the scatterplot, is strongly determined by the values for small $r_{\max}$, and 3. for large $r_{\max}$ the scatterplot includes too many points making interpretation difficult.

In order to facilitate the interpretation the mark-mark scatterplot is complemented by two contour lines, i.e. the (curved) contour line corresponding to mark pairs

(m_i, m_j) which satisfy $m_i m_j = \overline{m}^2$, thus dividing the mark-mark scatterplot into two regions of mark pairs (m_i, m_j) resulting in contributions $m_i m_j / \overline{m}^2$ less or larger than one. This is helpful when discussing certain values of the mark correlation function $k_{mm}(r)$ (see the following paragraphs in this section and Eq. 4.31). The second contour line (a pair of straight lines) corresponds to mark pairs (m_i, m_j) which satisfy $0.5(m_i - m_j)^2 = \sigma_m^2$, where σ_m^2 denotes the variance of the marks. This contour line is a boundary between comparatively similar and comparatively dissimilar mark pairs, likewise separating small and large contributions of $0.5(m_i - m_j)^2$ to the mark variogram $\gamma_m(r)$ (see Eq. 4.33). These contour lines were devised to match the test functions of $k_{mm}(r)$ and $\gamma_m(r)$. If other correlation functions were used, different contour lines would apply.

The mark-mark scatterplot magnifies the information on interactions between the marks of point pairs at short inter-point distances: It uncovers more crucial ecological information on the association of marks than the second-order summary functions, since the mark-mark scatterplot displays the original marks before averaging. This provides an opportunity to identify extreme pairs, with very big or very small mark differences, which leads to a better understanding of the summary characteristics for small r. Furthermore, the mark-mark scatterplot yields detailed information on the type of association between marks for short inter-point distances r (Ballani et al. 2019).

Here various values of $r_{\max}$ should be tried iteratively to find a good balance between too few data points and a chaotic plot with too many data points that make interpretation difficult. The visual assessment of mark-mark scatterplots gives a good impression of the type of spatial interactions at short distances, which are of particular ecological interest: Positive or negative association and the influence of mark size and correlation on these relationships. A good way to start is to check whether the points of the plot are located close to the diagonal $m_i = m_j$ or far from it (Ballani et al. 2019). Next, one could check how many point pairs are located outside the red and blue boundary lines relative to those inside.

The mark distributions in Fig. 4.42 are very different and correspond to types (b) and (a) in Fig. 4.41. The analyst may come to the conclusion that plot 1 in the Alex Fraser Research Forest represents an unevenaged forest whilst plot 1 at Clocaenog Forest is typical of an even-aged plantation stand. The mark distribution of plot 1 in the Alex Fraser Research Forest may even tempt the analyst to do a logarithmic transformation of the marks (Ballani et al. 2019).

Mark-mark scatterplots are clearly influenced by the mark distributions. In both plots, there are many mark pairs near the diagonal $m_i = m_j$ suggesting similar size. Whilst in the Douglas fir forest this is predominantly true for trees smaller than 20 cm in stem diameter, this relates to almost all sizes at Clocaenog (plot 1). In fact, the mark-mark scatterplot for Clocaenog looks similar to the result of a random labelling simulation, where the marks are randomly assigned to tree locations. This can be seen from the core square $[25, 25] \times [45, 45]$, which is nearly uniformly filled with points. In the Alex Fraser Research Forest, many extreme pairings of very large and very small trees occur, which are much rarer at Clocaenog Forest. The scatterplots therefore suggest that plot 1 in the Douglas fir forest should produce graphs of second-order characteristics with some positive and some negative associations, whilst the Sitka spruce forest at Clocaenog, plot 1, is probably not far from mark independence.

The mark-mark scatterplots can be applied using the R package mmsc Ballani et al. 2019. With the help of the remotes package mmsc can be downloaded from the first author's GitHub using the commands

```
> library(remotes)
> install_github('fballani/mmsc')
> library(mmsc)
> help(mmsc)
```

Details of how to use the package are provided in the help file, which can be called upon by using the last command of the above listing.

The *mark correlation function* $k_{mm}(r)$ is a conditional second-order characteristic assessing the similarity and dissimilarity of marks at given distances r (Penttinen et al. 1992; Stoyan and Penttinen 2000; Pommerening 2002; Illian et al. 2008). The function uses the mark-product principle (see Table 4.1) in the construction of its test function, i.e. marks m_i and m_j are multiplied. From the single values of the test function for each pair of marked points a mean is calculated for each r. Thus the function $k_{mm}(r)$ is conceived, which is dependent on r. It is advisable to divide the function by the square of the mean mark, μ^2, in order to make interpretation easier. The function can be interpreted as the conditional mean of $m(o) \cdot m(\mathbf{r})$ under the condition that at locations o and $\mathbf{r}$ there are points of the point process:

$$k_{mm}(r) = \frac{\mathbf{E}_{or}(m(o) \cdot m(\mathbf{r}))}{\mu^2}$$

Illian et al. (2008, p. 354f.) gave the estimator of the mark correlation function as

$$\hat{k}_{mm}(r) = \frac{1}{\overline{m}^2} \sum_{\xi_i, \xi_j \in W}^{\neq} \frac{m(\xi_i) m(\xi_j) k_h(\|\xi_i - \xi_j\| - r)}{2\pi r A(W_{\xi_i} \cap W_{\xi_j})}. \tag{4.31}$$

Here ξ_i and ξ_j are arbitrary points of the point pattern in the observation window W. k_h is the Epanechnikov kernel function (Eq. 4.28) but can also be another kernel, $A(W_{\xi_i} \cap W_{\xi_j})$ is the area of intersection of W_{ξ_i} and W_{ξ_j}, see Illian et al. (2008, p. 481f. and p. 188), relating to the translation edge correction (Ohser and Stoyan 1981), see Sect. 4.4.8.

Often points at close proximity tend to have small marks as a result of mutual growth inhibition in clusters. This typically causes mark correlation functions smaller than 1. In ecological applications, $k_{mm}(r) = 0$ is hardly possible for biological variability. For $k_{mm}(r) > 1$ both points at close proximity need to have marks larger than the mean mark. When tree stem diameters are used as marks, $k_{mm}(r) > 1$ is virtually impossible and therefore the mark correlation function can only use a limited range of values. However, $k_{mm}(r) > 1$ can occur with tree height (Suzuki et al. 2008) and fruits such as pine nuts (Gonçalves and Pommerening 2011). With $r \to \infty$ the mark correlation function tends towards the limit of 1, although like for other second-order functions the actual limit may differ from 1 because of statistical fluctuations and spatial inhomogeneity (Ballani et al. 2019).

For the implementation of the mark correlation function in R we again make use of spatstat and the markcorr() function. However, in defining the ppp object we now pass on stem diameter dbh as quantitative marks (line 1f.). The test function determined in line 4 is that of the mark correlation function $k_{mm}(r)$.

```
1  > myDataP <- ppp(myData$x, myData$y, window = xwindow, marks =
2  + myData$dbh)
3  > myR <- seq(0, 12, 0.25)
4  > kmm <- markcorr(myDataP, f = function(m1, m2) { m1 * m2 },
5  + r = myR, correction = "translate", method = "density",
6  + kernel = "epanechnikov", bw = 0.8)
```

The *mark variogram* $\gamma_m(r)$ is a characteristic similar to the mark correlation function, which was defined in analogy to geostatistical variograms. It is defined as the conditional expectation of the mark difference given that at locations o and $\mathbf{r}$ there are points of the point process:

$$\gamma_m(r) = \frac{1}{2}\mathbf{E}_{or}(m(o) - m(\mathbf{r}))^2; \qquad r \geq 0 \tag{4.32}$$

The function uses the mark difference construction principle (see Table 4.1) in its test function, i.e. marks m_i and m_j are subtracted from one another. If marks of points at close proximity are similar, $\gamma_m(r)$ has small values for small r. However, in ecological applications the case $\gamma_m(r) = 0$ at $r = 0$ cannot occur, since this would imply that points close in space have exactly the same mark, which is hardly possible because of biological variability. Therefore in ecological analyses, mark variograms always show a so-called nugget effect, i.e. a positive value of $\gamma_m(r)$ at $r = 0$. With increasing r a mark variogram tends towards a limit, often referred to as "sill", which is the mark variance σ_m^2. Similarly as for the mark correlation function, the corresponding limit of an empirical mark variogram may differ from the empirical mark variance because of statistical fluctuations and spatial inhomogeneity (Ballani et al. 2019; Pommerening and Särkkä 2013). Like with any other second-order characteristic, the point marking the end of the correlation range, r_{corr}, where $\gamma_m(r) = \sigma_m^2$ for $r > r_{\text{corr}}$, is an interpretable interaction characteristic (see Fig. 4.43). Large values of r_{corr} indicate a large interaction range. In addition there is the upper limit of the mark variogram for very small values of r, $\gamma_m(0+)$. With certain point patterns $\gamma_m(0+)$ can be larger than σ_m^2, i.e. large values of $\gamma_m(0+)/\sigma_m^2$ express large size differences between points at close proximity and are usually assumed to imply strong interaction (see Fig. 4.43, right). The mark variogram has small values, if the marks of the points in a pair with interpoint distance r are similar (regardless whether they are both small or large), and large values, if the marks differ strongly.

The definition of the mark variogram appears to be very similar to the definition of the geostatistical variogram, which is used to study the variability of regionalised

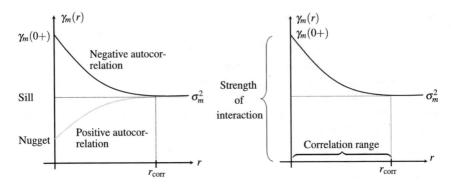

Fig. 4.43 Shape of a mark variogram, $\gamma_m(r)$, influenced by interaction between plants (negative autocorrelation variograms, black curve) compared to the standard shape of a geostatistical variogram $\gamma(r)$ (grey). r is the interpoint distance, r_{corr} the correlation range and σ^2 the field variance or variance of marks (also referred to as sill). Nugget is related to the inherent variability in the studied pattern at very small scale (Pommerening and Särkkä 2013)

variables taking values in the whole space and not only at specific plant locations (Cressie 1993; Chilès and Delfiner 1999; Wackernagel 2003), see Eq. (4.1). The typical shape of geostatistical variograms is shown by the grey curve in Fig. 4.43 (left). Regionalised variables measured at short distances are similar and therefore lead to typical geostatistical variograms, which increase with increasing distance. Such a trend is often termed *positive autocorrelation* or simply *positive association*.

The mark variogram, however, is based on measurements at specific plant locations and can have different shapes. If there is no correlation between the marks, the mark variogram is just a horizontal line, i.e. $\gamma_m(r)$ is constant. If trees of similar size are arranged in clusters, the mark variogram has a shape similar to a geostatistical variogram even though the marks are tree characteristics and not geostatistical observations. However, occasionally there are many close pairs of trees with one large tree and one small tree in a tree pattern leading to mark variograms with the shape of the black curve in Fig. 4.43. This shape is very different from the shape of a geostatistical variogram (see also Wälder and Stoyan 1996; Stoyan and Wälder 2000; Suzuki et al. 2008) reflecting *negative autocorrelation* or simply *negative association* with large size differences between neighbouring trees, i.e. large individuals are likely to be close to small ones and vice versa (Suzuki et al. 2008). Negative autocorrelation is therefore also an expression of high small-scaled diversity of tree sizes. Pommerening and Särkkä (2013) identified five processes causing negative autocorrelation in mark variograms applied to spatial forest data:

• Natural self-thinning during the stem exclusion phase (Oliver and Larson 1996),
• Selective thinnings as part of forest management promoting size differentiation,
• Selective thinnings and harvesting promoting birth processes,
• Natural competition processes leading to a differentiation of tree sizes (understory reinitiation and old growth stages according to Oliver and Larson 1996),

Fig. 4.44 Research plot
41–194 of the Swiss beech
thinning experiment at
Embrach. Point size is
proportional to stem
diameter. The filled circles
highlight pairs of trees with
the largest values of
$\frac{1}{2}\left(m(\xi_i) - m(\xi_j)\right)^2 r^{-2}$ that
are chiefly responsible for
the effect of negative
autocorrelation in the mark
variogram (modified from
Pommerening and Särkkä
(2013))

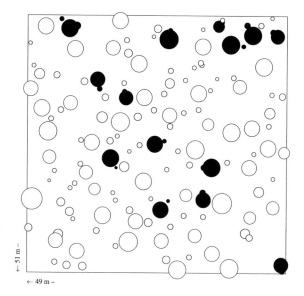

- Natural/human disturbances leading to the retention of a few old large trees which
  gives rise to mass colonisation by small trees followed by self-thinning among
  small trees (understory reinitiation and old growth stages according to Oliver and
  Larson 1996).

The authors' study particularly highlighted that disturbances, either natural or man-
made or a combination of both, are major causes of patterns with negative autocorrelation. Therefore, this summary characteristic is an important tool in the analysis
of disturbance ecology. Disturbances lead to a removal (death) of trees, and later to
an increase of small trees followed by death of some of the small trees. Therefore,
they can induce the development of local size hierarchies and negative autocorrelation and create temporary situations of high size diversity. Birth processes increase
the mark variance and are the most important processes leading to negative autocorrelation which is a temporary expression of high small-scaled diversity of tree
sizes. Beyond this point in time some of the smaller trees are outcompeted and die
and others approach the size of their larger neighbours. Sometimes also new waves
of incoming small regeneration trees destroy the pattern of negative autocorrelation
(Pommerening and Särkkä 2013).

   In addition to using mark-mark scatterplots for a better understanding of observed
mark variogram plots it is also possible to highlight pairs of trees with high test
function values for small r to check up on plausibility but also to find clues for
ecological interpretation (see Fig. 4.44).

   In analogy to the mark correlation function the estimator of the mark variogram
can be written as

$$\hat{\gamma}_m(r) = \sum_{\xi_i, \xi_j \in W}^{\neq} \frac{\frac{1}{2} \left(m(\xi_i) - m(\xi_j) \right)^2 k_h(\|\xi_i - \xi_j\| - r)}{2\pi r A(W_{\xi_i} \cap W_{\xi_j})}. \tag{4.33}$$

Here ξ_i and ξ_j are arbitrary points of the point pattern in the observation window W. k_h is an appropriate kernel function, e.g. the Epanechnikov kernel (Eq. 4.28), $A(W_{\xi_i} \cap W_{\xi_j})$ is the area of intersection of W_{ξ_i} and W_{ξ_j}, see Illian et al. (2008, p. 481f. and p. 188), relating to the translation edge correction (Ohser and Stoyan 1981), see Sect. 4.4.8. It is possible to normalise $\hat{\gamma}_m(r)$ by dividing the term on the right hand side of Eq. 4.33 by σ_m^2. This results in curves that can be compared to horizontal lines through 1 denoting situations where there is no spatial correlation between marks. However, as a result of this normalisation graphical information on σ_m^2 is lost.

For the implementation of the mark variogram in R we again employ `spatstat`, but this time the `markvario()` function (line 4). Again, in defining the `ppp` object we pass on stem diameter `dbh` as quantitative marks (line 1f.). The test function in this case does not have to be specified.

```
1  > myDataP <- ppp(myData$x, myData$y, window = xwindow, marks =
2  + myData$dbh)
3  > myR <- seq(0, 12, 0.25)
4  > mv <- markvario(myDataP, r = myR, correction = "translate",
5  + method = "density", kernel = "epanechnikov", bw = 1.3,
6  + normalise = TRUE)
```

For an easier comparison with the mark correlation function the aforementioned option `normalise = TRUE` was selected (line 6) and as a consequence the mark variogram curve was normalised as explained above (Fig. 4.45).

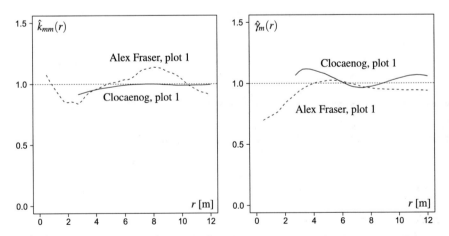

Fig. 4.45 Left: Mark correlation function $\hat{k}_{mm}(r)$ estimated for the two example forests from Fig. 4.42 with bandwidth $h = 0.8$ m. Right: The corresponding mark variograms $\hat{\gamma}_m(r)$ with bandwidth $h = 1.3$ m. In both cases the Epanechnikov kernel (Eq. 4.28) and stem diameters as marks were used

To advance the analysis of plot 1 at Clocaenog Forest and plot 1 at the Alex Fraser Research Forest (see Fig. 4.42), we can now interpret the mark correlation functions and the mark variograms for both plots (Fig. 4.45).

Whilst the mark correlation function for Clocaenog, plot 1 is a little "unspectacular", there is clearly a more complex spatial size structure at Alex Fraser. At Clocaenog we understand that there is a tendency for pairs of trees to be both smaller than the average at distances up to 6 m. The correlation range extends to 8 m. According to $\hat{k}_{mm}(r)$, the first 8 m describe the space in which weak interactions take place at Clocaenog, plot 1, as the mark-mark scatterplot suggested. At Alex Fraser at small r there is the rare situation of large mark values which quickly leads to a minimum at around 3 m, where both marks are smaller than the mean mark. There is a local maximum at $r = 8$ m indicating pairs of large trees. This reflects the structural heterogeneity with clusters of small trees interspersed by individual mature trees, where also some pairs of larger trees at close proximity occur (see Fig. 4.34, bottom left). The correlation range appears to extend beyond 12 m at Alex Fraser, plot 1.

The mark variogram at Clocaenog, plot 1, indicates a weak effect of negative autocorrelation up to 6 m. Around $r = 7$ m pairs of trees occur with similar small or large marks. Beyond this there is a tendency again for marks that increasingly differ. According to $\hat{\gamma}_m(r)$ the correlation range extends beyond 12 m. Switching to Alex Fraser, plot 1, we observe a tendency of similar marks (either both small or large) up to $r = 4$ m followed by a small local maximum at $r = 5$ m and configurations where tree marks are again similar. Also at Alex Fraser, plot 1, the correlation range appears to extend beyond 12 m.

Both $\hat{k}_{mm}(r)$ and $\hat{\gamma}_m(r)$ have largely produced results we expected from the preliminary analysis based on the mark-mark scatterplots (Fig. 4.42). The differences in the function shapes originate from the different test functions and any interpretation has to consider these closely. Whilst the mark variogram only accounts for mark similarity of difference (regardless of whether the marks are actually both large or small), the mark correlation function makes a distinction between large or small marks at the two point locations. It is therefore useful to consider both functions side by side in the interpretation (see also Suzuki et al. 2008).

An alternative to both mark correlation function and mark variogram is the *mark differentiation function* $\tau_m(r)$ (Pommerening et al. 2011; Hui and Pommerening 2014). In this function, the mark ratio contruction principle (see Table 4.1) is used in the test function, see also the size differentiation NNSS in Sect. 4.4.7.1. It is defined as the mean of the complement of the mark ratio under the condition that at locations o and $\mathbf{r}$ there are points of the point process:

$$\tau_m(r) = 1 - \mathbf{E}_{or} \frac{\min(m(o), m(\mathbf{r}))}{\max(m(o), m(\mathbf{r}))}; \quad r \geq 0 \qquad (4.34)$$

In analogy to the mark correlation function and to the mark variogram the estimator of the mark differentiation function can be written as

$$\hat{\tau}_m(r) = \sum_{\xi_i,\xi_j \in W}^{\neq} \frac{1 - \frac{\min\left(m(\xi_i),m(\xi_j)\right)}{\max\left(m(\xi_i),m(\xi_j)\right)} k_h(\|\xi_i - \xi_j\| - r)}{2\pi r A(W_{\xi_i} \cap W_{\xi_j})}. \qquad (4.35)$$

The symbols and notation used here are the same as for the other characteristics in this section. Like with the mark variogram it is possible to normalise $\hat{\tau}_m(r)$ by dividing the term on the right hand side of Eq. 4.35 by ET (Eq. 4.19), which is the limit of the mark differentiation function. This also results in curves that can be compared to horizontal lines through 1 denoting situations where there is no spatial correlation between marks. Normalising the mark differentiation function facilitates comparisons between different patterns, however, as a result of this normalisation graphical information on ET itself is lost.

For the implementation of the mark differentiation function in R we use the spatstat markcorr() function (line 4). Again, in defining the ppp object we pass on stem diameter dbh as quantitative marks (line 1f.). The test function of the mark differentiation function needs a bit more sophisticated programming this time.

```
1 > myDataP <- ppp(myData$x, myData$y, window = xwindow, marks =
2 + myData$dbh)
3 > myR <- seq(0, 12, 0.25)
4 > tau <- markcorr(myDataP, function(m1, m2) {ifelse(m1 / m2 >
5 + 1, 1 - m2 / m1, 1 - m1 / m2)}, r = myR, correction =
6 + "translate", method = "density", kernel = "epanechnikov",
7 + bw = 0.8, normalise = TRUE)
```

Up to $r = 5$ m stem diameter differentiation in plot 1 of the Alex Fraser Research Forest is lower than expected in a situation of uncorrelated marks (Fig. 4.46).

This is also the case for the Sitka spruce trees at Clocaenog 1 at distances around 2 m, however, between $2.5 \leq r \leq 6$ differentiation is larger than expected followed by a local minimum and another local maximum. Clusters of different and similar

Fig. 4.46 Mark differentiation function $\hat{\tau}_m(r)$ estimated for the two example forests from Fig. 4.42 with bandwidth $h = 0.8$ m. The Epanechnikov kernel (Eq. 4.28) and stem diameters as marks were used

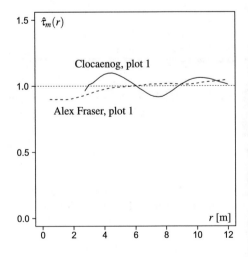

Fig. 4.47 Schematic example of a circular observation window W where the points inside W (filled circles) may have interactions with those outside (open circles) near the boundaries of the observation window

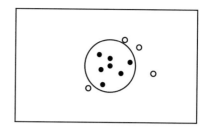

sized trees appear to alternate in this forest. Also for the mark differentiation functions the correlation ranges appear to extend beyond 12 m.

Overall the curves of $\hat{\tau}_m(r)$ are reminiscent of those of $\hat{\gamma}_m(r)$ suggesting that apart from minor differences both functions perform in a similar way (Pommerening et al. 2011; Hui and Pommerening 2014). Which to prefer depends on the nature of the marks used and on personal taste. The mark differentiation function can, for example, not be used in situations, where both marks can have a value of zero.

Stoyan (1987) introduced the *cross-mark correlation function* $k_{lm}(r)$ which considers the correlation between two quantitative marks l and m. The principle of this function can, of course, also be applied to the mark variogram and the mark differentiation function. In `spatstat`, the cross-mark correlation function can be estimated using the function `markcrosscorr()` (Baddeley et al. 2016, p. 660).

4.4.8 Edge Effects

Edge effects arise in spatial analysis when the observation window W, in which the pattern is observed, is part of a larger region. The essential problem is that unobserved objects outside W may interact with observed objects within W, but cannot be included in the estimation of important summary characteristics (Diggle 2014), because they have not been accounted for in the survey (Fig. 4.47). Ignoring these effects is understood to result in biased statistical estimations.

In point process statistics, the precise mathematical formulation of methods to address edge effects leading to a bias in the estimation of spatial characteristics (commonly in short referred to as *edge bias*) are dependent on the summary characteristic to be estimated and there are different edge-correction methods for nearest neighbour summary statistics and second-order characteristics. Edge-bias issues of competition indices and second-order characteristics have been frequently discussed in the statistical and forest-science literature (Finney and Palca 1949; Monserud and Ek 1974; Martin et al. 1977; Radtke and Burkhart 1998; Chiu et al. 2013; Illian et al. 2008). Comparatively little attention has been paid to structural indices, but Pommerening and Stoyan (2006) have addressed this problem.

There are two main categories of edge correction or edge mitigation: *plus-sampling* and *minus-sampling* (Chiu et al. 2013; Illian et al. 2008, p. 133 and p. 183ff., respectively, see Fig. 4.48). Plus-sampling makes full use of all data within

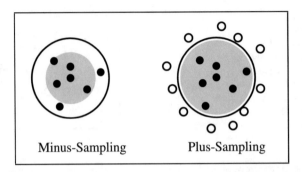

Fig. 4.48 The principles of minus- and plus-sampling. Filled circles—points inside the circular observation window W, open circles—points additionally surveyed outside W having interactions with points inside. Shaded area: Set of points used for calculating spatial summary characteristics

the observation window in the summary characteristic estimators either by recording additional objects outside the observation window or by simulating them, if needed.

Minus-sampling only makes use of an inner sub-set of the observation window in the summary statistic estimators, i.e. those objects that have no potential interaction with objects outside the observation window. Minus-sampling therefore usually leads to a loss of data, which is particularly crucial in small observation windows because of the unfavourable ratio of area to circumference. Pommerening and Stoyan (2006) could for example show that large 1-ha plots often do not even require an edge-bias compensation at all when estimating NNSS, as edge effects are very small. Table 4.6 summarises general edge-correction methods according to the two main categories. Plus-sampling can be realised by translation and reflection (Figs. 4.49 and 4.50), which are traditional methods used in many spatial approaches. Both methods extrapolate the spatial structure from within W to an infinite plane and join parts of the spatial pattern that do not occur so close together in nature. This can lead to unrealistic spatial patterns near the boundaries of the observation window. Particularly the

Table 4.6 An overview of general plus- and minus-sampling methods. Explanations are given in the text (adapted from Lilleleht et al. 2014)

Plus-sampling	Minus-sampling
Translation (= periodic boundary conditions, toroidal wrapping, torus)	*Internal buffer*
	• Fixed buffer
Reflection	• Flexible buffer
• Across an axis (e.g. plot boundary)	+ NN1
• Through a point (e.g. arbitrary point near plot boundary)	+ NN2
External buffer	
• Additional measurements	
• Conditional simulation (= reconstruction)	

Fig. 4.49 Illustration of the translation principle of edge correction, also referred to as periodic boundary conditions and toroidal wrapping. The observation window W is in the centre. Modified from Pommerening and Stoyan (2006)

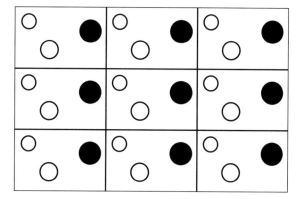

Fig. 4.50 Illustration of the reflection principle of edge correction. The observation window W is in the centre. Modified from Pommerening and Stoyan (2006)

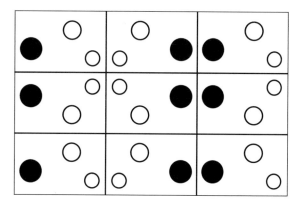

reflection method has the reputation of often performing badly and therefore cannot be recommended (Pommerening and Stoyan 2006).

Such periodic continuation is, however, a standard in spatial and spatio-temporal simulations, where the method is referred to as *periodic boundary conditions* or *torus correction* (Illian et al. 2008, p. 184). The term "torus" is used, because the correction is based on distances defined by torus metrics. Periodic boundary conditions are easy to implement in computer code by redefining the calculation of Euclidean distances.

Assuming a (xmax) and b (ymax) to be the side lengths of the observation window, the distance between two points ξ_1 and ξ_2 is defined as

$$\|\xi_1 - \xi_2\| = \sqrt{(\min\{|\Delta x|, a - |\Delta x|\})^2 + (\min\{|\Delta y|, b - |\Delta y|\})^2}. \qquad (4.36)$$

The listing below gives the function euclideanDistance implementing Eq. (4.36). The function takes the side lengths of the rectangular observation window as arguments as well as coordinates x_1 and y_1 of point ξ_1 and coordinates x_2 and y_2 of point ξ_2, respectively.

```
1 > euclideanDistance <- function(xmax, ymax, x1, y1, x2, y2) {
2 +   dx <- abs(x1 - x2)
```

```
3  +  dy <- abs(y1 - y2)
4  +  dx <- min(dx, xmax - dx)
5  +  dy <- min(dy, ymax - dy)
6  +  dz <- sqrt(dx * dx + dy * dy)
7  +  return(dz)
8  +}
```

The *external buffer* method can include the measurement of additional objects outside the observation window, which might interact with those inside. Determining the optimal width of the buffer is difficult; if it is too small, residual edge effects will remain; if it is too large, unnecessary sampling effort is applied. However, with nearest neighbour summary statistics in forest inventories, it is often sufficient to sample the nearest off-plot neighbours of trees near the plot boundaries, although this precludes retrospect analyses including changes to the number of neighbours of a structural measure (Lilleleht et al. 2014).

An alternative to measuring additional objects and another variant of the external buffer method is *conditional simulation* outside W. This method involves a structural analysis of the spatial pattern inside W and a simulation of this pattern outside W based on the results of the structural analysis. The *spatial reconstruction* method discussed in Sect. 5.1.2 can be used for this purpose. "Conditional" means that the simulation does not modify the spatial pattern within the observation window but only generates new patterns outside W which are statistically similar to those inside and have statistically correct ties to the inner objects (see Lilleleht et al. 2014; Illian et al. 2008).

The *internal buffer* method is a minus-sampling method. Like all minus-sampling methods the *fixed buffer* method only uses a subset of the objects in the observation window W. Again the choice of the buffer width is difficult (see Diggle 2014, p. 8f.) and refined versions have been developed which create a *flexible buffer* by addressing each object's potential relation to off-plot objects individually.

These methods are known as *nearest-neighbour edge correction methods* for NNSS (see Sect. 4.4.7.1) and have been proposed and investigated as NN1 and NN2 methods in Pommerening and Stoyan (2006). They are based on Hanisch (1984) and can be applied to any structural index that is based on the nearest-neighbour principle. The estimator NN1 includes more points than the unbiased buffer zone estimator, which as noted earlier, has the additional disadvantage that buffer-zone width is statistically difficult to determine.

The basic idea of NN1 and NN2 is to use variable buffer zones for points close to the boundaries of the observation window. NN1 and NN2 also include buffers but, in contrast to the traditional buffer method with a constant buffer width, the decision to exclude points close to the window's edge is made individually, based on the spatial configuration of the points.

In the statistical estimation of an NNSS, point ξ_i is used as a reference point only if its distance c_i to the boundary of window W is further than or equal to its distance $dist_i$ from its kth nearest neighbour in W. However, if the distance from the boundary is shorter than that from the kth neighbour, then it is possible that points nearer to point ξ_i occur outside W. In this case it is uncertain whether the window provides

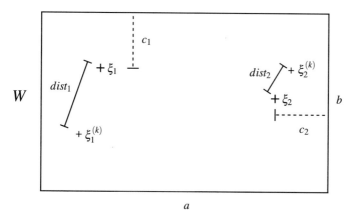

Fig. 4.51 Illustration of the working principle of the indicator function $\mathbf{1}(dist_i < c_i)$. For point ξ_1, $\mathbf{1}(dist_1 < c_1) = 0$ (since its distance c_1 to the boundary of W is smaller than distance $dist_1$ to the nearest neighbour $\xi_1^{(k)}$ in the window) and for point ξ_2, $\mathbf{1}(dist_2 < c_2) = 1$. Modified from Pommerening and Stoyan (2006)

all the necessary information for NNSS estimation, and therefore these points are rejected in the analysis.

An indicator function $\mathbf{1}(dist_i < c_i)$ returns 1, if point ξ_i is to be accepted for analysis and 0, if it is to be rejected (Fig. 4.51). Points ξ_1 and ξ_2 have the same distance $c_1 = c_2$ to the boundary of the observation window W. Points $\xi_1^{(k)}$ and $\xi_2^{(k)}$ are the corresponding kth nearest neighbours in W. Because $dist_1 > c_1$, $\mathbf{1}(dist_1 < c_1) = 0$ and point ξ_1 is not accepted. Point ξ_2, however, is accepted, since $dist_2 < c_2$ and $\mathbf{1}(dist_2 < c_2) = 1$.

As in the buffer or guard method, there is an inevitable loss of a number of data points. To compensate for this loss when applying NN approaches, the accepted points are weighted to obtain an unbiased estimator. In statistical theory, such weights are referred to as Horvitz-Thompson weights (Horvitz and Thompson 1952) and the idea is to give rare events larger weights than the more common ones. The weights in this case are inverses of the reduced areas F_i of W. The reduced area F_i is a function of $dist_i$ and W. For the two important shapes of observation windows it is

$$F_i = \begin{cases} (a - 2\,dist_i)\,(b - 2\,dist_i) & \text{for rectangular } W, \\ (R - dist_i)^2\,\pi & \text{for circular } W, \end{cases} \tag{4.37}$$

where $dist_i$ is again the distance between point i and its kth nearest neighbour. a and b are the side lengths of a rectangular observation window and R is the radius of a circular observation window. Theoretically F_i can also be defined for windows of irregular shape.

If $dist_i$ is small, it is probable that $dist_i < c_i$, F_i is large and point i receives only a small weight. For larger $dist_i$ it is increasingly unlikely that $dist_i < c_i$, F_i is small and therefore larger weights are given.

The species mingling NNSS introduced in Sect. 4.4.7.1 is used as an example here to explain and demonstrate NN1 and NN2. The NN1 estimators of the mean species mingling NNSS, $\hat{M}$, and of the mingling NNSS class z (see Sect. 4.4.7.1), $\hat{m}_z$, are

$$\hat{M} = \frac{1}{\hat{\lambda}} \sum_{i=1}^{N} \frac{M_i \, \mathbf{1}(dist_i < c_i)}{F_i} \tag{4.38}$$

and

$$\hat{m}_z = \frac{1}{\hat{\lambda}} \sum_{i=1}^{N} \frac{\mathbf{1}_i(z) \, \mathbf{1}(dist_i < c_i)}{F_i}. \tag{4.39}$$

Here instead of the intensity standard estimator N/F (F—area of W) the estimator

$$\hat{\lambda} = \sum_{i=1}^{N} \frac{\mathbf{1}(dist_i < c_i)}{F_i} \tag{4.40}$$

is used because this estimator is likely to reduce fluctuations of the NN1 estimator (Pommerening and Stoyan 2006). The estimator NN1 is ratio-unbiased. NN2 is closely related to NN1, but it is simpler and not ratio-unbiased. In the NN2 estimator, the sum of all M_i of all accepted points (those for which $\mathbf{1}(dist_i < c_i)$ returns 1) is simply divided by the number of accepted points:

$$\tilde{M} = \frac{1}{\hat{\lambda}} \sum_{i=1}^{N} \frac{M_i \, \mathbf{1}(dist_i < c_i)}{\sum_{i=1}^{N} \mathbf{1}(dist_i < c_i)} \tag{4.41}$$

and

$$\tilde{m}_z = \frac{1}{\hat{\lambda}} \sum_{i=1}^{N} \frac{\mathbf{1}_i(z) \, \mathbf{1}(dist_i < c_i)}{\sum_{i=1}^{N} \mathbf{1}(dist_i < c_i)} \tag{4.42}$$

Pommerening and Stoyan (2006) identified the NN1 method as a reliable and robust option. NN1 is also a common edge-correction method used in the nearest-neighbour distance distribution function, $G(r)$. However, for large observation windows with ≥ 150 points no edge correction is also a good choice. NNSS accounting for tree-location patterns, particularly those based on angles, always require edge correction. For very small observation windows, such as the small circular observation windows often used in forest inventory, minus-sampling methods including NN1 and NN2 can cause considerable variance.

Minus-sampling methods are not suitable for measures of competition (see Sect. 4.4.7.1), because an unbiased mark must be constructed for every tree location in the observation window and not only for a subset. Numerical edge-mitigation methods like linear expansion (Martin et al. 1977) and plus-sampling offer alternatives.

The listing below shows how NN1 can be implemented in R drawing on the spatstat package. After defining the ppp object in lines 1 and 2 the four nearest neighbours need to be determined in line 3. These are passed on to our own calcMingling() function (line 4) that we have previously defined in this chapter. Then we need a vector of the distance between reference tree and the fourth nearest neighbour, which is implemented in line 5. In line 6, we calculate the distance between each point and its nearest point on the boundary of the observation window using the spatstat function bdist.points().

```
1  > myDataP <- ppp(myData$x, myData$y, window = xwindow,
2  + marks = myData$species)
3  > neighbours <- nnwhich(myDataP, k = 1 : 4)
4  > mi <- calcMingling(myData$species, neighbours, 4)
5  > dist <- nndist(myDataP, k = 4)
6  > ci <- bdist.points(myDataP)
7  > Fi <- (xmax - 2 * dist) * (ymax - 2 * dist) / 10000
8  > HT <- (dist < ci) * 1 / Fi
9  > (mm <- sum(mi * HT) / sum(HT))
```

F_i for rectangular observation windows is calculated in line 7. d_i, c_i and F_i are now combined to calculate the Horvitz-Thompson weights (line 8). Here $\mathbf{1}(d_i < c_i)$ is simply expressed by (dist < ci). This expression returns boolean values (true, false) which in R are automatically turned into 1 and 0 by type coercion, see Appendix C, Sect. C.1. Line 9 gives the final estimator for $\hat{M}$ (Eq. 4.38).

The calculation of the mingling mark distribution according to Eq. 4.39 can be coded using the lines below. In line 1, the mingling mark distribution is initialised. k is the number of nearest neighbours (line 2). In the for loop of lines 3 and 4, the Horvitz-Thompson weights that are accounted for in class z are summed up.

```
1  > mh <- NA
2  > k <- 4
3  > for (z in 1 : (k + 1))
4  + mh[z] <- sum(HT[mi == c((z - 1) / k)])
5  > sumHT <- sum(mh)
6  > (mh <- mh / sumHT)
```

Finally the sum of Horvitz-Thompson weights in each class is divided by the total sum of Horvitz-Thompson weights (line 5) in line 6.

Edge-correction methods used for second-order characteristics are fundamentally different from those applied to NNSS. This is related to the fact that pairs of points are considered. For a given point ξ_i and interpoint distance r many partner points ξ_j are not in the observation window W. In order to construct an unbiased estimator, a large weight is assigned to pairs of points ξ_i and ξ_j with large interpoint distance (Illian et al. 2008).

When the assumption of stationarity holds, *stationary* or *translational* edge correction can be applied to the second-order characteristics. It is based on the weight $1/A(W_{\xi_i} \cap W_{\xi_j})$. Here $A(W_{\xi_i} \cap W_{\xi_j})$ is the area of the intersection of W_{ξ_i} and W_{ξ_j} where W_ξ is the translated window of W.

In the case that even the assumption of isotropy holds, *isotropic* or *rotational* edge correction can be applied to eliminate edge-bias effects when estimating the second-oder characteristics. This correction is based on the weight $1/w(\xi_i, \xi_j)$, where $w(\xi_i, \xi_j)$ is the boundary length of the circle with radius $\|\xi_i - \xi_j\|$ centred at ξ_i divided by the circle perimeter length $2\pi\|\xi_i - \xi_j\|$. More details can be found in Illian et al. (2008). Edge-correction methods for second-order characteristics are implemented and readily available in software packages such as spatstat (see Baddeley et al. 2016).

4.4.9 Hypothesis Testing

In natural sciences, research questions are usually answered by subjecting experimental or observational data to statistical tests. Since a quantity under study is affected by random variability, observations may show a trend or change or difference which is not real, but is simply due to this random variability. An apparent trend in the observed data does not necessarily indicate a real trend in the underlying variable, i.e. it is not necessarily significant in the statistical sense. The purpose of statistical tests is to decide whether findings can or cannot be attributed to chance (Baddeley et al. 2016, p. 369). This also applies to individual-based research in forest ecology and management using methods of point process statistics: The concept of patterns in data in general goes beyond random variation and therefore the rejection of a null hypothesis indicates that there is an underlying process that generates a pattern (Janssen et al. 2009).

Often graphical tests are preferred and the corresponding envelopes show regions around the estimated characteristics in which the null hypothesis is valid. Usually such tests are applied to cumulative summary characteristics, particularly to the L-function and the mark-weighted L-function. However, it is also possible to apply envelopes to probability density functions such as the pair or mark correlation function, although the interpretation of deviations is different then. In many cases hypothesis testing in point process statistics also involves simulations.

Important research problems in individual-based forest ecology and management relate to the question whether observed point patterns are just a realisation of *complete spatial randomness* (CSR) or whether they significantly deviate from a *Poisson process*. In a similar way, with marked point patterns we are interested in the question whether the marks are independent or whether the marks are positively or negatively correlated. Another interesting question in the case of marked point patterns is whether marks and points are correlated, e.g. whether marks depend on local point density (Illian et al. 2008, p. 460). Wiegand and Moloney (2014) referred to these null hypotheses as *null models*. Should the analyst conclude that the null hypotheses of CSR or independent marking cannot be rejected, a further analysis of interactions between trees is not useful. Still a lack of correlation is also an important benchmark result.

The homogeneous Poisson point process is a model of "randomness", i.e. points do not interact and the intensity of points does not vary in space. To distinguish this model from other random models, the model is referred to as *complete spatial randomness*

(CSR). An important property of the homogeneous Poisson point process, which has lent its name to the model, is that the number of points in a region B, $N(B)$, follows the Poisson distribution,

$$P(N(B) = k) = \frac{\mu^k}{k!}e^{-\mu} \text{ for } k = 0, 1, 2, ..., \tag{4.43}$$

where $\mu = \lambda$ area(B). λ is the only parameter of the homogeneous Poisson point process and it also is the intensity of the point process. In the particular case of rectangular B,

$$\mu = \lambda ab, \tag{4.44}$$

where a and b are the lengths of the sides of a rectangle. The homogeneous Poisson point process is the simplest and best investigated point process model for the homogeneous case. In applying the model, points are simulated independently from each other and distributed uniformly over a simulation plot. As a result these points form a Poisson pattern. The Poisson process is an important null or benchmark model for testing against any other point processes.

For a homogeneous Poisson process $R' = 1$ (Eq. 4.4), $\overline{\theta} = 90°$ (Eq. 4.5), $\overline{R} = 1.799$ (Eq. 4.7, for four neighbours), $L(r) = r$ (Eq. 4.24), $L(r) - r = 0$ and $g(r) = 1$ (Eq. 4.25). A realisation of a homogeneous Poisson process can easily be simulated in R using the code listed below. In line one, point density or intensity is specified followed by the definition of the rectangular observation window using xmax (a in Eq. 4.44) and ymax (b in Eq. 4.44) as the lengths of the rectangular sides.

```
1 > lambda <- 0.025
2 > xmax <- 100
3 > ymax <- 100
4 > N <- rpois(1, lambda * xmax * ymax)
5 > x <- runif(N, min = 0, max = xmax)
6 > y <- runif(N, min = 0, max = ymax)
```

In line 4, the number of points is calculated as a Poisson distributed random number using parameters λ, xmax and ymax. Finally the coordinates of N points are determined by drawing random numbers between 0 and xmax and 0 and ymax from a uniform distribution (lines 5 and 6). The spatstat package also provides the shortcut function

```
> pp <- rpoispp(lambda = 0.025, win = owin(c(0, xmax),
+ c(0, ymax)), nsim = 1)
```

where pp is a spatstat point process object and nsim is the number of realisations to be simulated.

When testing the *independence of marks* (*test of association*) two important null or benchmark hypotheses are considered which go back to work published by Goreaud and Pélissier (2003):

1. *A priori marking*, *random superposition* or *population independence* involves modelling separate, independent univariate point processes for each mark type (e.g. species) and to merge them by a process referred to as random superposition in the literature (Shen et al. 2009; Wiegand and Moloney 2014; Illian et al. 2008; Diggle 2014), see Fig. 4.12.
2. An alternative and traditional method of assigning marks is to use *a posteriori marking* or *random labelling*. Simulations under this mark independence hypothesis are typically based on fixed point locations and the marks are either permutated or they are determined independently by sampling from a specific mark distribution. A more general procedure includes two steps: First, a point process model is selected, which can be used to simulate plant locations and then marks are assigned to the simulated points using specific marking models (Illian et al. 2008, p. 296f.) in a second step.

A priori marking is for example associated with plant patterns involving two or more different species or genders. Typical examples for situations where a posteriori marking applies include tree patterns where some trees are affected by disease or damaged by wind or frost. Live and dead trees also relate to this group of examples. The same marking model applies to cases where a formerly continuous mark such as size is transformed to a categorical one, e.g. small and large trees of a monospecies forest. For quantitative marks only the null hypothesis of random labelling is considered a valid model (Grabarnik et al. 2011).

The examples suggest that a choice between the two hypotheses only applies to qualitative or categorical marks. They also show that a good understanding of underlying ecological processes is crucial for making a correct decision. The first approach is based on the understanding that most interactions between plants take place within species populations, i.e. between conspecific individuals. The composite pattern of the whole forest stand is then mainly the result of merging the point patterns of the component species, which are described by independent point process models. Therefore this approach implies population independence (Goreaud and Pélissier 2003; Grabarnik et al. 2011).

The second approach using marking models by contrast stresses the role of inter-action between species (contrary to the statements in Goreaud and Pélissier 2003) and implicitly hypothesises that the composite spatial pattern of a forest stand is mainly the result of a co-evolution of interactions between the species populations involved. The marking method reflects events affecting a posteriori the individuals of a single population.

If, for example, two species have very different seed dispersal mechanisms (e.g. animal dispersal versus wind dispersal) and the currently observed plant locations are largely determined by the seed dispersal mechanisms involved, superposition of random point patterns is a suitable approach (Howe 1989; Wiegand et al. 2009). Also, recent research has suggested that intraspecific competition plays a greater role in

4.4 Point Process Statistics

185

terms of growth and survival than interspecific competition (Anderson and Whiteman 2015). On the other hand in the long-term development of forest ecosystems there are certainly tree communities with a spatial species dispersion, which is mainly influenced by the interaction between heterospecific individuals. In that case the second approach is clearly more appropriate.

The recommendations for applying the two null or benchmark hypotheses are naturally only "rules of thumb" (see also Table 2 in Goreaud and Pélissier 2003), boundaries are fuzzy and more research is required. In any case, the details of the underlying processes such as the seed dispersal and competition mechanisms need to be taken into account. The main point is knowing whether we study two or more a priori different populations corresponding to two different main processes or whether we study an event occurring a posteriori on a single population. Unfortunately this is not always easy to know and also combinations of a priori and a posteriori processes can apply. Heterogeneous environments can add to the complication (Goreaud and Pélissier 2003). Another example highlighting the complexity of this research question involves young and old individuals of the same species. They sometimes have to be considered as two different populations because they result from different processes in time. Therefore young and old individuals of the same species would usually be modelled like different species using a priori marking.

For simulating random superposition the `spatstat` function `superimpose()` can be used, whilst random labelling can be achieved through random permutations based on the R function `sample()`, see Sect. C.1 in Appendix C.

Monte Carlo Tests for NNSS

Monte Carlo tests use a fixed number of simulations based on a null hypothesis. Typically patterns according to CSR or mark independence are simulated and for each replication the corresponding realisation is reduced to a single number and compared with the other numbers obtained (Baddeley et al. 2016). The basic idea is that the $n + 1$ patterns (n simulated patterns and 1 observed pattern) should be statistically equivalent, if the null hypothesis were true. The test procedure involves 1. simulating n independent point patterns under the assumption that the null hypothesis is true, 2. calculating the NNSS for each (marked) point pattern as a test statistic and 3. calculating the corresponding p-value.

Assuming that exceptionally large as well as small NNSS values are of interest in most cases, two-sided tests are recommended. Baddeley et al. (2016, p. 386f.) give the equations of the corresponding partial p-values for large positive and small (or large negative) simulated values, respectively, favourable to the alternative hypothesis H_1 as

$$p_+ = \frac{1 + \sum_{j=1}^{n} \mathbf{1}(\text{NNSS}_j \geq \text{NNSS}_{\text{obs}})}{n + 1} \qquad (4.45)$$

and

$$p_- = \frac{1 + \sum_{j=1}^{n} \mathbf{1}(\text{NNSS}_j \leq \text{NNSS}_{\text{obs}})}{n+1}. \tag{4.46}$$

Here NNSS_{obs} is the NNSS estimated from the observed pattern and the p-value of the two-sided test is $p = 2 \ \min(p_+, p_-)$.

This procedure can for example be applied to the species mingling NNSS $\overline{M}$ introduced in Sect. 4.4.7.1 and by Eq. (4.9). Because we are dealing with tree species, random superposition is used in the simulation of the $n = 999$ patterns with independent marks. Using the Manderscheid forest as an example (see Fig. 4.16, left), we fix the oak pattern and shift the entire beech pattern by a random value u (Illian et al. 2008, p. 462). To make this possible we use a variant of periodic boundary conditions (see Sect. 4.4.8).

The code listing below assumes that observed mean mingling was previously calculated and stored in variable mm. The simulated mean mingling values are stored in vector mmsim, which is initialised in line 2.

```
1   > n <- 999
2   > mmsim <- NA
3   > for (i in 1 : n) {
4   + cat("Random superposition simulation #", i, "out of", n,
5   + "\n")
6   + zx <- runif(1, min = 0, max = xmax)
7   + zy <- runif(1, min = 0, max = ymax)
8   + SimTreeList <- read.table(paste(dataPath, "Mand1.txt",
9   + sep = ""), header = TRUE)
10  + for (j in 1 : length(SimTreeList$x)) {
11  + if(SimTreeList$species[j] == 2) {
12  + SimTreeList$x[j] <- SimTreeList$x[j] + zx
13  + if(SimTreeList$x[j] > xmax)
14  + SimTreeList$x[j] <- SimTreeList$x[j] - xmax
15  + SimTreeList$y[j] <- SimTreeList$y[j] + zy
16  + if(SimTreeList$y[j] > ymax)
17  + SimTreeList$y[j] <- SimTreeList$y[j] - ymax
18  + }
19  + }
20  + simDataP <- ppp(SimTreeList$x, SimTreeList$y,
21  + window = xwindow, marks = factor(SimTreeList$species))
22  + neighbours <- nnwhich(simDataP, k = 1 : 4)
23  + mi <- calcMingling(SimTreeList$species, neighbours, k)
24  + mmsim[i] <- mean(mi)
25  + rm(SimTreeList)
26  + rm(simDataP)
27  + rm(neighbours)
28  + }
29  > (p_plus <- (1 + sum(mm > mmsim)) / (n + 1))
30  [1] 0.002
31  > (p_minus <- (1 + sum(mm < mmsim)) / (n + 1))
32  [1] 0.998
33  > (peither <- 2 * min(p_plus, p_minus))
34  [1] 0.004
```

At the beginning of the main `for` loop (lines 4f.) a message is passed on to the console showing the simulation progress. This is always a good idea for computational procedures that need more time like this one. In lines 6 and 7, the random variables are determined by which to shift x and y coordinates. In the nested `for` loop of lines 10–19, the x and y coordinates of the entire species 2 (beech, line 11) is shifted by `zx` and `zy`. In the case of multivariate patterns with multiple species or types it is possible to select as many species as required to shift approximately half of all points in the observation window. The `if` statements in lines 13f. and 16f. provide periodic boundary conditions. Once all trees of species 2 have been shifted mean mingling for the simulated pattern is calculated as before using `spatstat` functions (lines 20–24). The simulated mean mingling values are saved in vector `mmsim`. Finally for safety reasons the main data objects are then deleted in lines 25–27. The p-values are computed in lines 29, 31 and 35. For the two-sided test we see that the observed mean mingling of 0.44 in the Manderscheid woodland is very significant, i.e. the null hypothesis of independent marking has to be rejected.

For NNSS targeting quantitative marks, the random labelling hypothesis applies. This is easier to compute and in this case we use the mean size differentiation NNSS (Eq. 4.16) and Clocaenog (plot 1, see Fig. 4.16, right) as examples.

```
 1  > n <- 999
 2  > mtsim <- NA
 3  > for (i in 1 : n) {
 4  +   cat("Random labelling simulation #", i, "out of", n, "\n")
 5  +   SimTreeList <- read.table(paste(dataPath, "Clg1.txt",
 6  +   sep = ""), header = TRUE)
 7  +   SimTreeList$dbh <- sample(SimTreeList$dbh)
 8  +   simDataP <- ppp(SimTreeList$x, SimTreeList$y,
 9  +   window = xwindow, marks = SimTreeList$dbh)
10  +   neighbours <- nnwhich(simDataP, k = 1 : 4)
11  +   ti <- calcDiff(SimTreeList$dbh, neighbours, k)
12  +   mtsim[i] <- mean(ti)
13  +   rm(SimTreeList)
14  +   rm(simDataP)
15  +   rm(neighbours)
16  + }
17  > (p_plus <- (1 + sum(mt > mtsim)) / (n + 1))
18  [1] 0.617
19  > (p_minus <- (1 + sum(mt < mtsim)) / (n + 1))
20  [1] 0.384
21  > (peither <- 2 * min(p_plus, p_minus))
22  [1] 0.768
```

Stem diameter (dbh) is used to compute size differentiation in this case. The code listing above shares similarities with the previous listing, but this time we only have one `for` loop (lines 3–16). The coordinates of all trees remain the same in all n simulations, however, the size marks are permutated (line 7). All other computations are the same or similar compared to the previous listing. We see here that the mean differentiation of 0.17 estimated from the observed data is not significant, i.e. the null hypothesis of independent marks cannot be rejected. When testing for several NNSS applied to the same data, the multiple testing problem may apply and potentially need adjustments (Westfall and Young 1993). The speed of the simulations can be considerably increased when programming the `for` loops of the two listings in C++ and calling the C++ functions from inside R by using the `Rcpp` package.

Monte Carlo Tests for Summary Functions

Monte Carlo tests for summary functions including second-order characteristics are based on simulation envelopes. Any summary function can be used for this purpose, but cumulative characteristics have been preferred in the past. Like for NNSS (structural indices) the Monte Carlo tests here also involve simulations from a model related to the null hypothesis (null model), e.g. for the hypothesis of complete spatial randomness simulations using the Poisson point process model are appropriate. The procedure to follow is similar to that we have used for NNSS, i.e. 1. we estimate an arbitrary but suitable summary function $S_{\text{obs}}(r)$ for the observed data, 2. simulate n independent point patterns corresponding to the null hypothesis and 3. calculate their S-function estimates $S^{(1)}(r), \ldots, S^{(n)}(r)$ (Baddeley et al. 2016, p. 390f.).

The traditional tests for summary functions uses *pointwise envelopes*. Here $\max(S^{(1)}(r), \ldots, S^{(n)}(r))$ and $\min(S^{(1)}(r), \ldots, S^{(n)}(r))$ for each r of the n simulated patterns form the upper and lower envelopes. Envelopes and $S_{\text{obs}}(r)$ are then plotted together.

If any part of an observed function $S_{\text{obs}}(r)$ is outside the envelope the null hypothesis is rejected at the significance level $2/(n+1)$. This level is referred to as a local significance level (Wiegand et al. 2016). Strictly speaking the pointwise version of this test is only valid for an a priori chosen distance r which is hard to know beforehand (Grabarnik et al. 2011; Baddeley et al. 2016). If applied to the whole range of distances r the type I error probability is related to a so-called global test and can be too high, because multiple testing causes an inflation of the type I error probability (Westfall and Young 1993; Grabarnik et al. 2011). Grabarnik et al. (2011) proposed to increase the number of simulations to at least $n = 999$. As a consequence the (global) type I error probability has a reasonable value and therefore the envelope test can be employed as a rigorous statistical tool. Both cumulative and density functions can be used as test summary functions when testing the null hypothesis, however, the interpretation of the test result may be different. The distances r, where a density function (e.g. pair correlation function) crosses an envelope, can be directly attributed to the scales of the investigated pattern, which leads to a deviation from the null hypothesis. For cumulative functions (e.g. Ripley's L-function) such distances r may be far beyond the real inter-point distances which contribute to the null hypothesis violation.

As examples we use Clocaenog (plot 1, see Fig. 4.16 and the mark-weighted L-function, $L_\gamma(r)$, weighted by the test function of the mark variogram $\gamma_m(r)$. $L_\gamma(r)$ is the cumulative equivalent of $\gamma_m(r)$ used for testing. Since we found that horizontal graphs of L-functions are more useful for spotting deviations from reference curves or envelopes (see Fig. 4.30), we centre the $L_\gamma(r)$ function by computing $L_\gamma(r) - L(r)$, because $L(r)$ represents the null hypothesis of mark independence

Table 4.7 Characteristics representing the null hypothesis of mark independence for random labelling and random superposition (modified from Illian et al. (2008), p. 461ff.)

Random labelling	Random superposition
$L(r) = L_{ii}(r) = L_{ij}(r) = L_{jj}(r)$	$L_{ij}(r) = r$
$g(r) = g_{ii}(r) = g_{ij}(r) = g_{jj}(r)$	$g_{ij}(r) = 1$
$p_{ij}(r) = 2p_i p_j$	$p_{ij}(r) = 2p_i p_j$
$p_{ii}(r) = p_i^2$	$p_{ii}(r) = \frac{\lambda_i^2 g_i(r)}{\lambda_i^2 g_i(r) + \lambda_j^2 g_j(r) + 2\lambda_i \lambda_j}$
$L(r) = L_{mm} = L_\gamma = L_\tau$	–

when random labelling is considered (see Table 4.7). Now we can compare the data curve with a horizontal reference line through zero and with the envelopes, see Fig. 4.52, left. Whilst the data curve is more difficult to interpret than the mark variogram (Fig. 4.52, right), we can clearly see that $\hat{L}_\gamma(r) - \hat{L}(r)$ is well inside the envelopes of $\max(\hat{L}_\gamma(r) - \hat{L}(r))$ and $\min(\hat{L}_\gamma(r) - \hat{L}(r))$ for all r.

This implies that the null hypothesis of mark independence cannot be rejected. Our results using the mark variogram and stem diameters as marks confirm the test results we previously received from the NNSS-based test using size differentiation. A commonly used alternative is to plot the mark variogram along with the corresponding 95% pointwise envelopes from the same number of random labelling simulations (Fig. 4.52, right).

The listing below for the first approach in Fig. 4.52 (left) gives the `for` loop used for simulating random labelling and calculating $\hat{L}_\gamma(r)$ of the simulated patterns.

```
 1  > orgmarks <- myData$dbh
 2  > n <- 999
 3  > for (i in 1 : n) {
 4  +    cat("Random labelling simulation #", i, "out of", n, "\n")
 5  +    myData$dbh <- sample(orgmarks)
 6  +    myDataP <- ppp(myData$x, myData$y, window = xwindow,
 7  +    marks = myData$dbh)
 8  +    L_gamma_sim <- Kmark(X = myDataP, f = function(m1, m2)
 9  +    { (m1 - m2)^2 / 2 }, returnL = TRUE, r = myR,
10  +    correction = "translate")
11  +    lines(L_gamma_sim$r, L_gamma_sim$trans - Lr$trans, lwd = 2,
12  +    col = "gray")
13  + }
```

As before the actual random labelling is performed in line 5 using a copy of the original marks saved in line 1. A new `ppp` object now needs to be created that includes the permutated marks (lines 6f.). $\hat{L}_\gamma(r)$ is calculated using the `spatstat` function `Kmark` for the mark-weighted K-function. Here the test function is defined as that of the mark variogram and an L-function is returned. Finally the new simulated $\hat{L}_\gamma(r) - \hat{L}(r)$ function is added to an existing graph (line 11f.).

The alternative of Fig. 4.52 (right) can be programmed along the lines of the listing below. In line 5, a matrix is defined that serves as a container for observed $\hat{\gamma}(r)$ and

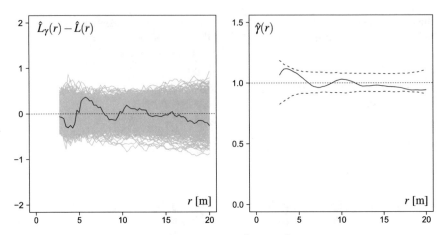

Fig. 4.52 Left: Centred mark weighted L-function $\hat{L}_\gamma(r) - \hat{L}(r)$ for Clocaenog Forest (plot 1) including the corresponding pointwise curves of 999 random labelling simulations (grey). Right: Normalised mark variogram $\hat{\gamma}(r)$ with the corresponding 95% pointwise envelopes from 999 random labelling simulations

the 999 simulation curves. The observed function is then deposited at index 1 of this container (line 6). The random labelling simulations are again carried out in the `for` loop and the mark variograms of the simulated patterns are stored to `funcs`. Finally the lower and upper pointwise 95% pointwise envelopes are calculated in lines 18–21.

```
1  > mv <- markvario(myDataP, r = myR, correction = "translate",
2  + method = "density", kernel = "epanechnikov",
3  + bw = 1.3, normalise = TRUE)
4  > n <- 999
5  > funcs <- matrix(nrow = length(myR), ncol = rep + 1)
6  > funcs[, 1] <- mv$trans
7  > orgmarks <- myData$dbh
8  > for (i in 1 : n) {
9  +   cat("Random labelling simulation #", i, "out of", n, "\n")
10 +   myData$dbh <- sample(orgmarks)
11 +   myDataP <- ppp(myData$x, myData$y, window = xwindow,
12 +   marks = myData$dbh)
13 +   mv_sim <- markvario(myDataP, r = myR,
14 +   correction = "translate", method = "density",
15 +   kernel = "epanechnikov", bw = 1.3, normalise = TRUE)
16 +   funcs[, i + 1] <- mv_sim$trans
17 + }
18 > lo <- apply(funcs, MARGIN = 1, FUN = quantile,
19 + probs = 0.025)
20 > hi <- apply(funcs, MARGIN = 1, FUN = quantile,
21 + probs = 0.975)
```

A more rigid alternative to pointwise envelope tests are *rank envelope tests* or more specifically *global envelope tests* (Myllymäki et al. 2018). A non-parametric global

Fig. 4.53 Centred mark-weighted L-function $\hat{L}_\gamma(r) - \hat{L}(r)$ for Clocaenog Forest (plot 1) including the corresponding envelopes of 2499 random labelling simulations using the GET package (grey)

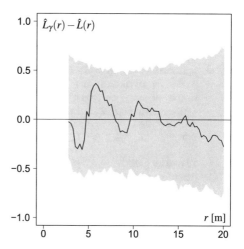

envelope test rejects the null hypothesis, if the observed characteristic (data curve) is not completely inside the 95% envelopes. In this approach, the observed and simulated functional characteristics are ranked.

The idea is to define the kth upper and lower rank curves, where k is the largest number to allow the observed characteristic to be positioned between lower and upper envelope. A p-value is calculated based on the position of the observed curve within the k envelopes. The test also provides information on which values of r lead to the rejection of the null hypothesis and thus helps to identify reasons why the data contradict the null hypothesis. The global envelope test requires a large number of simulations ($n = 2499$) and can be computed using the GET package, which can be downloaded from https://github.com/myllym/GET. The results from applying the global envelope test to Clocaenog (plot 1) and the function $\hat{L}_\gamma(r) - \hat{L}(r)$ confirms the results we previously obtained, see Fig. 4.53. The p-value is 0.516 in this case.

The corresponding code listing starts with the estimation of observed $\hat{L}_\gamma(r)$ and $\hat{L}(r)$ in lines 2–5. In line 7, again a matrix is defined that serves as a container for observed $\hat{L}_\gamma(r) - \hat{L}(r)$ and the 2499 simulation curves. The observed function is then deposited at index 1 of this container (line 8). The for loop carrying out the random-labelling simulations is in lines 10–19. At the end of each simulation the simulated $\hat{L}_\gamma(r) - \hat{L}(r)$ function values are stored to the container funcs. A specific function of the GET package, create_curve_set prepares the function data and in line 23 the global envelope test is carried out.

```
1 > myR <- seq(0, 20, 0.25)
2 > L_gamma_obs <- Kmark(X = myDataP, f = function(m1, m2) {
3 + (m1 - m2)^2 / 2 }, returnL = TRUE, r = myR,
4 + correction = "translate")
5 > Lr <- Lest(myDataP, correction = "translate", r = myR)
6 > n <- 2499
7 > funcs <- matrix(nrow = length(myR), ncol = rep + 1)
8 > funcs[, 1] <- L_gamma_obs$trans - Lr$trans
```

```
 9  > dummy <- myData$dbh
10  > for (i in 1 : n) {
11  + cat("Random labelling simulation #", i, "out of", n, "\n")
12  + myData$dbh <- sample(dummy)
13  + myDataP <- ppp(myData$x, myData$y, window = xwindow,
14  + marks = myData$dbh)
15  + L_gamma_sim <- Kmark(X = myDataP, f = function(m1, m2) {
16  + (m1 - m2)^2 / 2 }, returnL = TRUE, r = myR,
17  + correction = "translate")
18  + funcs[, i + 1] <- L_gamma_sim$trans - Lr$trans
19  + }
20  > library(GET)
21  > cset <- create_curve_set(list(r = x, obs = funcs[,1],
22  + sim_m = funcs[,-1]))
23  > res <- global_envelope_test(cset)
24  > plot(res)
```

References

Abellanas B, Abellanas M, Pommerening A, Lodares D, Cuadros S (2011) A forest simulation approach using weighted Voronoi diagrams. an application to Mediterranean fir Abies pinsapo Boiss stands. For Syst 25:e062

Aguirre O, Hui GY, Gadow K, Jiménez J (2003) An analysis of spatial forest structure using neighbourhood-based variables. For Ecol Manag 183:137–145

Albert M (1999) Analyse der eingriffsbedingten Strukturveränderung und Durchforstungsmodellierung in Mischbeständen. [Analysis of thinning-induced changes in stand structure and modelling of thinnings in mixed-species stands] PhD thesis, Göttingen University. Hainholz Verlag Göttingen, 195 p

Anderson TL, Whiteman HH (2015) Asymmetric effects of intra- and interspecific competition on a pond-breeding salamander. Ecology 96:1681–1690

Armas C, Ordiales R, Pugnaire FI (2004) Measuring plant interactions: a new comparative index. Ecology 85:2682–2686

Assunção R (1994) Testing spatial randomness by means of angles. Biometrics 50:531–537

Baddeley A, Rubak E, Turner R (2016) Spatial point patterns. methodology and applications with R. CRC Press, Boca Raton, 810 p

Bagchi R, Illian JB (2015) A method for analysing replicated point patterns in ecology. Methods Ecol Evol 6:482–490

Ballani F, Pommerening A, Stoyan D (2019) Mark-mark scatterplots improve pattern analysis in spatial plant ecology. Ecol Inform 49:13–21

Bella IE (1971) A new competition model for individual trees. For Sci 17:364–372

Berger U, Hildenbrandt H (2000) A new approach to spatially explicit modelling of forest dynamics: spacing, ageing and neighbourhood competition of mangrove trees. Ecol Model 132:287–302

Besag J (1977) Contribution to the discussion of Dr Ripley's paper. J R Stat Soc Ser B 39:193–195

Biging GS, Dobbertin M (1992) A comparison of distance-dependent competition measures for height and basal area growth of individual conifer trees. For Sci 38:695–720

Biging GS, Dobbertin MS (1995) Evaluation of competition indices in individual tree models. For Sci 41:360–377

Bitterlich W (1984) The relascope idea. relative measurements in forestry. Commonwealth Agricultural Bureaux, Norwich, 242 p

Boyden S, Binkley D, Senock R (2005) Competition and facilitation between Eucalyptus and nitrogen-fixing Falcataria in relation to soil fertility. Ecology 86:992–1001

Bravo F, Guerra B (2002) Forest structure and diameter growth in maritime pine in a Mediterranean area. In: Gadow K, Nagel J, Saborowski J (eds) Continuous cover forestry. assessment, analysis, scenarios. Kluwer Academic Publishers, Dordrecht, pp 123–134

Brunner A (1998) A light model for spatially explicit forest stand models. For Ecol For Ecol Manag. 107:19–46

Burkhart HE, Tomé M (2012) Modeling forest trees and stands. Springer, New York, p 457

Burrough PA, McDonnell RA (1998) Principles of geographical information systems, 2nd edn. Oxford University Press, Oxford, p 356

Burton PJ (1993) Some limitations inherent to static indices of plant competition. Can J For Res 23:2141–2152

Canham CD, LePage PT, Coates KD (2004) A neighbourhood analysis of canopy tree competition: effects of shading versus crowding. Can J For Res 34:778–787

Chilès J-P, Delfiner P (1999) Geostatistics: modeling spatial uncertainty. Wiley, New York, p 695

Chiu SN, Stoyan D, Kendall WS, Mecke J (2013) Stochastic geometry and its applications, 3rd edn. Wiley, Chichester, p 544

Clark PhJ, Evans FC (1954) Distance to nearest neighbour as a measure of spatial relationships in populations. Ecology 35:445–453

Clutter JL, Fortson JC, Pienaar LV, Brister GH, Bailey RL (1983) Timber management: a quantitative approach. Wiley, New York, p 329

Coates KD, Canham CD, Beaudet M, Sachs DL, Messier C (2003) Use of a spatially explicit individual-tree model (SORTIE/BC) to explore the implications of patchiness in structurally complex forests. For Ecol Manag 186:297–310

Comas C, Mateu J (2007) Modelling forest dynamics: a perspective from point process methods. Biom J 49:176–196

Corral-Rivas JJ (2006) Models of tree growth and spatial structure for multi-species, uneven-aged forests in Durango (Mexico). PhD thesis University of Göttingen (Germany), 80 p

Cressie N (1993) Statistics for spatial data, Revised edn. Wiley, New York, p 900

Dale MRT, Fortin M-J (2014) Spatial analysis: a guide for ecologists, 2nd edn. Cambridge University Press, Cambridge, p 438

Dalgaard P (2008) Introductory statistics with R, 2nd edn. Statistics and computing, Springer, New York, p 363

Damgaard C (2011) Measuring competition in plant communities where it is difficult to distinguish individual plants. Comput Ecol Softw 1:125–137

Davies O, Pommerening A (2008) The contribution of structural indices to the modelling of Sitka spruce (Picea sitchensis) and birch (Betula spp.) crowns. For Ecol Manag 256:68–77

Degenhardt A (1999) Description of tree distribution patterns and their development through marked Gibbs processes. Biom J 41:457–470

Díaz-Sierra R, Verwijmeren M, Rietkerk M, Resco de Dios V, Baudena M (2012) A new family of standardized and symmetric indices for measuring the intensity and importance of plant neighbour effects. Methods Ecol Evol 8:580–591

Diggle PJ, Heagerty P, Liang K-Y, Zeger SL (2014) Analysis of longitudinal data, 2nd edn. Oxford University Press, Oxford, Oxford statistical science series, p 379

Diggle PJ (2014) Statistical analysis of spatial and spatio-temporal point patterns, 3rd edn. CRC Press, Boca Raton, p 267

Diggle PJ (1981) Binary mosaics and the spatial pattern of heather. Biometrics 37:531–539

Dungan JL, Perry JN, Dale MRT, Legrendre P, Citron-Pousty S, Fortin M-J, Jakomulska A, Miriti M, Rosenberg MS (2002) A balanced view of scale in spatial statistical analysis. Ecography 25:626–640

Finney D, Palca H (1949) The elimination of bias due to edge-effects in forest sampling. Forestry 23:31–47

Kv Gadow (1999) Waldstruktur und Diversität [Forest structure and diversity]. Allgemeine Forst-
    und Jagdzeitung 170:117–122
Kv Gadow, Hui GY, Albert M (1998) Das Winkelmaß-ein Strukturparameter zur Beschreibung
    der Individualverteilung in Waldbeständen [The neighbourhood pattern–a new parameter for
    describing forest patterns]. Centralblatt für das gesamte Forstwesen 115:1–10
Gadow Kv, Zhang CY, Wehenkel C, Pommerening A, Corral-Rivas J, Korol M, Myklush S, Hui
    GY, Kiviste A, Zhao XH (2012) Forest structure and diversity, 29–83. In: Pukkala T, Gadow Kv
    (eds) Continuous cover forestry. managing forest ecosystems, 2nd edn. Springer, Dordrecht, 296
    p
Kv Gadow (1993) Zur Bestandesbeschreibung in der Forsteinrichtung [New variables for describing
    stands of trees]. Forst und Holz 48:602–606
Gadow Kv, Hui G (2002) Characterising forest spatial structure and diversity. In: Bjoerk L (ed)
    Proceedings IUFRO international workshop on sustainable forestry in temperate regions. Lund,
    pp 20–30
Gavrikov V, Stoyan D (1995) The use of marked point processes in ecological and environmental
    forest studies. Environ Ecol Stat 2:331–344
Gavrikov V, Grabarnik P, Stoyan D (1993) Trunk-top relations in a Siberian pine forest. Biom J
    35:487–498
Gerrard DJ (1969) Competition quotient—a new measure of the competition affecting individual
    forest trees. agricultural experiment station. Mich State Univ Res Bull 20
Gonçalves AC, Pommerening A (2011) Spatial dynamics in cone production in Mediterranean
    climates: a case study of Pinus pinea L. in Portugal. For Ecol Manag 266:83–93
Goreaud F, Pélissier R (2003) Avoiding misinterpretation of biotic interactions with the intertype
    K_{12}-function: population independence versus random labelling hypothesis. J Veg Sci 14:681–
    692
Grabarnik P, Myllymäki M, Stoyan D (2011) Correct testing of mark independence for marked
    point patterns. Ecol Model 222:3888–3894
Gspaltl M, O'Hara KL, Sterba H (2012) The relationship between available area efficiency and
    area exploitation index in an even-aged coast redwood (Sequoia sempervirens) stand. Forestry
    85:567–577
Hanisch K-H (1984) Some remarks on estimators of the distribution function of nearest neighbour
    distance in stationary spatial point processes. Mathematische Operationsforschung und Statistik
    - Statistics 15:409–412
Hegyi F (1974) A simulation model for managing jack-pine stands. In: Fries J (ed) Growth models
    for tree and stand simulation. Royal College of Forest, Stockholm, pp 74–90
Horvitz DG, Thompson DJ (1952) A generalization of sampling without replacement from a finite
    universe. J Am Stat Assoc 47:663–685
Howe HF (1989) Scatter- and clump-dispersal and seedling demography: Hypothesis and implica-
    tions. Oecologia 79:417–426
Hu Y, Hui G (2015) How to describe the crowding degree of trees based on the relationship of
    neighboring trees [In Chinese]. J Beijing For Univ 37:1–8
Hui GY, Albert M, Kv Gadow (1998) Das Umgebungsmaß als Parameter zur Nachbildung
    von Bestandesstrukturen [Diameter dominance as a parameter for simulating forest structure].
    Forstwissenschaftliches Centralblatt 117:258–266
Hui G, Pommerening A (2014) Analysing species and size diversity patterns in multi-species
    uneven-aged forests of northern China. For Ecol Manag 316:125–138
Hui G, Wang Y, Zhang G, Zhao Z, Bai C, Liu W (2018) A novel approach for assessing the
    neighborhood competition in two different aged forests. For Ecol Manag 422:49–58
Illian J, Penttinen A, Stoyan H, Stoyan D (2008) Statistical analysis and modelling of spatial point
    patterns. Wiley, Chichester, p 534
Jansen M, Judas M, Saborowski J (eds) (2002) Spatial modelling in forest ecology and management.
    A case study, Springer, Heidelberg, p 225

Janssen MA, Radtke NP, Lee A (2009) Pattern-oriented modeling of commons dilemma experiments. Adapt Behav 17:508–523

Keddy PA (1989) Competition. Chapman and Hall, London, p 552

Kleinn C (2000) Estimating metrics of forest spatial pattern from large area forest inventory cluster samples. For Sci 46:548–557

Kramer H (1988) Waldwachstumslehre [Forest growth and yield science]. Verlag Paul Parey, Hamburg, p 374

Krebs CJ (1999) Ecological methodology, 2nd edn. Addison Wesley Longman, New York, p 620

Kunstler G, Falster D, Coomes DA, Hui F, Kooyman RM, Laughlin DC, Poorter L, Vanderwel M, Vieilledent G, Wright SJ, Aiba M, Baraloto C, Caspersen J, Cornelissen JHC, Gourlet-Fleury S, Hanewinkel M, Herault B, Kattge J, Kurokawa H, Onoda Y, Peñuelas J, Poorter H, Uriarte M, Richardson S, Ruiz-Benito P, Sun I-F, Ståhl G, Swenson NG, Thompson J, Westerlund B, Wirth C, Zavala MA, Zeng H, Zimmermann JK, Zimmermann NE, Westoby M (2016) Plant functional traits have globally consistent effects on competition. Nature 529:204–218

LeMay V, Pommerening A, Marshall P (2009) Spatio-temporal structure of multi-storied, multi-aged interior Douglas fir (Pseudotsuga menziesii var. glauca) stands. J Ecol 97:1062–1074

Lewandowski A, Pommerening A (1997) Zur Beschreibung der Waldstruktur: Erwartete und beobachtete Arten-Durchmischung [On the description of forest structure: expected and observed mingling of species]. Forstwissenschaftliches Centralblatt 116:129–139

Lewandowski A, Kv Gadow (1997) Ein heuristischer Ansatz zur Reproduktion von Waldbeständen [A method for reproducing uneven-aged forest stands]. Allgemeine Forst- und Jagdzeitung 168:170–174

Lilleleht A, Sims A, Pommerening A (2014) Spatial forest structure reconstruction as a strategy for mitigating edge-bias in circular monitoring plots. For Ecol Manag 316:47–53

Loetsch F, Zöhrer F, Haller KE (1973) Forest inventory, vol 2. BLV Verlagsgesellschaft, Munich, p 469

Lotwick HW, Silverman BW (1982) Methods for analysing spatial processes of several types of points. J R Stat Soc Ser B 44:406–413

Martin GL, Ek AR (1984) A comparison of competition measures and growth models for predicting plantation red pine diameter and height growth. For Sci 30:731–743

Martin GL, Ek AR, Monserud RA (1977) Control of plot edge bias in forest stand growth simulation models. Can J For Res 7:100–105

Mason WL, Kerr G, Pommerening A, Edwards C, Hale S, Ireland D, Moore R (2004) Continuous cover forestry in British conifer forests. In: Forest research, 2004. annual report and accounts, pp 38–53

Matérn B (1960) Spatial variation. Medd Fran Statens Skogsforskningsinstitut 49:1–144

McElhinny C, Gibbons P, Brack C, Bauhus J (2005) Forest and woodland stand structural complexity: its definition and measurement. For Ecol Manag 218:1–24

Miina J, Pukkala T (2002) Application of ecological field theory in distance-dependent growth modelling. For Ecol Manag 161:101–107

Moeur M (1993) Characterizing spatial patterns of trees using stem-mapped data. For Sci 39:756–775

Moffiet T, Mengersen K, Witte C, King R, Denham R (2005) Airborne laser scanning. exploratory data analysis indicates potential variables for classification of individual trees or forest stands according to species. Photogramm Remote Sens 59:289–309

Møller J, Waagepetersen RP (2007) Modern statistics for spatial point processes. Scand J Stat 34:643–684

Monserud RA, Ek AR (1974) Plot edge bias in forest stand growth simulation models. Can J For Res 4:419–423

Montgomery DC (2013) Design and analysis of experiments, 8th edn. Wiley, New Delhi, p 726

Motz K, Sterba H, Pommerening A (2010) Sampling measures of tree diversity. For Ecol Manag 260:1985–1996

Myllymäki M, Mrkvička T, Grabarnik P, Seijo H, Hahn U (2018) Global envelope tests for spatial processes. J R Stat Soc Ser B 79:381–404

Næsset E, Økland T (2002) Estimating tree height and tree crown properties using airborne scanning laser in a boreal nature reserve. Remote Sens Environ 79:105–115

Neumann M, Starlinger F (2001) The significance of different indices for stand structure and diversity in forests. For Ecol Manag 145:91–106

Ohser J, Stoyan D (1981) On the second-order and orientation analysis of planar stationary point processes. Biom J 23:523–533

Oliver CD, Larson BC (1996) Forest stand dynamics, Update edn. Wiley, New York, p 520

Payn TW, Hill RB, Höck BK, Skinner MF, Thorn AJ, Rijkse WC (1999) Potential for the use of GIS and spatial analysis techniques as tools for monitoring changes in forest productivity and nutrition, a New Zealand example. For Ecol Manag 122:187–196

Penttinen A, Stoyan D, Henttonen HM (1992) Marked point process in forest statistics. For Sci 38:806–824

Pielou EC (1977) Mathematical Ecology. Wiley, New York, p 385

Pommerening A (2002) Approaches to quantifying forest structures. Forestry 75:305–324

Pommerening A (2006) Evaluating structural indices by reversing forest structural analysis. For Ecol Manag 224:266–277

Pommerening A, Maleki K (2014) Differences between competition kernels and traditional size-ratio based competition indices used in forest ecology. For Ecol Manag 331:135–143

Pommerening A, Murphy ST (2004) A review of the history, definitions and methods of continuous cover forestry with special attention to afforestation and restocking. Forestry 77:27–44

Pommerening A, Sánchez Meador AJ (2018) Tamm review: tree interactions between myth and reality. For Ecol Manag 428:164–176

Pommerening A, Särkkä A (2013) What mark variograms tell about spatial plant interactions. Ecol Model 251:64–72

Pommerening A, Stoyan D (2006) Edge-correction needs in estimating indices of spatial forest structure. Can J For Res 36:1723–1739

Pommerening A, Stoyan D (2008) Reconstructing spatial tree point patterns from nearest neighbour summary statistics measured in small subwindows. Can J For Res 38:1110–1122

Pommerening A, Uria-Diez J (2017) Do large trees tend towards high species mingling? Ecol Inform 42:139–147

Pommerening A, Gonçalves AC, Rodríguez-Soalleiro R (2011) Species mingling and diameter differentiation as second-order characteristics [German Journal of Forest Research]. Allgemeine Forst- und Jagd-Zeitung 182:115–129

Pommerening A, LeMay V, Stoyan D (2011) Model-based analysis of the influence of ecological processes on forest point pattern formation. Ecol Model 222:666–678

Pommerening A, Svensson B, Zhao D, Wang H, Myllymäki M (2019) Spatial species diversity in species-rich forest ecosystems: revisiting and extending the concept of spatial species mingling. Ecol Indic, in print

Pretzsch H (2009) Forest dynamics, growth and yield: from measurement to model. Springer, Heidelberg, p 664

Pretzsch H (1995) Zum Einfluss des Baumverteilungsmusters auf den Bestandeszuwachs [On the effect of the spatial distribution of trees on the stand growth]. Allgmeine Forst- und Jagdzeitung 166:190–201

Pretzsch H, Biber P, Durský J (2002) The single tree-based stand simulator SILVA: construction, application and evaluation. For Ecol Manag 162:3–21

Radtke PJ, Burkhart HW (1998) A comparison of methods for edge-bias compensation. Can J For Res 28:942–945

Rajala T, Illian J (2012) A family of spatial biodiversity measures based on graphs. Environ Ecol Stat 19:545–572

Rajala T, Olhede SC, Murrell DJ (2018) When do we have the power to detect biological interactions in spatial point patterns? J Ecol 107:711–721

Riaño D, Meier E, Allgöwer B, Chuvieco E, Ustin SL (2003) Modeling airborne laser scanning data for the spatial generation of critical forest parameters in fire behaviour modeling. Remote Sens Environ 86:177–186

Ripley BD (1976) The second-order analysis of stationary point processes. Journal of Applied Probability 13:255–266

Seifan T, Seifan M (2015) Symmetry and range limits in importance indices. Ecol Evol 5:4517–4522

Seifan M, Seifan T, Ariza C, Tielbörger K (2010) Facilitating an importance index. J Ecol 98:356–361

Shen G, Yu M, Hu X-S, Mi X, Ren H, Sun I-F, Ma K (2009) Species-area relationships explained by the joint effects of dispersal limitation and habitat heterogeinity. Ecology 90:3033–3041

Staupendahl K, Zucchini W (2006) Estimating the spatial distribution in forest stands by counting small angles between neighbours. Allg Forst-Und Jagdztg 177:160–168

Stoyan D (1987) Statistical analysis of spatial point processes: a soft-core model and cross-correlations of marks. Biom J 29:971–980

Stoyan D, Penttinen A (2000) Recent applications of point process methods in forestry statistics. Stat Sci 15:61–78

Stoyan D, Wälder O (2000) On variograms in point process statistics, II: models of markings and ecological interpretation. Biom J 42:171–187

Stoyan D, Stoyan H (1994) Fractals, random shapes and points fields. Wiley, Chichester, p 406

Suzuki SN, Kachi N, Suzuki J-I (2008) development of local size hierarchy causes regular spacing of trees in an aven-aged abies forest: analyses using spatial autocorrelation and the mark correlation function. Ann Bot 102:435–441

Szmyt J (2014) Spatial statistics in ecological analysis: from indices to functions. Silva Fenn 48:1008

Tomé M, Burkhart HE (1989) Distance-dependent competition measures for predicting growth of individual trees. For Sci 35:816–831

Torquato S (2002) Random heterogeneous materials: microstructure and macroscopic properties. Springer, New York, p 701

Uria-Diez J, Pommerening A (2017) Crown plasticity in Scots pine (Pinus sylvestris L.) as a strategy of adaptation to competition and environmental factors. Ecol Model 356:117–126

Vogt DR, Murrell DJ, Stoll P (2010) Testing spatial theories of plant coexistence: no consistent differences in intra- and interspecific interaction distances. Am Nat 175:73–84

Vovides A, Berger U, Grueters U, Guevara R, Pommerening A, Lara-Domínguez AL, López-Portillo J (2018) Change in drivers of mangrove crown displacement along a salinity stress gradient. Funct Ecol. https://doi.org/10.1111/1365-2435.13218

Wackernagel H (2003) Multivariate geostatistics: an introduction with applications. Springer, Heidelberg, p 387

Wälder O, Stoyan D (1996) On variograms in point process statistics. Biom J 38:895–905

Weigelt A, Jolliffe P (2003) Indices of plant competition. J Ecol 91:707–720

Weiskittel AR, Hann DW, Kerschaw JA, Vanclay JK (2011) Forest growth and yield modeling. Wiley Blackwell, Chichester, p 415

Westfall PH, Young SS (1993) Resampling-based multiple testing: examples and methods for p-value adjustment. Wiley, New York, p 368

Wiegand T, Huth A, Martínez I (2009) Recruitment in tropical tree species: revealing complex spatial patterns. Am Nat 174:E106–E140

Wiegand T, Grabarnik P, Stoyan D (2016) Envelope tests for spatial point patterns with and without simulation. Ecosphere 7:e01365

Wiegand T, Moloney KA (2014) Handbook of spatial point-pattern analysis in ecology. CRC Press, Boca Raton, p 538

Zawadzki J, Ciezewski ChJ, Zasada M, Lowe RC (2005) Applying geostatistics for investigations of forest ecosystems using remote sensing imagery. Silva Fenn 39:599–617

Chapter 5
Spatial and Individual-Based Modelling

Since its beginnings in the late 18th century the result of modelling in forest science has always been intriguing, because it allows studying plant populations as they travel through space and time in a time-lapse mode, whereas field and lab-based studies of plant development usually take much time. On the other hand models can only approximate reality. For individual-based forest ecology and management models are of particular importance, since this field involves large, complex ecological systems with slow dynamics, where the main lessons can only be learned from simulations based on agent- or individual based models that pull theory and experimental results together and synthesise them.

This chapter starts off by briefly reviewing methods of spatial modelling, e.g. parametric and non-parametric point process models, and then continues with spatio-temporal agent/individual-based models including a discussion about their components, analysis and implementation.

5.1 Modelling of (Marked) Point Patterns

Modelling in point process statistics can serve two purposes, 1. to confirm and further explore the data analysis and 2. for simulation. In the first case, models aid in the interpretation and understanding of empirical patterns and their summary characteristics by showing theoretical forms and information on statistical variation. The process of modelling often reveals further information that leads to a better understanding of the evolution of certain structures. Simulation of spatial patterns is based on models and can serve the following general purposes (Illian et al. 2008) which are briefly explained with examples in the paragraphs below:

© Springer Nature Switzerland AG 2019
A. Pommerening and P. Grabarnik, *Individual-based Methods*
in Forest Ecology and Management, https://doi.org/10.1007/978-3-030-24528-3_5

- Hypothesis testing (see Sect. 4.4.9),
- Investigation of the performance of statistical methods,
- Visualisation of spatial models or results,
- Simulation of plant dispersal for regeneration processes,
- Reconstruction, see Sect. 5.1.2,
- Spatio-temporal simulation, see Sect. 5.2.

In Sect. 4.4.9, we demonstrated that the simulation of the Poisson process and different marking models is very important for hypothesis testing. In a similar way, point process models can be used to test new sampling designs thus complementing mapped data (Motz et al. 2010). Often patterns simulated from point process models help to reveal valuable, additional insights, because their theoretical properties are known and the simulated patterns are realisations of these models.

In the same way visualising realisations of a point process model estimated from observed data is useful for validating the analysis and for becoming inspired by new ideas for further analysis.

As we will briefly see in the next section, Neyman–Scott point process models are often applied to modelling clustered patterns of regenerated forests while hard-core processes are preferred for more mature forest patterns (Batista and Maguire 1998; Stoyan and Penttinen 2000; Boyden et al. 2005).

When new summary statistics are developed, modelling can help to evaluate them by answering the question of how much they contribute to a synthesis of forest structure (Pommerening 2006; Pommerening and Stoyan 2008). In this example, simulation is used as a way of investigating the performance of statistical methods.

Spatially explicit growth models, simulators for sampling research and landscape visualisation tools require spatial data for their initialisation (Pommerening 2000). Despite advances in surveying technology spatial data involving mapped tree locations are still expensive to gather and model simulations can help with data imputation.

Finally reconstruction of spatial woodland structure (see Sect. 5.1.2) offers the opportunity to re-establish patterns within large observation windows where no samples have been taken, for example outside smaller subwindows, such as those used in forest surveys (Pommerening and Stoyan 2008). As part of this process, the analyst improves his understanding of plant interactions. Also, reconstruction can be used as a plus-sampling edge-correction method (Lilleleht et al. 2014, see Sect. 4.4.8). Such methods can extrapolate potential plant locations and other attributes for missing plants outside the observation window through simulation.

Approaches to modelling spatial structure can be subdivided into *parametric* and *non-parametric* methods (Pommerening and Stoyan 2008).

5.1.1   *Parametric Point Process Models*

A number of point process models with only few parameters have been developed for modelling spatial patterns. They are based on model assumptions with local or regional parameters and in contrast to modelling applications in forest growth and yield (Burkhart and Tomé 2012; Weiskittel et al. 2011) usually applied to only one or several replicated point patterns from the same ecosystem. From the point of view of spatial relationships between plants, in analogy to point-pattern types two main groups of point processes can be distinguished, cluster and hard-core processes (see Stoyan and Penttinen 2000). Another important family are Gibbs or Markov process models (see Tomppo 1986; Degenhardt and Pofahl 2000; Grabarnik and Särkkä 2009). Comas and Mateu (2007) provided an overview.

Cluster processes are a broad family of point process models describing point aggregation or clustering resulting from environmental variability and interaction (Illian et al. 2008) and include Cox and Neyman–Scott point processes. Cluster processes in general represent models where the local density of the points (i.e. the number of points in small areas) fluctuates across the observation window more markedly than it is common for a homogeneous Poisson process. This, for example, occurs when trees regenerate in canopy gaps or other plants colonise patches with favourable soil conditions. A particular variant of the Neyman–Scott point process model is the *Matérn cluster process* (Matérn 1960). Here the parent points form a stationary Poisson process with intensity λ_p and the offspring points in each cluster are random in number and scattered independently and uniformly around the parent point. The latter only have an auxiliary role and are removed before the end of the simulation.

Consider a homogeneous Poisson process with intensity λ_p. Each point ξ_i of this process is considered as the centre of a disc $b(\xi_i, R)$ with radius R and a finite Poisson process (offspring process) with intensity λ_c is generated within the disc (see Fig. 5.1, left). The superposition of all these offspring points within circular clusters is the Matérn cluster process. This model can be interpreted as a Cox process with distributional properties determined by the underlying random field $\Lambda(\xi)$. In the case of the Matérn cluster process the random field is given as

$$\Lambda(\xi) = \lambda_c \sum \mathbf{1}_{b(\xi_i, R)}(\xi). \tag{5.1}$$

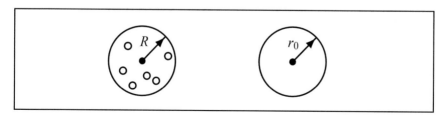

Fig. 5.1   General principle of a cluster process (left) as opposed to a hard-core process (right). R is the cluster radius (left) and r_0 the hard-core distance (right). Filled circles: parent points, open circles: offspring points

The model parameters are the intensity of offspring λ_c, the intensity of centres of clusters λ_p and the radius of the clusters R (Illian et al. 2008). A simulation of the Cox/Matérn cluster process can be carried out by calculating the intensity field $\hat{\Lambda}(\xi)$, which is a realisation of the random field $\Lambda(\xi)$, followed by a simulation of the inhomogeneous Poisson process with intensity $\lambda(\xi) = \hat{\Lambda}(\xi)$. Thus, the cluster process is a kind of Poisson process with a random intensity and therefore cannot be used as a model for interactions between points.

In a case study in tropical forests, Batista and Maguire (1998) modelled the distribution of regeneration trees in former clear cut areas with a homogeneous Neyman–Scott process. Shimatani and Kubota (2004) developed a new non-stationary approach, which is a combination of an inhomogeneous Poisson process and a Neyman–Scott process, and applied it to an *Abies sachalinensis* (FR. SCHMIDT) MAST. population in the boreal region of northern Japan. spatstat provides functions for fitting and simulating Matérn cluster processes. More refined and realistic models for describing cluster processes have been developed over the years (Stoyan and Penttinen 2000) and the aforementioned textbooks (Illian et al. 2008; Diggle 2014; Baddeley et al. 2016) provide details.

Hard-core or inhibition point processes by contrast simulate regular patterns by explicitly modelling the hard-core distance r_0 (see Fig. 5.1, right). The hard-core distance is the allowable minimum distance between any two points, or in other words, r_0 is the radius of the circle drawn around a point that no other point is allowed to penetrate. Point patterns resulting from such models describe repulsion effects between points, which can be the result of competition, natural self-thinning processes in plant communities or thinnings of trees in forest management.

Interestingly, the term "thinning" is also defined as an operation in point process statistics. More specifically, thinnings are operations carried out to transform one point process to another one by deleting points according to specified rules (Illian et al. 2008). As such they are a wonderful mathematical expression and metaphor of what happens in nature (e.g. self-thinning) and as part of forest management activities. Thinnings in point process statistics can, for example, be employed to transform a homogeneous to an inhomogeneous point process (see Sect. 4.4.3): Lewis and Shedler (1979) suggested a generic location-dependent thinning method that can be applied to any homogeneous point process. Assuming a homogeneous point process with intensity λ the thinning proposed by Lewis and Shedler (1979) leads to a new, location-dependent intensity $\lambda(\xi)$, where ξ is any location in the observation window. $P(\xi) = \lambda(\xi)/\lambda$ is the thinning function and hence each point ξ_i of the homogeneous point process is retained with probability $P(\xi_i) = \lambda(\xi_i)/\lambda$ independent of the fate of any other point (Illian et al. 2008, p. 119). A possible thinning strategy could, for example, be to introduce a linear trend in the direction of x coordinates to simulate a linear trend in soil conditions, e.g. soil moisture becoming more favourable with increasing x. Such a linear trend can be described with the intensity function $\lambda(\xi) = \lambda(x, y) = a \cdot x$, where a is a model parameter and ξ has coordinates x and y. The R code below illustrates the thinning procedure:

```
 1  > lambda <- 0.05
 2  > xmax <- 100
 3  > ymax <- 100
 4  > xwindow <- owin(c(0, xmax), c(0, ymax))
 5  >
 6  > nPoints <- rpois(1, lambda * xmax * ymax)
 7  > x <- runif(nPoints, min = 0, max = xmax)
 8  > y <- runif(nPoints, min = 0, max = ymax)
 9  > myData <- data.frame(x, y)
10  >
11  > a <- 0.0005
12  > pxy <- a * myData$x / lambda
13  > myData <- myData[pxy > runif(length(myData$x)),]
```

In lines 1–4, density λ of the homogeneous Poisson process and the observation are set. The homogeneous Poisson process is simulated in lines 6–8 in the same way as shown in Sect. 4.4.9. The linear trend is defined in lines 11–12 and the thinning is carried out in line 13. For illustration purposes, Fig. 5.2 gives one realisation of a homogeneous Poisson process using the above R code (left) and the corresponding result of a thinning with linear trend (right).

Naturally any other homogeneous point process could be used instead of a Poisson process and it is also possible to use other trend functions, see Illian et al. (2008, p. 119). In practical applications, λ(x, y) is often given and λ has to be adjusted so that λ(x, y) results from the thinning.

Thinnings also allow transforming a homogeneous Poisson process to a homogeneous hard-core process. A special case is the sequential inhibition processes that builds hard-core processes iteratively (Diggle 2014). Matérn (1960) suggested two hard-core models and we refer to one of them here for illustrating the general princi-

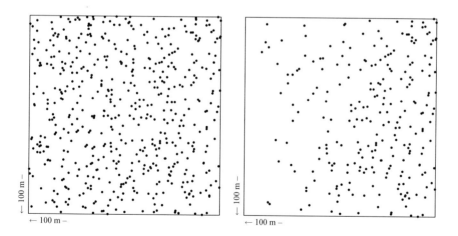

Fig. 5.2 Left: Realisation of a homogeneous Poisson process with λ = 0.05 and 536 points. Right: Result of a thinning of the same realisation with a linear trend in the direction of x coordinates, intensity function λ(x, y) = 0.0005 · x and 254 remaining points

ple of these types of models. The basic idea of the homogeneous *Matérn hard-core process* is to carry out a dependent thinning on a stationary Poisson process with intensity λ_b. The points of this process are independently marked by uniformly distributed random numbers in [0, 1] (Illian et al. 2008). These random numbers are often interpreted as times of birth or arrival and a point is removed, if it lies within a certain distance of an "older" point (Diggle 2014). For example the points can describe the locations of seeds and the marks reflect the time (year, week, day) of germination.

Let $b(\xi, r_0)$ be the circle around a point ξ with a radius r_0. Then the resulting hard-core process includes the locations ξ of those plants that were the earliest to germinate within circles $b(\xi, r_0)$. Thus the hard-core process is the result of a dependent thinning which retains a point ξ of the stationary Poisson process with mark $m(\xi)$, if the disc $b(\xi, r_0)$ contains no points with marks smaller than $m(\xi)$, i.e. points that are older than ξ. The intensity λ of the resulting hard-core process is $\lambda = p\lambda_b$, where p is a so-called retention probability. The simulation of a Matérn hard-core process follows the principles outlined in this paragraph: 1. Simulate a homogeneous Poisson process with intensity λ_b and 2. apply the thinning rule explained above. Care has to be taken, since points earmarked for deletion can still cause the deletion of other points, i.e. the actual removal of points should happen simultaneously after the marking for thinning is complete in the entire observation window. Again spatstat provides functions for fitting and simulating Matérn hard-core processes and Illian et al. (2008, p. 391ff.) offer details of more refined hard-core process models. The summary characteristics for such processes typically show $L(r) < r$ and $g(r) < 1$, i.e. there is a negative interaction between points with less points at short distances than expected under Poisson conditions. Hard-core models are typically applied to mature forests with a long history of competition, self-thinning or intensive forest management. A visual example is given in Fig. 5.3 (right).

By contrast, in a soft-core point process model, the minimum interpoint distance is not constant but follows a distribution, i.e. certain inhibitory forces increase continuously with decreasing interpoint distance (Ogata and Tanemura 1985; Stoyan 1987). As a consequence the core condition over all pairs of points is not as strong as in the hard-core model and the corresponding pair correlation function $g(r)$ slowly increases with r unlike $g(r)$ for a hard-core process. Soft-core models are important in biology and ecology. More realistically they describe an interaction between points that continuously decreases in a "soft" way rather than interaction that ends abruptly in a "hard" fashion. Stoyan (1987) introduced a soft-core point process model as a generalisation of the aforementioned Matérn hard-core process.

A flexible family of point process models relevant to individual-based forest ecology and management are *Gibbs point processes with pairwise interactions* (Stoyan and Penttinen 2000; Illian et al. 2008; Grabarnik and Särkkä 2009). An important part of these models is a pair-potential function $\Phi(\|\xi_i - \xi_j\|)$, which depends on distance $r = \|\xi_i - \xi_j\|$ between two points ξ_i and ξ_j of a point process $\Xi = \{\xi_1, \xi_2, \dots, \xi_N\}$ and is interpreted as the strength of interaction between these points. Gibbs processes are versatile models, in particular for describing point patterns with repulsion

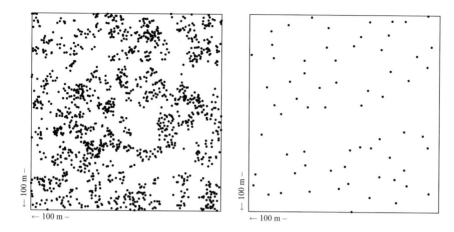

Fig. 5.3 Left: Realisation of the Matérn cluster process with $\lambda_p = 0.03$, $R = 3$ m and $\bar{c} = 5$ simulated using the `spatstat` function `rMatClust`. Right: Realisation of the Matérn hard-core process II with $\lambda_b = 0.01$ and $r_0 = 5.5$ m simulated using the `spatstat` function `rMaternII`. After Pommerening and Stoyan (2006)

or inhibition but also for patterns with moderate clustering (Grabarnik and Särkkä 2001).

Advantages of Gibbs processes include that they are so-called likelihood-based models and therefore can be treated by the well-established likelihood theory and also allow modelling mixed regular to clustered patterns (Grabarnik and Särkkä 2001), which may be relevant to spatial patterns of natural tree regeneration.

In the literature, two forms of Gibbs point processes are used. One of them includes a random number of points in a sample or observed window and the second is based on a fixed number of points which is the conditional (on the number of points) form of the previously mentioned unconditional case. For a given number of points N in an observed window W a Gibbs point process with pairwise interactions is defined through the density function

$$f(\xi_1, \ldots, \xi_N) = C \, \exp\left(-\sum_{i=1}^{N-1} \sum_{j=i+1}^{N} \Phi(\|\xi_i - \xi_j\|) \right), \qquad (5.2)$$

where C is a normalising constant. $\Phi(r) = 0$, if ξ_i and ξ_j are not mutually interacting and if $\Phi(r) = 0$ for all r, then a pattern of N uniform points in W is obtained (Stoyan and Penttinen 2000). Positive values of $\Phi(r)$ indicate inhibition whilst negative values show attraction at corresponding r. Many different pair-potential functions have been suggested and Illian et al. (2008) and Diggle (2014) provided details.

Iterative Markov chain Monte Carlo (MCMC) methods are used for simulating Gibbs processes. They are often implemented as spatial discrete time *birth-and-death processes*. Below an algorithm for simulating a Gibbs process with a random number of points is sketched:

1. Start with a suitable pattern, e.g. a Poisson point pattern.
2. Randomly choose either a death or birth "proposal" and correspondingly proceed either with step 3 or 4.
3. Pick a random point and tentatively delete it (death). Then proceed with step 5.
4. Tentatively simulate a new point at a random location in W (birth).
5. Accept, if the changed point pattern after either deleting one point or including a new point satisfies the so-called Hastings ratio based on the pair-potential function, otherwise decline.
6. Repeat steps 2–5 until the monitored statistics have stabilised or a maximum number of iterations has been reached.

The procedure is reminiscent of the *rejection method* in general simulation theory (Illian et al. 2008). Seemingly similar birth-and-death processes are also employed in spatial reconstruction that is discussed in the next section. Naturally also the application of Gibbs process models is supported by spatstat (Baddeley et al. 2016).

Stoyan and Stoyan (1998) combined an inhomogeneous Poisson process and a Gibbs process to model a hickory woodland in North Carolina. Degenhardt (1999) modelled the time series of a mixed lime-ash research plot in North–East Germany by a series of Gibbs processes with time dependent parameters. Picard et al. (2009) applied a multi-scale marked area-interaction point process for modeling locations of kimboto trees (*Pradosia cochlearia* (LECOMTE) TDPENN.) in French Guiana.

The principles of Gibbs processes are in many ways not too different from individual-based modelling and the ecological field theory (Wu et al. 1985). Based on interaction kernel functions the ecological field theory models plants in terms of sizes and spatial context (see Sect. 5.2). By contrast Gibbs processes as such do not model the growth of individuals based on size and spatial information. However, in modelling the spatial locations of individuals they may be considered as modelling the survival of individuals given their locations and relationship with neighbouring trees and their properties (Illian et al. 2008, p. 159). The kernel functions used in ecological field theory and in individual-based modelling are in fact quite similar to the pair potential function of the Gibbs point process model. A crucial problem in creating a spatio-temporal point process model is that point process models in contrast to individual-based models are not capable of accounting for asymmetric (size-dependent) interaction between individuals within a plant community, i.e. they do not discriminate between one- or two-sided interaction between different plant sizes (see Sect. 2.1.1). To overcome this limitation of traditional Gibbs models, Grabarnik and Särkkä (2009) extended a Gibbs model with hierarchical interactions introduced by Högmander and Särkkä (1999). The main idea in Grabarnik and Särkkä (2009) is that information on the size of trees allows building a partial ordering among them corresponding to the natural size hierarchy of trees in a given forest ecosystem. The ecologically justified assumption that large trees influence smaller trees but not vice versa, can be modelled as a sequence of Gibbs point processes, eventually leading to size-dependent competition effects. In a first attempt, trees can, for example, be divided into three groups, large trees, medium-sized trees and small trees, resulting in a multitype point pattern with three types of points. The largest trees would then form the highest level of hierarchy, the medium-sized trees the next highest level of hierarchy and the smallest trees the lowest level of hierarchy. The locations of large trees (highest hierarchy level) only depend on the locations of neighbouring large trees while the locations of medium-sized trees depend on the locations of neigh-bouring medium-sized trees as well as of neighbouring large trees. Consequently the locations of the smallest trees depend on the locations of all neighbouring trees.

5.1.2 Non-parametric Modelling Methods

A general strategy for decreasing model uncertainty when aiming at producing stochastic copies of observed patterns is to simulate spatial patterns from summary characteristics. In such non-parametric approaches, the step of estimating model parameters is skipped and replaced by estimating summary characteristics. These are then directly used in a simulation algorithm known as *reconstruction*. Thus in this approach, no assumptions on model parametrisation are made. Both homogeneous and inhomogeneous plant patterns can be reconstructed (Wiegand and Moloney 2014). The idea here is that meaningful summary characteristics include sufficient information on plant interactions so that they can be used for reversing the analy-sis and reconstructing observed patterns (Fig. 5.4). Therefore such non-parametric modelling methods are also referred to as methods of *spatial reconstruction*.

Reconstruction in this context is the process and result of re-establishing some-thing from partially known information represented by characteristics which are the result of an analysis of the original full information.

Fig. 5.4 Schematic principle of reconstruction as a process of reversing the analysis in an attempt to reinstate an observed pattern through simulation

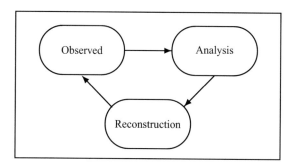

Spatial reconstruction is a technique that had previously only been used in physics and materials science (Torquato 2002). Torquato described the method as an intriguing inverse problem: From the knowledge of limited information provided by statistical summary characteristics the observed structures are re-established. Spatial reconstruction can be used to test alternative summary characteristics (Crawford et al. 2003; Pommerening 2006), e.g. several competing functions that take qualitative marks and points into account. Reconstruction can answer the question how much a newly proposed structural characteristic contributes to the synthesis of a given forest structure.

If, for example two competing or alternative summary characteristics are separately used for the reconstruction of spatial forest structure, that one is to be preferred that leads to a better synthesis. Another important purpose of reconstruction is data initialisation or imputation: Growth models, sampling simulators and landscape visualisation tools require mapped tree data, which may only partly exist and reconstruction can help to simulate the missing data. A special variant of data imputation is the use of reconstruction for plus-sampling in edge correction: Here missing off-plot information is simulated outside the observation window based on the analysis of the structure within the observation window. Another important field of application is habitat modelling at landscape level, where habitats suitable for certain key animal species can be reconstructed on the basis of summary characteristics that describe the species requirements.

The last consideration in the previous paragraph leads to the concept of *spatial construction*. It is naturally also possible to synthesise plant or landscape patterns that do not exist or have not been observed yet based on theoretical or desirable shapes of spatial summary characteristics. This is useful for exploring the limits or uniqueness of spatial plant patterns (Torquato 2002) or to simulate patterns required in a habitat simulator or for testing. As such construction can also be considered a useful alternative to *marking models* that are used to assign qualitative or quantitative marks to the points of a simulated point pattern (Wiegand and Moloney 2014). Construction can also be applied to thinnings in forest management and conservation: In the spirit of structure-based forest management (Li et al. 2014), summary characteristics can be set to describe the desired forest structure after thinning and the construction algorithm attempts to approach this target structure by removing trees conditional on a certain residual basal area. After for example 1000 construction replications those trees could be identified from the results that are most frequently selected by the construction algorithm. These trees are likely to be the trees that would induce great changes if removed.

Reconstruction and construction are not limited to point process data but can also be applied to random set data, e.g. image data from remote sensing. In some way reconstruction inter- and extrapolates spatial information similar to the interpolation methods in geostatistics, e.g. kriging (Chilès and Delfiner 1999).

An effective reconstruction based on summary characteristics enables one to synthesise accurate structures at will which can be used for multiple analyses. The method was first introduced by Torquato (Yeong and Torquato 1998; Crawford et al. 2003; Torquato 2002) and applied to simulating point processes by Tscheschel and

Stoyan (2006) from correlation functions. Pommerening and Stoyan (2008) reconstructed spatial forest structure based on NNSS.

5.1.3 Reconstruction Algorithm

The general procedure of spatial reconstruction has been well described by Torquato (2002, Chap. 12.6) and Illian et al. (2008, p. 408 ff.) and is based on the *simulated annealing* optimisation method (Kirkpatrick et al. 1983; Chen and Gadow 2002). The method can be considered as an application of the so-called Joshi–Quiblier–Adler (JQA) device, which was originally applied in physics for heterogeneous microstructures (Rice 1945). For a given spatial pattern suitable summary characteristics are selected that can include any of those introduced in Chap. 4 or others. These are set as *target functions*. Starting from some initial realisation of a forest or landscape pattern (e.g. using a Poisson, cluster or hard-core point process model), the reconstruction method proceeds to find a realisation in which the summary functions calculated from the simulations, $\hat{f}(x_i)$, best match the target functions, $f(x_i)$, i.e. observed summary characteristics. This is achieved by minimising the sum of squared differences between the summary functions calculated from the simulations and the target functions (Torquato 2002).

At any particular time step, an *energy* or *contrast function* E is defined such that

$$E = \sum_{x_i}^{c} \left(\hat{f}(x_i) - f(x_i) \right)^2, \tag{5.3}$$

where the sum is over all discrete classes of an empirical NNSS distribution or the discrete values of distance r. $f(x)$ is a suitable summary function, e.g. an empirical NNSS mark distribution or a second-order characteristic (Torquato 2002; Pommerening and Stoyan 2008; Lilleleht et al. 2014; Pommerening et al. 2019). In practice, often complex energy or contrast functions E_T are used that include partial energy functions for several (z) summary characteristics, i.e.

$$E_T = \sum_{i=1}^{z} E_i \cdot w_i, \tag{5.4}$$

where the weights add up to 1 and can be determined by trial and error (Pommerening and Stoyan 2008). The weights reflect the relative contribution of the individual summary characteristic to the reconstruction.

To evolve the simulation towards $f(x)$ (i.e. minimising E) in the simplest case we randomly select a marked point and move it to a new random candidate location. With image data we simply interchange the states of two arbitrarily selected pixels of different phases (e.g. black and white), thus automatically preserving the proportions of the phases (Torquato 2002). After the change is performed, the new energy E' and the energy difference $\Delta E = E' - E$ between two successive states are calculated. Changes leading to $E' < E$ are always accepted, however, to avoid getting caught in a local energy minimum, a change with $E' \geq E$ is only accepted and made permanent with some probability $P(\Delta E)$ that depends on ΔE, using the Metropolis acceptance rule, i.e.

$$P(\Delta E) = \begin{cases} 1 & \text{for } E' < E, \\ \exp(-\Delta E/T) & \text{for } E' \geq E, \end{cases} \tag{5.5}$$

where T is a fictitious temperature. This draws on an analogy with physics where it is well-known that a system heated to a high temperature T and then slowly cooled down to zero equilibrates to its ground state. In each iteration, temperature T is reduced by a cooling factor so that the system evolves to the desired state not too slowly whilst not getting trapped in any local energy minima (Torquato 2002). A change with an inferior $E' \geq E$ is accepted, if a uniform random number in the interval [0, 1] is less than the corresponding Metropolis probability $P(\Delta E)$. The higher the initial temperature T, the greater the value of $P(\Delta E)$, i.e. the greater the probability that a state with $E' \geq E$ is accepted.

Tscheschel and Stoyan (2006) found that for reconstructing point processes it was more efficient, faster and had better convergence properties when T was set to $T = 0$ and therefore the Metropolis acceptance rule was bypassed. They referred to this simulated annealing variant as the so-called *improvements-only* or *relaxation algorithm*. This setting was also successfully used in Pommerening and Stoyan (2008) and Lilleleht et al. (2014).

The random selection of marked points and their random move subject to the energy or contrast function is clearly reminiscent of the birth-and-death algorithm of simulation of Gibbs point processes, see Sect. 5.1, although in the latter Markov chains are used to approach the equilibrium state which generates point patterns that can be considered as having been sampled from a Gibbs point process of interest (Illian et al. 2008). By contrast, patterns resulting from spatial reconstruction using inhomogeneous Markov chains can be regarded as realisations of a general class of point processes with specified target functions. There are a number of alternatives to the algorithm of birth-and-death processes described above which can be used alternatively or additionally and the choice depends on the nature of reconstruction and the research question. Instead of moving points (i.e. letting them die at one location and be reborn at another) you can theoretically also

- Delete a marked point without replacement,
- Add a completely new marked point,
- Swap marked points.

In the reconstruction simulation, it is important to use periodic boundary conditions for simulations. This should be included in the function calculating Euclidean distance, see Sect. 4.4.8.

In some situations, where the reconstruction method is supposed to inter- or extrapolate plant or landscape structure between or outside observed, mapped plant or landscape patterns, the *conditional simulation* technique applies: Conditional simulation maximises the use of observed data by retaining them in the simulation process, whilst any reconstructed marked points are simulated conditional on this known information which must remain unchanged. Practically this can, for example, mean that in a reconstruction of the structure of a large forest from trees measured in circular sample plots (Pommerening and Stoyan 2008), these trees remain unchanged and the reconstruction simulation only affects the space outside those circular sample plots. However, the reconstruction ensures that simulated trees outside the sample plots have correct interaction relationships with the observed trees inside the plots, because the trees inside the sample plots contribute to the energy function. The same applies to edge-correction applications: Here off-plot trees are simulated based on structural information from inside the observation window and conditional on all observed trees, i.e. in contrast to other plus-sampling edge-correction methods conditional simulation ensures correct interaction relationships between simulated and observed marked points.

It is also possible to include additional conditions. For faster convergence Pommerening and Stoyan (2008), for example, included the condition that any point moved did not produce a simulated hard-core distance $\hat{r}_0$ smaller than observed r_0.

The following listing is based on Tscheschel and Stoyan (2006) and Pommerening and Stoyan (2006) and gives the coding for a simple construction example. The objective here is to construct patterns that correspond to a certain value of the aggregation index by Clark and Evans (1954), see Eq. (4.4), which is set in line 1 as CEtarget. The initial point pattern is a Poisson process (see the code in Sect. 4.4.8) and stored to initialData. In line 2, the aggregation index by Clark and Evans (1954) is calculated for the initial data. This is achieved using a self-built function calcCE() (not shown) here, because the calculation of the index involves the calculation of distances to the first point neighbours and this calculation needs to include the aforementioned periodic boundary conditions as shown in the function euclideanDistance() in Sect. 4.4.8. energyAim and maxSimSteps are abort criteria for the while loop which is the framework of the reconstruction code (line 10).

```
 1  > CEtarget <- 0.5
 2  > CE <- calcCE(xmax, ymax, initialData)
 3  > E0 <- calcEnergy(CE, CEtarget)
 4  > energyAim <- 5E-15
 5  > maxSimSteps <- 10000
 6  > simData <- initialData
 7  > coolingFactor <- 0.9
 8  > Te <- 0
 9  > j <- 1
10  > while ((E0 > energyAim) & (j < maxSimSteps)) {
11  +   i <- round(runif(1, min = 1, max = length(simData$x)), 0)
```

```
12  +  choice <- round(runif(1, min = 1, max = 3), 0)
13  +  if(choice == 1) { # Delete point
14  +    rememberX <- simData$x[i]
15  +    rememberY <- simData$y[i]
16  +    simData <- simData[-i,]
17  +  }
18  +  else if(choice == 2) { # Add point
19  +    x <- runif(1, min = 0, max = xmax)
20  +    y <- runif(1, min = 0, max = ymax)
21  +    simData <- rbind(simData, cbind(x, y))
22  +  }
23  +  else { # Move point
24  +    rememberX <- simData$x[i]
25  +    rememberY <- simData$y[i]
26  +    simData$x[i] <- runif(1, min = 0, max = xmax)
27  +    simData$y[i] <- runif(1, min = 0, max = xmax)
28  +  }
29  +  CE <- calcCE(xmax, ymax, simData)
30  +  E1 <- calcEnergy(CE, CEtarget)
31  +  Accepted <- TRUE
32  +  if(E1 >= E0) {
33  +    if(Te > 0) {
34  +      u <- runif(1, min = 0, max = 1)
35  +      p <- exp((E0 - E1) / Te)
36  +      if(u < p) # Accept
37  +        E0 <- E1
38  +      else { # Reject
39  +        Accepted <- FALSE
40  +        if(choice == 1) {
41  +          x <- rememberX
42  +          y <- rememberY
43  +          simData <- rbind(simData, cbind(x, y))
44  +        }
45  +        else if(choice == 2) {
46  +          simData <- simData[-length(simData$x),]
47  +        }
48  +        else {
49  +          simData$x[i] <- rememberX
50  +          simData$y[i] <- rememberY
51  +        }
52  +      }
53  +    }
54  +    else { # If T == 0 we accept only improvements
55  +      Accepted <- FALSE
56  +      if(choice == 1) {
57  +        x <- rememberX
58  +        y <- rememberY
59  +        simData <- rbind(simData, cbind(x, y))
60  +      }
61  +      else if(choice == 2) {
62  +        simData <- simData[-length(simData$x),]
63  +      }
64  +      else {
```

```
65  +        simData$x[i] <- rememberX
66  +        simData$y[i] <- rememberY
67  +      }
68  +    }
69  +  }
70  +  else # If E1 < E0 always accept
71  +    E0 <- E1
72  +  Te <- Te * coolingFactor
73  +  cat("Iteration: ", j, "Point #: ", i, " E0: ", E0,
74  +  " E1: ", E1, " CE: ", CE, "T: ", Te, "Choice: ", choice,
75  +  "Number of points: ", length(simData$x), "Accepted: ",
76  +  Accepted, "\n")
77  +  j <- j + 1
78  + }
```

In line 6, the initial point pattern consisting of two vectors for x and y coordinates is passed on to the data frame simData for use in the simulation process while initialData remains unchanged. The settings in lines 7 and 8 are for the afore-mentioned Metropolis rule (Eq. 5.5), i.e. temperature and cooling factor. In this case temperature is set to 0, i.e. the improvements-only variant of the algorithm is applied. However, this can easily be changed by setting a temperature larger 0 in this line.

At the beginning of the while loop a random point is selected and its index stored to i (line 11). Now also randomly one out of three choices is made (line 12): Either the previously selected point is deleted (lines 13–17), a new point with random, uniformly distributed coordinates x and y is added to the point pattern (lines 18–22) or the previously selected point with index i is moved to a new candidate location (birth-and-death step of reconstruction algorithm, lines 23–28). In the first and the third case the old coordinates of the selected point i are stored to the dummy variables rememberX and rememberY (lines 14f. and 24f.) in case the change is not accepted and needs to be undone later.

Following this the change in the simulated pattern is tested by 1. calculating the aggregation index for the altered data (line 29) and then by 2. calculating the resulting new energy function E' (E1, line 30).

Once the new energy E1 is calculated the change in the pattern has to pass a complex system of acceptance/rejection rules. This system is divided into two main parts for the cases that 1. $E' \geq E$ (E1 > = E0, lines 32–53) and 2. $E' < E$ (E1 < E0, lines 54–71). In case of rejecting the deletion or move of a point (choice == 1 and choice == 3), the previous point coordinates need to be reinstated using the dummy variables rememberX and rememberY (lines 41f., 49f., 57f. and 65f.).

In the case of acceptance the current energy value in E0 is overwritten by the new one stored to E1, see lines 37 and 71. Finally the temperature is decreased in line 72 and the results of each iteration are written into the R console (lines 73–76). In line 77, the iteration index j is incremented. This simple algorithm naturally will run faster if implemented in C++, but it may be easier to understand the code when written in R. The implementation of the energy function is given in the following lines:

```
calcEnergy <- function(CEcurrent, CEtarget) {
  return((CEcurrent - CEtarget)^2)
}
```

The two listings here should be understood as a simple, instructive example. For more serious applications the energy function needs to include a clever combination of several, more sophisticated functional summary characteristics and the choice always depends on the point pattern and on the research question. For second-order characteristics it is also important to select an appropriate range of distance r in order to give due consideration to relevant scales (see also Wiegand and Moloney 2014, p. 276ff.).

5.1.4 Applications of Reconstruction

In an early attempt, Lewandowski and Gadow (1997) constructed a three-phase reconstruction approach using nearest neighbour summary statistics (NNSS). After randomly permuting the original locations of trees for initialisation, in the first phase, tree locations were optimised towards empirical distance distributions by moving points in the plane. In the second phase, the species mingling mark distribution of the marked point pattern was optimised by swapping both qualitative and quantitative marks for trees with unequal species marks. Finally the size differentiation mark distribution of the simulated pattern was improved by swapping both qualitative and quantitative marks for trees with the same species (see Fig. 5.5), thus automatically preserving species mingling. In each independent phase, a number of iterations applied before moving on to the next. Pommerening (2006) improved on this approach by using more and different NNSS in combination with cellular automata. Interestingly the author also used simultaneous or bivariate NNSS distributions by combining the marginal distributions of for example species mingling and size dominance in order to preserve observed correlations between NNSS. Tscheschel and Stoyan (2006) for the first time applied the reconstruction method to point processes. Pommerening and Stoyan (2008) reconstructed spatial tree point patterns from NNSS sampled in small circular subwindows. They selected NNSS for the energy function so that all three aspects of spatial tree diversity, location, species and size diversity (see Fig. 1.3) were represented in the energy function. An important gain was achieved by using several variants of the same summary characteristic with different numbers of k nearest neighbours (as an approximation of ∞ in Eq. 5.6). An interesting by-product of this study was a method for estimating Ripley's K-function and other second-order characteristics from standard forest inventories based on the close relationship between Ripley's K-function and the nearest neighbour distribution functions:

$$\lambda K(r) = \sum_{k=1}^{\infty} D^{(k)}(r), \qquad (5.6)$$

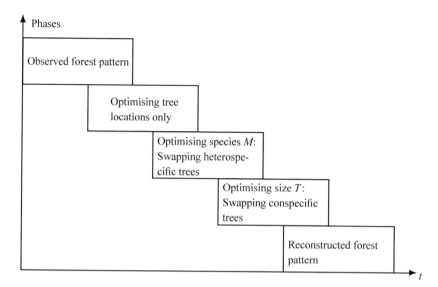

Fig. 5.5 Schematic principle of the reconstruction algorithm by Lewandowski and Gadow (1997) and Pommerening (2006). M—mingling, T—differentiation

where $D^k(r)$ are the cumulative distribution functions of the distance to the kth neighbours briefly mentioned in Chap. 4 (see also Illian et al. 2008). The good performance of the reconstruction method in this study was explained by the fact that the NNSS used in the energy function took care of small-scale local variation while the systematically placed sample plots controlled global variation. The study also revealed that for some NNSS the total error (difference between observed forest pattern before sampling and reconstructed pattern) was smaller than the sampling error. This suggests that reconstruction even has the potential to offer improved estimators for forest inventory.

Nothdurft et al. (2010) came to a similar conclusion when using the reconstruction method for mitigating the bias of a biased sampling design, the k-tree point-to-tree distance sampling. Reconstruction was used here to develop a new reconstruction-based density estimator. The authors included the cumulative versions of the spherical contact and the nearest neighbour distance distribution in the energy function. Also here the functions were computed for several k neighbours like in Tscheschel and Stoyan (2006) and Pommerening and Stoyan (2008). Instead of moving trees according to birth-and-death processes the authors only included the two options of randomly adding or deleting points which were used in alternating sequence (in contrast to our listing). Bäuerle and Nothdurft (2011) applied a similar approach to reconstructing habitat trees from transect samples.

Strîmbu et al. (2016) developed a data imputation method similar to the reconstruction method for remotely sensed tree data where they used a geostatistical variogram model (see Sect. 4.2) in the energy function. Another data imputation study in a wider sense was carried out by Lilleleht et al. (2014). In the spirit of plus-sampling the authors employed spatial reconstruction for mitigating the edge bias arising from the use of small circular observation window as typically applied in forest inventory. The basic idea of this study was to simulate off-plot tree neighbours of plot trees in such a way that the whole point pattern had NNSS as close as possible to those estimated from the core area of the plot. In their reconstruction algorithm, the authors used adding, deleting and moving trees in the simulation. In addition they swapped the stem diameters of trees of the same species to improve size mingling as in Lewandowski and Gadow (1997). The mean directional index, species mingling and size differentiation (see Sect. 4.4.7.1) were used in the energy function, whilst the Hegyi competition index (see Table 4.1) was the validation statistic. The results suggested that the reconstruction method considerably reduced the edge bias of the Hegyi index. The authors also noted that reconstruction can be used to expand observed point patterns or to convert them to other shapes of observation windows, e.g. from circular observation windows to rectangular ones. For practical use in model-based growth projections, off-plot neighbour trees would be independently reconstructed in every growth simulation run.

In a wider sense parametric methods as briefly discussed in Sect. 5.1.1 can also be considered as methods of spatial reconstruction. Pretzsch (1997) for example developed an approach for imputing data for a spatially explicit individual-oriented tree growth simulator which was based on an empirical function, estimating the distance to the nearest neighbour, and a set of probability functions (a combination of an inhomogeneous Poisson process and a hard-core process) to model the spatial pattern of mixed beech-larch forests in Lower Saxony (Germany).

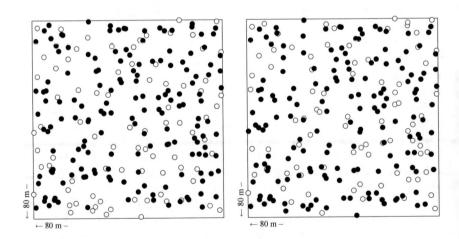

Fig. 5.6 Original map (left) of the mixed oak-beech woodland Manderscheid (see Fig. 4.16) and map of a partial reconstruction realisation (right) after 100,000 iterations using the species segregation function $\Psi'(r)$ (Eq. 4.14) in the energy function (Eq. 5.3) and the improvements-only algorithm. Quantitative marks were ignored and tree locations were fixed. Oak—open circles, beech—filled circles

Finally, Fig. 5.6 presents one result taken from partial reconstruction simulations using the Manderscheid woodland from Fig. 4.16 in Chap. 4 and the species segregation function $\Psi'(r)$ (Eq. 4.14). Here a special variant of the improvements-only algorithm was applied where only the species marks mattered. To change and potentially improve the simulated spatial species configuration, a pair of points with different species marks was randomly selected and the marks are swapped following Lewandowski and Gadow (1997). For the specific purpose of this study the tree locations were fixed in the simulation and consequently remained unchanged. The objective of this reconstruction application was to test the species segregation function $\Psi'(r)$ (Pommerening et al. 2019). We can see that although the locations of beech patches and individual oak are different in both maps, the general pattern is visually and statistically very similar (Fig. 5.6).

5.2 Individual-Based Modelling

Starting at the beginning of the 1990s (according to others in the 1980s) individual-based modelling has shown considerable growth over the past decades. It parallels the growth of related agent-based models of economics, social science and artificial intelligence and of particle-based models in physics (DeAngelis and Mooij 2005). An early review of individual-based models (IBM) in ecology even predicted that IBM would eventually provide a unified approach to applied and theoretical questions in ecology (Huston et al. 1988).

Individual-based or agent-based models simulate populations and communities as being composed of discrete agents that represent individual organisms with sets of traits that vary among the agents following a strict bottom-up approach rather than modelling distributions of individual properties and predictions based on regression analyses and general equations. Each agent (e.g. organism, human, organisation) has a unique history of complex interactions with its environment and other agents and is described as unique and autonomous entity. Agents have goals (e.g. survival, fitness, profit) and base their behaviour on adaptive decisions. IBMs attempt to capture the variation among individuals that is relevant to the questions in need of addressing. Each individual has a set of state variables and behaviour. State variables can include spatial location and physiological traits. Behaviour can include growth, reproduction, habitat selection, foraging and dispersal. State variables and behaviour vary among the individuals and can change over time (DeAngelis and Mooij 2005; Grimm and Railsback 2005; DeAngelis and Grimm 2014). Individual-based models are strict bottom-up models in which population-level behaviour emerges from the interactions among autonomous individuals with each other and their abiotic environment. Important reasons for the IBM approach include the complexity, size and slow dynamics of ecological systems, which usually prevent the use of controlled experiments (Stillman et al. 2015; Grimm and Railsback 2012).

As briefly discussed in Chap. 1, emergence in this context means that behaviour results from the individuals' behavioural decisions, which are based on fitness-related decision rules. Adaptive behaviour can also be modelled by artificially evolving successful decision strategies (Grimm and Railsback 2005; Stillman et al. 2015).

Individual-based models are mechanistic, explanatory models aimed at answering theoretical as well as practical questions in forest ecology and management (Bugmann 2001; Stillman et al. 2015; Pommerening et al. 2011). They are mechanistic in terms of the explicitness this type of models considers interactions.

Some researchers claim that individual-based or agent-based models have their origins in gap-phase replacement models such as JABOWA (Botkin et al. 1972; DeAngelis and Grimm 2014; Bugmann 2001). Although this view is contentious, many IBMs share model elements with gap models (Berger and Hildenbrandt 2000; Grüters et al. 2014).

Often agent or individual-based modelling is mentioned in the context of *game theory* and vice versa. Both concepts are not the same, but can certainly be combined. Founded by Neumann and Morgenstern (1944) and Nash (1950), game theory is a mathematical framework applied to the dynamics of conflicts and rivalry between two or more opponents (Adami et al. 2016). In game theory, the objective is to find an appropriate strategy to resolve arising conflicts or alternatively to find the optimal sequence of decisions that leads to the highest payoff. Maynard Smith (1982) coined the term *evolutionary game theory* (EGT) denoting a system capable of simulating observed evolutionary strategies and principles (see also O'Sullivan and Perry 2013, p. 91ff.). Falster and Westoby (2003) reviewed EGT in terms of plant science and specifically for plant height. The authors concluded that the benefits of height are related to total leaf area per unit area and to the potential plant heights that can be achieved with other strategies. In applying EGT they found confirmation that the vertical structure of ecosystems and the large amount of carbon fixed in vertical stems are outcomes of an evolutionary "arms race". McNickle and Dybzinski (2013) reviewed applications of game theory to plant ecology and concluded that this mathematical framework produces interesting predictions quite different from conventional ideas in plant ecology and are especially important when frequency-dependent processes occur. Although also explicitly dealing with behaviour and decision making, Adami et al. (2016) concluded that the limit where mathematical solutions for game-theoretic approaches are feasible represents rather unrealistic environments or involves other limiting assumptions and that individual-based simulations can often go where mathematics cannot. However, agent/individual-based modelling can certainly include elements of game theory.

IBMs are also an elegant way to describe the evolution of marked point patterns (Berger and Hildenbrandt 2000; Renshaw and Särkkä 2001; Grimm and Railsback 2005; Grabarnik and Särkkä 2011; Pommerening et al. 2011; Grüters et al. 2014) combining spatial and temporal processes, thus providing a link between an observed pattern and the processes influencing it, since this is currently not possible with point process models. Therefore point process analysis as outlined in Chap. 4 also acts as a preparation for model development and fitting. In an attempt to establish general spatio-temporal models for marked point processes, Renshaw and Särkkä (2001) and Särkkä and Renshaw (2006) independently of the IBM community suggested an intriguing, general growth interaction model (GI model) which in fact is very similar to individual-based models (Häbel et al. 2019). To a large degree individual-based modelling and point process statistics approximately at the same time started to head towards a similar direction in modelling with different original objectives in mind. However, IB modelling was positively influenced by point process statistics and one goal of this chapter is to show and emphasise the links.

Individual-based ecology is also envisaged as a research programme in which virtual laboratories—the IBMs—are set up, calibrated, tested and made to work. Once these laboratories exist, a wide range of specific and general questions can be efficiently answered (Stillman et al. 2015).

5.2.1 Interaction-Kernel Models

IBMs in plant ecology are often spatially explicit models and are then frequently associated with interaction fields (Fig. 5.7, right). The concept has origins in different fields of natural sciences including the ecological field theory (Wu et al. 1985; Li et al. 2000; Miina and Pukkala 2002), shot-noise fields in physics (Baccelli and Blaszczyszyn 2001), individual-based modelling (Snyder and Chesson 2004; Adams et al. 2011) and competition kernels (Vogt et al. 2010). Interaction fields are a result of aggregated signals at any point in the observation window. All kernel approaches have in common that every plant of a given community emits a signal (also termed impulse, response or effect), which is largest at or near the location of a plant and decreases with increasing distance from that plant. The signals or impulses are usually assumed to be homogeneous, i.e. they only depend on the mark and on the difference in location of a given plant and another point (Chiu et al. 2013). Spatial interaction kernels are functions that define how the strengths of biological processes change with distance (Snyder and Chesson 2004). At any point in the community the plants' interaction signals can be aggregated additively or multiplicatively to obtain the total amount of interaction at that point. This aggregation or superposition of local signals essentially results in an interaction or dispersal field for the entire plant community (Fig. 5.7, right). Kernel functions describe the contribution of point ξ_j with mark m_j to this field (Chiu et al. 2013). Like with competition/interaction indices, there is no evidence to support the question whether multiplicative or additive aggregation should be preferred, but there is a trend towards additive aggregation (Pommerening and Sánchez Meador 2018), although Miina and Pukkala (2002) reported statistical evidence in favour of multiplicative aggregation as used in ecological field theory. Different names have been attached to this model type,

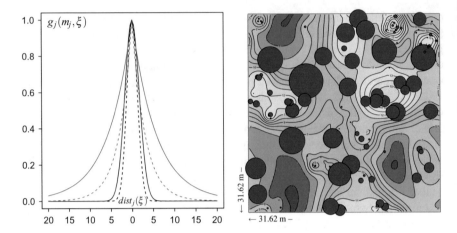

Fig. 5.7 Left: Gaussian (black) and exponential (red) kernels for trees with a stem diameter at breast height of 60 cm (continuous lines) and 20 cm (dashed lines). The unit of $dist_j(\xi)$ is metres. Right: Interaction map of a Douglas fir monitoring plot 2 in the Alex Fraser Research Forest (BC, Canada; see also Fig. 4.34, right) in 1988 based on the Gaussian kernel (Eq. 5.7). The filled brown circles represent tree locations, where the circle sizes are proportional to stem diameters. The colours represent the different intensities of the interaction field. The largest field values are indicated by yellow and pink colours, the lowest by blue colours. Modified from Pommerening and Sánchez Meador (2018)

e.g. the aforementioned ecological field theory (Wu et al. 1985; Li et al. 2000; Miina and Pukkala 2002), field of neighbourhood (FON) (Berger and Hildenbrandt 2000), (competition) kernel models (Schneider et al. 2006; Adams et al. 2011; Vogt et al. 2010), growth-interaction models and individual/agent-based models (Grimm 1999; Berger et al. 2002; Särkkä and Renshaw 2006; Fibich and Lepš 2011). We can unify these approaches by collectively referring to them as *interaction-kernel models*. They describe how biological processes such as competition, growth, survival and birth of an individual depend on its own size and the size of and distance to other individuals. Competition and dispersal kernels used in modelling seed dispersal (Nanos et al. 2010) are examples of such interaction kernels.

Interaction kernels are functions describing how ecological processes such as growth, survival and reproduction of an individual depend on the size of and distance to other individuals. The use of kernels has recently been much facilitated by the fast development of powerful computer technology. Interaction kernels are often preferred to competition indices in IBMs because they are based on more solid mathematical and ecological grounds, although Pommerening and Maleki (2014) could only find a small advantage in using kernel approaches and interaction fields for the estimation of growth rates as opposed to applying the traditional competition indices described in the previous chapter. The neighbourhood competition/crowding indices by Canham et al. (2004) can be interpreted as hybrid development between indices and kernel functions.

As mentioned before, Särkkä and Renshaw (2006) proposed an IBM with the intention to model spatio-temporal marked point processes. They termed their IBM *growth-interaction model*, which is a very good description for many if not all of these plant IBMs: They are a new interpretation of growth and other dynamics as a result of spatial interaction between plants and between plants and their environment.

5.2.2 Kernel Types and Components

Schneider et al. (2006) and Vogt et al. (2010) stated that little is known about the form and shape of kernel functions. The authors therefore revised a number of common kernel models and studied their properties and relation to estimating growth rates. Chiu et al. (2013) also referred to kernel functions as attenuation functions.

When discussing the merits of kernel functions, it is, of course, necessary to raise the question whether absolute or relative growth rates (AGR or RGR) really are appropriate dependent variables, see Chap. 6. Growth rates describe the change in mark and typically are non-spatial characteristics and have a high dependency on size. The contribution of spatial information to accurately estimating growth rates is comparatively small (Wenk et al. 1990). Cronie et al. (2013) for example fitted their growth-interaction model depending on interaction and time dependent marks $m(t)$ instead. One should also consider that the advantages of using IBMs lie elsewhere and do not necessarily include the optimisation of growth projections. Here other model types such as traditional, empirical growth models are more useful. Growth rates probably will continue to be an important response and target variable, however, when discussing the performance of kernel-based IBMs, one should clearly also consider other criteria such as biological and ecological realism, compliance with ecological theory and whether the model produces patterns that relate to multiple observations and ecological expectation. IBM modellers therefore often use *pattern-oriented modelling* (POM) by systematically deriving goodness-of-fit criteria from multiple patterns observed in real systems at different hierarchical levels and scales (Grimm et al. 2005; Piou et al. 2009). The combined use of multiple patterns or traits is recognised as an effective and powerful modelling strategy to optimise IBM complexity and to reduce uncertainty (Wiegand et al. 2003; O'Sullivan and Perry 2013).

Despite a mathematical similarity between kernel functions of IBM and the pair potential function of the Gibbs point process model (see Sect. 5.1.1), which is responsible for the interaction between plant locations, a functional relationship between them is very complicated. There were attempts going back to Law and Dieckmann (2000) to find how spatial moments (e.g. the pair correlation function) depend on dispersal and competition kernels (Adams et al. 2011). In its turn the connection between spatial moments and pair potential function of the Gibbs point process is also complicated and cannot be obtained in an explicit form (Diggle et al. 1987).

Schneider et al. (2006, Table 1) offered a detailed overview of different kernel functions and the majority of these functions model asymmetric interaction.

Frequently used basic functions include Gaussian (Eq. 5.7), exponential kernels (Eq. 5.8) and hyperbolic kernels (Eq. 5.9) (Adler 1996; Schneider et al. 2006):

$$g_j(m_j, \xi) = e^{\frac{-\delta\, dist_j^2(\xi)}{m_j^\beta}}, \tag{5.7}$$

$$g_j(m_j, \xi) = e^{\frac{-\delta\, dist_j(\xi)}{m_j^\beta}}, \tag{5.8}$$

$$g_j(m_j, \xi) = \frac{m_j^\beta}{1 + (dist_j(\xi)/\delta)^2}, \tag{5.9}$$

where $g_j(m_j, \xi)$ is the kernel function related to tree j, m_j is a quantitative mark associated with tree j, ξ is an arbitrary location in the forest, $dist_j(\xi)$ is the distance between tree j and ξ, and α and β are parameters of the kernel function (Fig. 5.7, left). For clarity, time is not considered here. The comparison between the kernels suggests that the power to which $dist_j(\xi)$ is raised can theoretically be another model parameter. In the Gaussian and exponential kernel model, parameters β and δ both scale the spatial range of the signal, i.e. the attenuation of the curve with distance. β has a stronger influence than the auxiliary parameter δ and both act conversely to one another. Large values of β stretch the range of interaction. With hyperbolic kernels, both an increase of β and δ enlarges the range of interaction.

The R functions implementing the three kernel functions are shown below. Function `impulse1()` (lines 1–3) implements the Gaussian kernel, whilst functions `impulse2()` (lines 4–6) and `impulse3()` (lines 7–9) give exponential and hyperbolic kernels, respectively. The meaning of the variables is indicated by their code names.

```
1  > impulse1 <- function(beta, delta, dist, mark) {
2  +   return(exp(-delta * dist^2 / mark^beta))
3  + }
4  > impulse2 <- function(beta, delta, dist, mark) {
5  +   return(exp(-delta * dist / mark^beta))
6  + }
7  > impulse3 <- function(beta, delta, dist, mark) {
8  +   return(mark^beta / (1 + dist / delta)^2)
9  + }
```

Kernel functions are not only a crucial part of individual-based modelling but also act as summary characteristics describing interactions similar to second-order characteristics of Chap. 4. Their parameters are interpretable and plotted functions such as in Fig. 5.7 (left) provide information about the influence range of a plant depending on size.

Using a Gaussian kernel function for estimating an interaction field for plot 2 in the Alex Fraser Research Forest Fig. 5.7 (right) shows a diverse mosaic of interaction hotspots (yellow-pink areas) separated by areas with less interaction activity (green-blue areas). These are partly a reflection of local densities and also suggest that hotspots are not so much caused by individual, large trees but more commonly by clusters of medium- and smaller-sized trees. These clusters were also indicated by the pair correlation function in Fig. 4.34 (right). Depending on what mark is used in the kernel function, the resulting interaction fields look different.

There are also other, rarer kernel types such as box-shaped kernels (Baptestini et al. 2009). Overall Schneider et al. (2006) concluded that the type of kernel functions (e.g. Gaussian, hyperbolic or exponential) was found to be of less importance, probably because all of them had sufficient flexibility to capture the interaction information present in the data. The authors stated that structural components of kernels (asymmetry, size, distance) were of greater importance than the kernel type. However, Baptestini et al. (2009) found in their work that the shape of interaction kernels can affect the likelihood of disruptive selection in genetics.

Adler (1996) put forward a framework generalising earlier plant interaction models that used particular forms of local competition. In line with his concept and for a better, systematic understanding it is helpful to distinguish between three hierarchies of kernel-based IBM functions:

- the *kernel function* $g_j(m_j, \xi)$ as discussed before,
- the *local effect* $p_j(m_j, \xi)$ and
- the *interaction function* $h_i(m_i, m_j, \xi_i)$.

The most basic level is the kernel function as in Eqs. (5.7)–(5.9) and has a maximum of 1. The local effects are the product of kernel function and mark of plant j. The mark of plant j is usually raised to the power of a model parameter. Finally the interaction function additionally includes the mark of plant i, i.e. the mark of the plant the competition/interaction load is calculated for. Whilst the first two functions only include the mark and location of plant j, in the interaction function additional information on the typical plant i, that plant j interacts with, is taken into account. The interaction field is usually constructed from the local effect that is the product of kernel function and size effect, m_j^α. An interaction field cannot be constructed from the interaction function, since m_i is only defined at the location of plant i, i.e. ξ_i. In the literature, these three hierarchical functions are not always clearly separated from each other and sometimes even used as quasi-synonyms causing confusion.

From a computing point of view the last two functions can also be considered as wrappers, i.e. they include preceding function hierarchies. In Adler's generalisation, the general local effect of a plant j at time t is defined in terms of its uptake of resources at any location ξ:

$$p_{j,t}(m_{j,t}, \xi) = m_{j,t}^\alpha \cdot g(m_{j,t}^\beta, dist_j(\xi)), \tag{5.10}$$

where $m_{j,t}$ is an arbitrary mark of plant j at time t, usually representing plant size or a composite mark involving more than one plant size attribute. The kernel

function $g(m, dist)$ increases with m and decreases with $dist$. It has a maximum of
1 at $dist = 0$. The exponent α scales maximum resource absorption as a function of
the mark selected and governs the strength of the interaction signal. β again scales
how the effect decreases or decays with distance, see previous paragraphs. A large
value of α enlarges the local effect of large plants and describes a form of asymmetric
interaction. A large value of β stretches the spatial extent of the local effects, particularly of large plants, and produces another form of asymmetry. These differences
are understood to correspond to differences in the resource exploitation profiles of
plants of different sizes (Adler 1996). For very large $dist_j(\xi)$, $g(m^\beta_{j,t}, dist_j(\xi)) = 0$
and consequently $p_{j,t}(m_{j,t}, \xi) = 0$, i.e. the local interaction effect decreases to a
value of zero if a point of interest, e.g. a plant location, is sufficiently far away
from plant j. At the location of plant j, the local effect $p_{j,t}(m_{j,t}, \xi) = m^\alpha_{j,t}$, since
$dist_j(\xi_j) = 0$.

The R listing for a local effect, for example using a Gaussian kernel, just needs
to be extended, by the term $m^\beta_{j,t}$:

```
> localEffect <- function(alpha, beta, delta, dist, mark) {
+     return(mark^alpha * exp(-delta * dist^2 / mark^beta))
+ }
```

An interaction field such as that in Fig. 5.7 (right) results from superimposing local
effects, i.e. $p_{j,t}(m_{j,t}, \xi)$ at any location ξ in the observation window at time t.

The definition of the interaction function or interaction term greatly varies from
model to model. Theoretically it is possible to define a pairwise interaction function
like in point process statistics. Often, however, in a first step the local effects are
additively aggregated at the location of the subject or typical plant i where the
"result" of total interaction for this individual is calculated:

$$h_{i,t} = \sum_{j \neq i} p_{j,t}(m_{j,t}, \xi_i) = \sum_{j \neq i} m^\alpha_{j,t} \cdot g(m^\beta_{j,t}, dist_j(\xi_i)) \qquad (5.11)$$

It is naturally also possible to aggregate the local effects of individuals subject to
certain conditions:

$$h^*_{i,t} = \sum_{j \neq i} m^\alpha_{1,j,t} \cdot g(m^\beta_{1,j,t}, dist_j(\xi_i)) \, \mathbf{1}(m_{2,j,t} > a \cdot m_{2,i,t}) \qquad (5.12)$$

Here two different marks $m_{1,j,t}$ and $m_{2,j,t}$, for example stem diameter and total tree
height, are considered and only the local effects of other trees j are summed up,
if their height is larger than that of subject tree i. Otherwise "neutral interaction"
applies. $\mathbf{1}(\ )$ is again an indicator function: The value returned by the function is 1,
if the condition inside the round brackets is fulfilled, otherwise it is 0. Parameter a
allows for some flexibility to define the critical mark difference (Miina and Pukkala
2002). In a similar way it is also possible to subtract the local effects of smaller
plants (instead of setting them to zero as in Eq. 5.12) whilst adding those of larger
plants. This strategy could help to take facilitation effects into account (see Tomé
and Burkhart 1989 and Table 4.1).

Fig. 5.8 Exploring $f_1(m_{i,t}, m_{j,t})$ with $m_{j,t}$ ranging between 0 and 80, $\alpha = 0.5$, $m_{i,t} = 30$ (solid curve), $m_{i,t} = 50$ (dashed curve). For the dotted curve $\alpha = 0.7$ and $m_{i,t} = 30$. The straight lines indicate $m_{j,t} = 30$ and $m_{j,t} = 50$

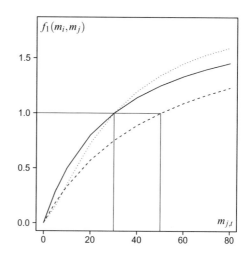

After aggregating local effects, in a second step the mark m_i of plant i is taken into consideration, since in the spirit of asymmetric interaction larger plants i tend to be less affected by the same amount of cumulative interaction $h_{i,t}$ than smaller plants. This also relates to the question of how available space or resources are shared (García 2014) and can be achieved in a number of different ways. A simple way to do this is to divide $h_{i,t}$ by $m_{i,t}^{\alpha}$, since $m_{i,t}^{\alpha}$ is the local effect of plant i at its own location ξ_i. As an alternative Schneider et al. (2006) and Adams et al. (2011) suggested a multiplicative term to account for mark differences:

$$f_1(m_{i,t}, m_{j,t}) = \tanh\left(\alpha \cdot \ln\left(\frac{m_{j,t}}{m_{i,t}}\right) + 1\right) \qquad (5.13)$$

When applying Eq. (5.13) the term $m_{j,t}^{\alpha}$ in Eq. (5.10) is replaced by $f_1(m_{i,t}, m_{j,t}) \times m_{j,t}$. Function $f_1(m_{i,t}, m_{j,t})$ increases the effect of $m_{j,t}$ for $m_{j,t} > m_{i,t}$ and decreases it otherwise (Fig. 5.8).

The model parameter α introduces ecological symmetry ($\alpha = 0$) or asymmetry ($\alpha \to \infty$), see Sect. 2.1.1. In a comparison of different kernel approaches conducted by Schneider et al. (2006), the inclusion of Eq. (5.13) led to a marked reduction in the summed root squared error.

Adler (1996) instead suggested the function

$$f_2(m_{i,t}, m_{j,t}) = \frac{m_i^{\alpha}}{m_i^{\alpha} + h_{i,t}}, \qquad (5.14)$$

whilst Fibich and Lepš (2011) proposed $f_3(m_{i,t}, m_{j,t}) = (m_j/m_i)^2$ for $m_i > m_j$, i.e. a plant i larger than plant j decreases the strength of interaction exerted by j.

When applying the concept of the ecological field theory, which is also based on interaction kernels, to spatial tree data, Miina and Pukkala (2002) argued that

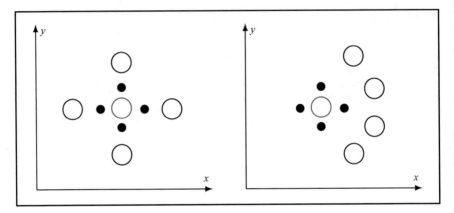

Fig. 5.9 Subject plant i (open red circle) interacting with different spatial configurations of four other plants j (open black circles). All plants have the same marks $m_i = m_j$. The filled black circles represent satellite locations around subject plant i where the interaction function (Eq. 5.11) is computed. Modified from Miina and Pukkala (2002)

not only proximity to subject tree i, size and size difference matters but also the directional context of interaction, i.e. how the other trees j, particularly those with a large influence on i, are spatially arranged around the subject trees (Fig. 5.9). The authors did not calculate the interaction function $h_{i,t}$ directly at the location of tree i but at four satellite locations in what can be described as an "orbit" around the tree (see Fig. 5.9). For simplicity the authors initially defined the orbit by multiplying stem diameter by 10. The values obtained from computing the interaction function at the fixed four satellite locations were summed and this method of computing total interaction explained growth rates better than a method that computed the interaction function at the location of the subject tree only. Later the authors optimised the multiplier used to obtain orbit radius and found that $9.8 \cdot$ dbh was best for Scots pine (*Pinus sylvestris* L.) and $133 \cdot$ dbh worked better for Norway spruce (*Picea abies* (L.) H. KARST.) in Finland.

For future work it can be recommended to apply a nonlinear estimator for such orbits similar to those used for crown-radius models or ZOIs. In fact a crown-radius model may actually be a plausible proxy for an unknown orbit radius (see Table 5.1). In the long run the four satellite locations require a generalisation so that for example the interaction function is computed for the whole circular area of the orbit or for its circumference line.

A particular variant of interaction-kernel models are those that are based on zones of influence (ZOI; Berger and Hildenbrandt 2000). As explained in Sect. 4.4.5 these are territories around a plant where the plant dominates and takes up resources. ZOIs can have irregular shapes, but simple geometric shapes such as circles or cylinders are preferred for simplicity. Usually ZOI size is a reflection of plant size, i.e. larger plants also have larger ZOIs compared to smaller plants. Interaction is defined in terms of overlap events, i.e. only those trees interact whose ZOIs overlap.

Table 5.1 Typical models for the radius of circular ZOIs used in the literature. $a_0, \ldots, a_2$ are model parameters, $R_t^{(m)} = \frac{m_t}{2}$ is the mark radius at time t

Model	Reference
$a_0 \cdot \sqrt{R_t^{(m)}}$	Berger and Hildenbrandt (2000)
$a_0 \cdot R_t^{(m)^{a_1}}$	Berger et al. (2002)
$a_0 + a_1 \cdot R_t^{(m)^{a_2}}$	Weiskittel et al. (2011)
$\frac{a_0 \cdot R_t^{(m)}}{a_1 + R_t^{(m)}}$	Pommerening and Maleki (2014)

Radii for circular ZOI have been modelled in various ways. For research involving trees good advice is to use (maximum) crown or root-plate radii models as proxies and reference, since the extension of tree crowns and roots for physiological reasons is most likely to be close to what can be perceived as a "real" ZOI. In general, nonlinear functions with saturation effects should be preferred to take environmental resistance into account, otherwise the size of ZOIs for large individuals can become unrealistic. Four models from the literature are listed in Table 5.1.

The model parameters relating to ZOI can theoretically be estimated simultaneously with other IBM parameters. However, in our experience this does not work well in situations where more than one ZOI model parameter occurs. Alternatively it is possible to assume parameter values based on the literature or to work with additional crown/root-plate data. With these data usually several radii were measured per tree and the quadratic mean per tree (Hasenauer 1997) is a good independent variable for applying the models in Table 5.1. Another option is to use quantile regression (Cade and Noon 2003) in order to approximate ZOIs of open-grown trees.

All individuals with intersecting ZOIs interact according to the ZOI logic (see Fig. 5.10). ZOIs can also be interpreted as uniform kernel density functions (Fig. 5.11). Most kernel-interaction models do not use ZOIs, since this is almost like using two systems of kernels at the same time. The logic of kernel approaches is that the local effect automatically approaches zero with increasing distance from a given plant.

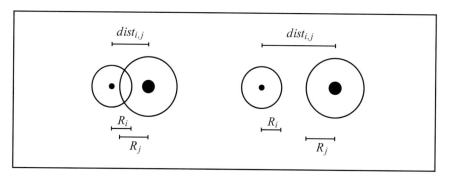

Fig. 5.10 ZOI principle of interaction: Plants interact (left) if $R_i + R_j > dist_{i,j}$. The two plants in each example are indicated by filled circles and their radii are proportional to plant size

In kernel-interaction models without ZOIs, from a theoretical point of view the size of ZOIs can be considered infinite (Häbel et al. 2019). Based on the ZOI concept and earlier work by Gerrard (1969) and Bella (1971), Särkkä and Renshaw (2006) suggested the interaction function

$$h_{i,t}^{(1)} = \sum_{j \neq i} \frac{p_{j,t}(\xi_i)}{\pi \, R_{i,t}^2} = \sum_{j \neq i} c \frac{|b_{\xi_i}(R_{i,t}) \cap b_{\xi_j}(R_{j,t})|}{\pi \, R_{i,t}^2}, \tag{5.15}$$

quantifying the overlap area of the ZOIs of trees i and j in relation to the area of the ZOI of subject tree i. $b_{\xi_i}(R_{i,t})$ and $b_{\xi_j}(R_{j,t})$ are ZOI disks around the location of trees i and j with radius $R_{i,t}$ and $R_{j,t}$, respectively. The interaction parameter c is a measure of the strength of interaction in the plant population. Although seemingly a simplification of kernel-interaction models, Schneider et al. (2006) found that ZOI-based models were among the most effective in reducing the summed root squared error when estimating growth rates. The interaction function in Eq. (5.15) is a key element of the *growth-interaction model* (Särkkä and Renshaw 2006; Cronie et al. 2013).

Berger and Hildenbrandt (2000) indeed suggested a combination of kernel-type and ZOI-based model which they termed *field of neighbourhood* (FON). In this approach, $g_j(m_j, \xi) = p_j(m_j, \xi)$:

$$g_j(m_j, \xi) = p_j(m_j, \xi) = \begin{cases} 1 & \text{for } 0 \leq dist_j(\xi) < \frac{m_{j,t}}{2}, \\ e^{-c\left(dist_j(\xi) - \frac{m_{j,t}}{2}\right)} & \text{for } \frac{m_{j,t}}{2} \leq dist_j(\xi) \leq R_{j,t}, \\ 0 & \text{otherwise.} \end{cases} \tag{5.16}$$

In this model, $c = |\ln g_{\min}| / (R_{j,t} - m_{j,t}/2)$, where $g_{\min}$ is a minimum local effect value near the ZOI boundary usually set as a model parameter. Common values include 0.1 and 0.2 (Berger and Hildenbrandt 2000; Fibich and Lepš 2011), but c can, of course, also be statistically estimated as a model parameter. Both $g_j(m_j, \xi)$ and $p_j(m_j, \xi)$ have a maximum of 1 not only for $dist_j(\xi) = 0$ but also for values of $dist_j(\xi)$ up to $dist_j(\xi) = \frac{m_{j,t}}{2}$ in all directions, i.e. the strength of the local effect (as defined in Fig. 5.11, left) is the same for all plants irrespective of their size and the maximum of the local effect is not only restricted to the point defined by a plant's coordinates. The decay of the interaction signal is modelled using an exponential kernel that is defined until the radius of the ZOI is reached (Fig. 5.11, right). As a consequence superimposing fields of neighbourhood only exist within the boundaries of ZOIs. In a sufficiently dense plant community, the overlapping ZOIs tend to cover the whole observation window with only few blank spots. As soon as the ZOIs of two or more individuals overlap, interaction occurs. To quantify interaction the summed values of $g_j(m_j, \xi)$ of plant j within the overlapping area are integrated instead of considering only the overlap area as in Eq. (5.15):

$$h_{i,t}^{(2)} = \frac{1}{\pi R_{i,t}^2} \int_{\pi R_{i,t}^2} \sum_{j \neq i} g_j(m_j, \xi) d\xi \tag{5.17}$$

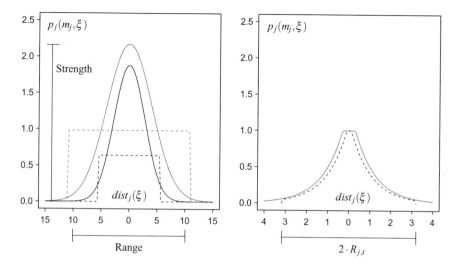

Fig. 5.11 Left: The shape of a local effect based on a Gaussian interaction kernel for hypothetical trees j with a stem-diameter mark of 40 cm (red) and 20 cm (black) and the uniform ZOI kernel for trees j of the same sizes. The height of the uniform interaction kernels is arbitrary here and additionally depends on the mark of tree i. Modified from Häbel et al. (2019). Right: The corresponding FON local effects for the same tree sizes with parameters taken from Berger and Hildenbrandt (2000)

If more neighbours interact with plant i, it is assumed that the corresponding $g_j(m_j, \xi)$ superimpose independently, i.e. they are all summed up in the overlapping areas (Bauer et al. 2004). The FON approach can be interpreted as a refinement of the growth-interaction model by Särkkä and Renshaw (2006). Grüters et al. (2014) published a recent update on the FON approach. Since the interaction function is based on the overlap areas, $h_{i,t}^{(2)}$ also includes directional information, see Fig. 5.9.

5.2.3 Species Representation

The representation of different species in mixed-species plant communities has been handled in different ways, although there is precious little detailed information in the literature on this topic (Vogt et al. 2010). In gap models, for example, only the growth potential is defined in a species-specific way, whilst interaction/competition between individual trees is calculated always in the same way regardless of species (Botkin et al. 1972). Also with individual-based models there appears to be a tendency not to modify the kernel type and respective model parameters directly. The growth-interaction approach and its refinement, the FON approach, offer the opportunity to make the FON radius $R_{j,t}$ dependent on both size and species, i.e. to estimate species-specific parameters for the calculation of $R_{j,t}$. Another possibility is to define

Fig. 5.12 Kernel shapes for intraspecific and interspecific interaction leading to heteromyopia. A *leptokurtic* kernel results in a short interaction range (interspecific interaction), while a *platikurtic* kernel results in a large interaction range (intraspecific interaction)

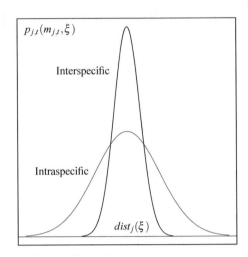

a species specific shade-tolerance parameter v to modify the interaction function $h_{i,t}$, e.g. by dividing $h_{i,t}$ by v_i of tree i (Berger et al. 2006; Fibich and Lepš 2011).

An interesting idea of species representation in interaction kernels is *heteromyopia*. Murrell and Law (2003) proposed the term heteromyopia for plant individuals that are "short-sighted" in sensing neighbours of other species and they showed how this concept may be sufficient to allow an otherwise weaker competitor to invade a population of a superior species. This term relates to a theory where interspecific competition occurs over shorter distances than intraspecific competition (Murrell and Law 2003), i.e. plant individuals are short-sighted in sensing neighbours of other species relative to their own. Also interspecific interactions are more intense than intraspecific interactions at short distances, whereas at longer distances this relationship should be reversed (Fig. 5.12). This pattern promotes coexistence by allowing conspecific clusters to build up whilst leaving gaps for other species to exploit. The interesting theory relates to the maintenance of biodiversity in ecosystems, see Sect. 2.1.2.4, but the relevance of this theory to real communities still needs to be explored in greater detail (Vogt et al. 2010). The concept points into a research direction where it is perhaps more important to distinguish between intra- and interspecific interaction than between different, concrete species.

Heteromyopia promotes coexistence by allowing conspecific clusters to build up leaving gaps for other species to exploit. In their study, Vogt et al. (2010) also found evidence that size difference matters more than species identity. Assuming a Gaussian or exponential kernel, a leptokurtic kernel can be transformed to a platikurtic kernel by increasing the range parameter β and multiplying $g_{j,t}(m_{j,t}, \xi)$ with a factor smaller than 1. This can be achieved with the multiplicative term $m_{j,t}^{\alpha}$ in the local effect function governing the strength of the interaction signal. To this end Brown et al. (2011), for example, introduced bivariate kernel functions with range parameters β for intraspecific and β_{ij} for interspecific interaction regardless of concrete species identities.

5.2.4 Seed and Offspring Dispersal

To complete the life cycle of plants represented in individual-based models the movement of seeds and establishment of seedlings and/or saplings have to be modelled. For seedlings and saplings the term *recruitment* process is very common in contrast to *seed dispersal* and *germination* processes (Vanclay 1994). A number of different modelling strategies have been employed to achieve this. They include the use of

- dispersal kernels,
- point process models,
- random fields.

Dispersal kernels are not fundamentally different from interaction kernels and Adams et al. (2011) even have applied the same kernel type with different parameters to both ecological processes. Like with interaction kernels any probability density distribution can be used and Bullock et al. (2017) provided a detailed overview. The authors pointed out that seed dispersal is notoriously difficult and resource-consuming to measure. The different methods and protocols used add to the variability of data and kernel types selected. Naturally it is also important to consider the dispersal mechanism and for representing total or overall dispersal of seeds a combination of kernels for multiple dispersal modes is necessary. Interestingly Gaussian dispersal kernels did not perform as well as exponential kernels in this study (Bullock et al. 2017).

Actual dispersal distances separating offspring from their parent tree cannot be directly measured in the field, since dispersal clouds of several parent trees overlap and the number of offspring per parent is unknown. Dispersal distances and fecundity of parent trees as well as the parameters of the dispersal kernels have therefore to be estimated by inverse modelling approaches (Nanos et al. 2010). A typical difference to interaction kernels that occurs with certain species is that the maxima of dispersal kernels are slightly offset from the stem centre, i.e. they occur at distances $dist_j(\xi) > 0$.

Because of the aforementioned difficulties with modelling seed dispersal and germination often recruitment is modelled instead. Berger and Hildenbrandt (2000) modelled seedling recruitment based on a Poisson process (see Sect. 4.4.9) which was thinned by the interaction field subject to a probability function. Technically this is a conditional thinning of a Poisson process with regard to an external field, i.e. the interaction field. Cluster processes are theoretically also an option here. Adams et al. (2011) used a Poisson process model and a Gaussian dispersal kernel as recruitment alternatives. Often combinations of the three options are applied for modelling offspring dispersal.

5.2.5 Growth Processes

The choice of functions for modelling growth processes is not specific to IBMs. As long as the selected function adheres to the established principles of tree growth including an upper asymptote any choice is possible (see for example Zeide 1993). Many growth functions selected for IBMs, however, have in common that they are independent of plant age, i.e. they model size-dependent growth, and they return absolute growth rates (AGR) in discrete annual steps. The reason for this is that plant age often varies a lot and cannot be easily established. Incidentally, the relationship between size and growth rate is an allometric relationship, see Sect. 6.2.4.

The growth function in Berger and Hildenbrandt (2000) as well as in Grüters et al. (2014) is based on the *maximum growth equation* of the JABOWA model (Botkin et al. 1972; Bugmann 2001):

$$\frac{\Delta(m_1^2 \, m_2)}{\Delta t} = r \cdot L \left(1 - \frac{m_1 \cdot m_2}{m_{1,\max} \cdot m_{2,\max}} \right), \tag{5.18}$$

where Δt is a discrete time step, r is a growth rate parameter and L is leaf area. Marks m_1 (stem diameter in JABOWA) and m_2 (total tree height in JABOWA) are allometrically related so that the resulting growth rate is an approximation of volume growth and linearly depends on leaf area (Bugmann et al. 1996; Botkin et al. 1972). For clarity, indices i and t (as in $m_{i,t}$) were omitted in Eq. (5.18).

Redenbach and Särkkä (2013) used the logistic growth function

$$\frac{\Delta m_{i,t}^{(1)}}{\Delta t} = \lambda m_{i,t} \left(1 - \frac{m_{i,t}}{K} \right), \tag{5.19}$$

where λ here is an intrinsic growth rate parameter and K is the carrying capacity. Equation (5.19) is a special case of

$$\frac{\Delta m_{i,t}^{(2)}}{\Delta t} = c_0 \, m_{i,t} - c_1 \, m_{i,t}^{p+1} \tag{5.20}$$

with $c_0 = \lambda$, $c_1 = \lambda/K$ and $p = 1$. Adler (1996) suggested

$$\frac{\Delta m_{i,t}^{(3)}}{\Delta t} = \frac{m_{i,t}^{\alpha}}{m_{i,t}^{\alpha} + h_{i,t}} m_{i,t}, \tag{5.21}$$

where α is the same strength parameter as in the local effect function of Eq. (5.10) and the fracture following the equal sign is relative growth rate (RGR, see Chap. 6).

Often the growth function used expresses *potential* or *maximum growth*, i.e. the growth typically expected from dominant plants, which in a second step is reduced by the interaction function $h_{i,t}$. Dominant plants facing little competition accordingly achieve growth rates near the potential, whilst dominated plants have reduced or modified growth. This modelling principle is referred to as the *potential-modifier*

Fig. 5.13 Annual absolute stem-diameter growth rates (AGR) pooled from all six plots and survey years from interior Douglas fir in the Alex Fraser Research Forest (BC, Canada, see Fig. 4.34), modified from Pommerening and Maleki (2014). The red curve represents potential mark (stem diameter) growth rate using Eq. (5.22) and quantile regression (Cade and Noon 2003) with $\tau = 0.975$

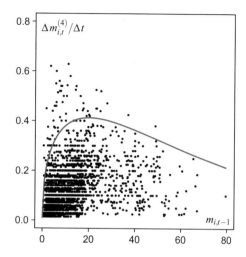

approach (Newnham 1964; Botkin et al. 1972, see Fig. 5.13). Pommerening and Särkkä (2013) for example applied a variant of the Chapman-Richards growth function (Pienaar and Turnbull 1973; Zeide 1993), where time was exchanged for size:

$$\frac{\Delta m_{i,t}^{(4)}}{\Delta t} = Akp \, e^{-k \cdot m_{i,t}} \cdot (1 - e^{-k \cdot m_{i,t}})^{p-1} \tag{5.22}$$

Here A, k and p are model parameters. In the original Chapman-Richards function, parameter A is an asymptote representing the maximum mark $m_{i,t}$ for all plants, parameter k scales the growth rate and p determines the location of the inflection point of the growth function (Pommerening et al. 2011).

Through quantile regression (Koenker and Park 1994; Cade and Noon 2003) it is possible to identify the growth rates of the most dominant trees of a forest stand based on a suitable growth function. In lines 1–4 in the R listing below, the Chapman-Richards growth function of Eq. (5.22) is implemented.

```
1  > dpot <- function(dbh, xA, xk, xp) {
2  +  return(xA * xk * xp * exp(-xk * dbh) *
3  +  (1 - exp(-xk * dbh)) ^ (xp - 1))
4  +  }
5  > library(quantreg)
6  > nlsout <- nlrq(AGR ~ dpot(dbh, A, k, p), data = TreeList,
7  +  start = list(A = 54.1, k = 0.01, p = 1.19),
8  +  tau = 0.975, trace = TRUE)
```

Then the library `quantreg` (based on Koenker and Park 1994) is called in line 5. The actual quantile-regression routine `nlrq` is coded in lines 6–8. It uses the growth function `dpot` from lines 1–4 and requires a list of starting values for the growth function provided in `start`. `tau` specifies the quantile and `trace = TRUE` indicates that we want to see the iteration steps.

A consequence of this approach is that growth rates can never exceed an upper threshold, i.e. the potential, which makes the model more robust and allows an easier adaptation of the model to different environmental conditions. Potential growth rates are then modified by the interaction function and other additional modifiers representing environmental conditions. The general approach (Grabarnik and Särkkä 2011) commonly is

$$\frac{\Delta m_{i,t}^{\times}}{\Delta t} = \frac{\Delta m_{i,t}}{\Delta t} \times (1 - h_{i,t}), \tag{5.23}$$

where $h_{i,t}$ sometimes needs to be transformed to lie between 0 and 1. In the last term, it is also possible to modify $h_{i,t}$ further to take for example shade tolerance factor v of the species of plant i into account, i.e. $1 - \frac{h_{i,t}}{v}$ (Berger et al. 2006; Fibich and Lepš 2011).

Särkkä and Renshaw (2006) instead proposed an additive way of combining growth and interaction function, i.e.

$$\frac{\Delta m_{i,t}^{+}}{\Delta t} = \frac{\Delta m_{i,t}}{\Delta t} + h_{i,t}. \tag{5.24}$$

This method implies that marks can shrink in size, which is not possible in the multiplicative approach of Eq. (5.23). Usually small plants tend to be affected by shrinking. Särkkä and Renshaw (2006) consequently defined "death by shrinking" for those plants whose marks eventually equal zero or even become negative. This model feature may seem odd on first sight, but the shrinking is intriguing, because it can be thought of as mimicking failing tree health and performance due to diseases (Häbel et al. 2019).

5.2.6 Death Processes

A wide range of different approaches exist which are not specific to individual-based models. Obviously all four main processes, interaction, growth, death and birth are always closely related. However, the modeller has the choice whether to make plant death directly dependent on interaction or on growth. Naturally also combinations of both occur. Adams et al. (2011) for example modelled the probability of mortality based on the equation

$$P_m(t) = a_0 + a_1 \cdot h_{i,t}. \tag{5.25}$$

Here a_0 is a fixed baseline and a_1 causes individuals under intense competition to have an elevated mortality rate.

By contrast Fibich and Lepš (2011) considered the possibility of a slow death process dependent on the interaction function of the last l_i years. l_i is the number of

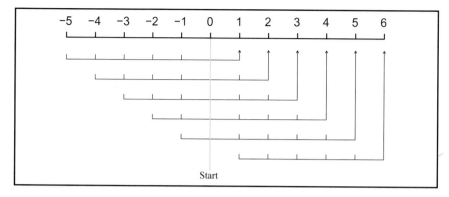

Fig. 5.14 General principle of temporal edge effect in IBM simulations that use memory effects. A memory of five years is assumed and the numbers denote simulation years

years a plant i can tolerate stress and it apparently differs from plant to plant. This model uses a *growth memory effect* that is also known from other models (Berger and Hildenbrandt 2000; Pommerening et al. 2011). According to Fibich and Lepš (2011) a plant dies, if

$$\sum_{t-l_i}^{t} 1 - \frac{h_{i,t}}{v} < 1. \tag{5.26}$$

Here v is the aforementioned shade tolerance factor or coefficient and t is current time. Small values of $1 - h_{i,t}/v$ mean heavy interaction/competition whilst values near 1 are typical of dominant, well-growing healthy plants. Death occurs, if the sum of the interaction function values (divided by v and subtracted from 1) is smaller than 1. Whilst this modelling approach is probably closer to reality than sudden death events from other mortality approaches, such memory effects require a *temporal edge correction* or *temporal boundary conditions*, since the values of the interaction function $h_{i,t}$ are not observed for the l_i years before the start of the simulation (see Fig. 5.14). This problem is related to spatial edge effects (see Sect. 4.4.8) but here the "edge" is given by the start of the simulation. Fibich and Lepš (2011) initialised these unknown values with 1 for the years before the simulation starts. This basically assumes maximum growth performance for all plants at the beginning of the simulation.

In a similar way, Berger and Hildenbrandt (2000) used a memory effect in their mortality model, however, here l was set to five years for all trees and the memory related to absolute growth rates. In their model a tree died, if the mean AGR during the last five years was less than half of AGR under optimal conditions. With this mortality model the authors also had to overcome the problem of temporal edge correction but they did not include their solution in the publication. Fibich and Lepš (2011) argued that their mortality although based on the values of the interaction

Fig. 5.15 Principle of a mortality model using five-years RGR and a model for critical RGR, see Sect. 5.2.10

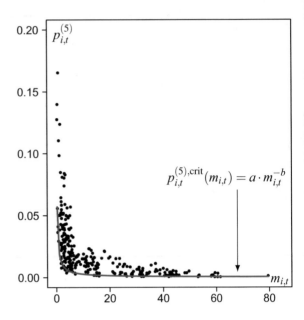

function is equivalent with the growth-based model in Berger and Hildenbrandt (2000). However, in other models, this depends on how growth exactly is modelled. If the growth model, for example, additionally includes environmental information that differs within the population, the outcomes of the two models may differ as well.

Häbel et al. (2019) found that temporal edge corrections have a considerable influence on simulation results of IBMs even much beyond the initial five years. In an attempt to solve this problem better, the authors grew the trees in their model back by five years in annual steps from the starting year. Thus reduced tree sizes were applied to the growth function and in the interaction model. During this process the authors assumed that the point pattern remained unchanged (with the exception that tree marks may be reduced to values of less than zero and then disappear) and consequently all interactions were largely based on the point pattern of the starting year.

Pommerening and Särkkä (2013) considered the memory effect of relative growth rates (RGR, see Chap. 6) instead of AGR, because small RGR values are indicative of imminent mortality (Gillner et al. 2013). Since RGR is a multiplicative concept, they compared the product of the previous five years with a critical value. Later Häbel et al. (2019) replaced the critical value by a power function to better take care of the size influence on RGR (Fig. 5.15).

Naturally it is possible to draw on the vast literature on mortality modelling reviewed in textbooks such as Burkhart and Tomé (2012) and Weiskittel et al. (2011).

5.2.7 Parameter Estimation

Apart from a few publications in general statistics the fitting of IBMs is largely a well-kept secret. In early and theoretical tree-IBM publications, model parameters were "assumed" on a trial-and-error basis (Berger and Hildenbrandt 2000; Fibich and Lepš 2011). Cronie and Särkkä (2011) detailed a simultaneous least squares method for fitting the parameters of the aforementioned growth-interaction model and tested three spatial edge-correction methods. Redenbach and Särkkä (2013) introduced a new parameter estimation process for the same model that not only considered the estimation of marks but also point locations by using Besag's L function (see Chap. 4). This is an interesting direction meriting more research, since IBMs are generally not developed for improving growth estimations but rather to understand the complex dynamics of forest structure and their dependency on growth interactions. Therefore it seems appropriate and in fact necessary to consider spatial structure already in the estimation of the model parameters.

The parameter estimation of interaction-kernel models is not an easy task, since it involves spatial calculations in every regression iteration. This is why standard regression routines provided in R or other software cannot be used without writing considerable extensions. Another important element of IBM parameter estimation concepts is the *simultaneous* estimation of all model parameters. This requires an estimation routine which includes the IBM itself and the model often is run several times in each iteration. Redenbach and Särkkä (2013) defined the original least-squares criterion as

$$S_m = \sum_{t=2}^{n} \sum_{i \in \Xi_t} (\hat{m}_{i,t} - m_{i,t})^2, \tag{5.27}$$

where Ξ_t denotes the marked point pattern at time t and n is the number of time points where data have been recorded. $t = 2$ is the time of first mark projection while $t = 1$ denotes the initial state. The model parameter values that minimise S_m are chosen as the estimates. In a similar way it is possible to use absolute mark growth rates:

$$S_{\Delta m} = \sum_{t=2}^{n} \sum_{i \in \Xi_t} (\hat{\Delta m}_{i,t} - \Delta m_{i,t})^2 \tag{5.28}$$

In modelling growth processes, it is important to account for spatial autocorrelation effects (Nord-Larson 2006; Nord-Larson and Johannsen 2007; Álvarez-González et al. 2010). Reporting a comparison of least-squares and maximum-likelihood estimation methods, Häbel et al. (2019) found that the latter usually is superior to the former. A good plausibility check includes plotting the kernel and other probability density functions with the newly estimated parameters. Changing the start parameters will reveal potential instabilities in the estimation, if the resulting model parameters greatly differ.

The R listing below shows the core of the spatial regression routine coded with
the function `optim()` (not shown here). `optim()` uses the function shown below as
part of the loss function.

```
1  > calcInteractIntensityforTrees <- function(xalpha, xbeta,
2  + xdelta, xnu, xdata) {
3  +   xdata$hi <- 0
4  +   for (i in 1 : length(xdata$dbh)) {
5  +     hi <- 0.0
6  +     for (j in 1 : length(xdata$dbh)) {
7  +     if((i != j) & (xdata$year[i] == xdata$year[j]) &
8  +       (xdata$Plotno[i] == xdata$Plotno[j])) {
9  +       dist <- euclideanDistance(xdata$xmax[i],
10 +       xdata$ymax[i], xdata$x[i], xdata$y[i],
11 +       xdata$x[j], xdata$y[j])
12 +       hi <- hi + localEffect(xalpha, xbeta, xdelta, dist,
13 +       xdata$dbh[j]) / xdata$dbh[i]^xalpha
14 +     }
15 +   }
16 +   hi <- exp(-xnu / hi)
17 +   xdata$ci[i] <- 1 - hi
18 + }
19 + return(xdata$hi)
20 + }
```

The function `calcInteractIntensityforTrees()` relates to the *TreeShotNoise*
model described in Sect. 5.2.10 and calculates the interaction function (Eq. 5.33) for
each tree. As part of the parameter estimation the function loops through a large
data set including several survey years and observation windows (plots). That is
why the `if` statement in lines 7–8 ensures that only pairs of different trees from the
same survey year and plot are used in the calculation. In line 9, Euclidean distance
is calculated and the local effects of trees other than tree i are summed in lines 12
and 13. The calculation of the interaction function is finalised in lines 16–17. An x
prefix is attached to the data-frame name (in `xdata`) as well as to the names of the
model parameters α, β, δ and ν to ensure that these variables are truly local so that
they cannot be influenced by global variables from outside the function. Since spatial
regressions rely on several loops, it is best to code the corresponding functions in
C++ and to call them from R through the `Rcpp` package (Eddelbuettel 2013).

5.2.8 Sensitivity Analysis

Studying the model behaviour based on sensitivity analysis has almost become a
standard in individual-based modelling. In their publications on transparent and comprehensive ecological modelling (TRACE), Schmolke et al. (2010) and Grimm et al.
(2014) integrated model conception, building, parametrisation, validation and sensitivity analysis as well as model documentation in a consistent modelling-cycle
framework.

Sensitivity analysis can be employed for tracing the contribution of model parameters and the corresponding processes in spatial pattern formation. The aim of sensitivity analysis in general is to explore for a given model the influence of model parameters X_i on an output variable Y. The output of a model is a deterministic function of the X_i (Pommerening et al. 2011; Saltelli et al. 2009),

$$Y = f(X_1, \ldots, X_z).$$

The vector $(X_1, \ldots, X_z)$ is considered a point in an z-dimensional parameter space. In *local* sensitivity analysis, parameters are separately varied within a neighbourhood centred at some point in the parameter space. Global methods try to simultaneously explore the model behaviour in the whole parameter space. As a consequence also parameter interaction is studied. This concerns the mutual influence of the X_i in such a way that, for example, a simultaneous increase of X_1 and X_2 leads to a larger effect on Y than a simple addition of the effects of a separate increase of X_1 and X_2 (Pommerening et al. 2011; Saltelli et al. 2009).

Often the extended Fourier Amplitude Sensitivity test, a variance-based global sensitivity method (Saltelli et al. 2009; Pianosi et al. 2016), is used. The Fourier Amplitude Sensitivity Test (FAST) was first devised in the 1970s by Cukier and others (see Cukier et al. 1978) and further developed by Saltelli et al. (1999) to become the extended FAST method (eFAST). eFAST is model-independent and is applicable irrespective of the degree of linearity or additivity of the model. The method is based on a variance decomposition of an arbitrary model output variable Y, i.e.

$$\text{Var}(Y) = D = \sum_{j=1}^{z} D_j + \sum_{1 \leq i < j \leq z} D_{ij} + \cdots + D_{1,2,\ldots,z}.$$

For the decomposition $z > 1$ individual input parameters are mathematically interpreted as random variables $\mathbf{X} = (X_1, \ldots, X_z)$. The first order contributions of the $j = 1, \ldots, z$ input parameters correspond to the variances of the expected value of Y given X_j, i.e. $D_j = \text{Var}_{X_j}(\mathbf{E}[Y|X_j = x_j])$. The contributions from higher-order interactions between the variables $D_{..}$ are defined accordingly. The eFAST method approximates main effects $S_j = D_j/D$, which are also known as Sobol' first order indices, and so-called Sobol' total order indices collecting the main effects and all interactions including j. From these approximations higher-order interaction terms can be obtained by subtracting the main effects from the corresponding total order indices. In this way, the eFAST results highlight, which input parameters have a significant influence on the simulation with respect to the output variable and give a measure for sensitivity or uncertainty (Saltelli et al. 2009; Saloranta and Andersen 2007; Pommerening et al. 2011).

In our context, the model parameters constitute the input. The sensitivity analysis helps to identify those parameters that have the largest influence on the outcome variable. Hence, if a researcher, for example, selects the model with the highest

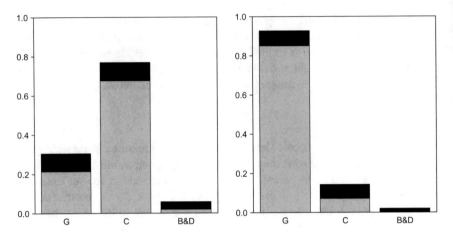

Fig. 5.16 Proportions of the total variance explained by groups of model parameter with regard to deviations of observed and simulated mark variograms (see Sect. 4.4.7.2) and analysed by the extended Fourier amplitude sensitivity test (eFAST). The orange area (main effect) denotes the portion of total variance explained by the particular model parameters alone and the black area the part explained by all parameter interactions. Left: Interior Douglas fir (*Pseudotsuga menziesii* var *glauca* (MIRB.) FRANCO) in the Alex Fraser Research Forest (BC, Canada). Right: Norway spruce (*Picea abies* (L.) KARST.) at Karlstift, Austria (Pommerening et al. 2011)

sensitivity to the interaction parameters, for example, the chance of describing the interaction process well is high. The variability of the input parameters should be representative of the observational error, e.g. 10% (Häbel et al. 2019).

Using a previous version of *TreeShotNoise* (see Sect. 5.2.10) Pommerening et al. (2011), for example, studied the relative importance of growth (G), competition (C) and birth and death processes (B&D) in three forest ecosystems. Analysing the relative importance of these processes was possible by grouping the model parameters driving these processes. The authors concluded that this relative importance as identified by the sensitivity analysis much depended on the forest ecosystem in question, e.g. its development stage, but also on the simulation length which coincided with the observation length (Fig. 5.16). Parameter interaction was comparatively low, however, while competition was more than twice more important than growth in the Canadian interior Douglas fir woodland, in Norway spruce (*Picea abies* (L.) KARST.) in Austria, growth was more than four times more important than competition. Birth and death processes in both ecosystems played a minor role.

Sensitivity analysis provides valuable information on the extent of the parameter space and on model behaviour. It is also useful when comparing different models for getting a deeper understanding and assessing their suitability. Methods of sensitivity analysis and related fields are also useful when identifying *tipping points* and *tipping elements* (Lenton et al. 2008; Grimm and Berger 2016). The term tipping point commonly refers to a critical threshold at which a tiny change can markedly modify the state or development of a system, see Sect. 2.1.2.2. Such threshold changes are triggered when the system's bounds of resilience are exceeded (Perry et al. 2008; Lenton et al. 2008). Tipping points can lead to abrupt changes and are particularly often discussed in the context of climate change, see Sect. 2.1.2.2. Tipping elements are broadly speaking components of a system that may pass a tipping point. Each model parameter represents or is at least associated with a model process that is the metaphor of an ecological process. Very sensitive parameters can act as tipping elements of tipping parameters by triggering abrupt system changes. Further analysis can then establish whether these thresholds coincide with observed changes or likely future changes in a forest ecosystem.

5.2.9 Model Implementation

Individual-based models can be implemented in any higher programming or script language. The choice of programming medium largely depends on existing skills and personal taste. If analyses and parameter estimation are carried out in R, it makes sense to implement the model in R, too. Because of its flexibility and ease of use R provides more opportunities for testing the model and experimenting with the new IBM. In complex models, loops and other model elements may slow down computations in R. Then it is recommended to outsource parts of the code in C++ (Eddelbuettel 2013). In fact it is a good idea to divide the tasks between R and C++ in such a way that in both languages those things are coded that they can process best. This implies implementing the majority of sub-models in C++ and handling input, output and statistical as well as graphical tasks in R. For successful model applications and publishing it is not necessary to implement your model as an R package, however, potential model users are sure to be grateful for this effort.

Uri Wilenski and colleagues have developed the NetLogo programming environment `https://ccl.northwestern.edu/netlogo/` for agent/individual-based models. This software uses a script language and a user-friendly user interface along with easy-to-use diagnostic tools (see Fig. 5.17). In addition all code written in Net-Logo is open and the software website has a model library promoting an exchange of modelling and programming experience. Grimm and Railsback (2012) published a NetLogo practical IBM book to go with their earlier theory book (Grimm and Railsback 2005). Thiele and Grimm (2010) developed an R extension for NetLogo that allows linking NetLogo with R.

There are also various Java-based specialised development packages such as JABM `http://jabm.sourceforge.net/` or JADE `http://jade.tilab.com/`. There are also websites comparing various development packages.

5.2.10 Example Model

Grimm et al. (2006, 2010) published a standard protocol (ODD—Overview, Design concepts and Details) for describing and communicating individual-based models. The protocol provides a common structure of presenting IBM information thus facilitating understanding and cooperation among other things. It is good practice

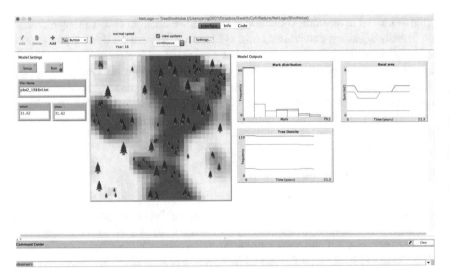

Fig. 5.17 Screenshot from an NetLogo implementation of the *TreeShotNoise* model described in the following section. In the centre of the screenshot the interaction map relating to the Douglas fir monitoring plot 2 in the Alex Fraser Research Forest (BC, Canada; see also Fig. 5.7, right) in 2004 is shown after 16 years of simulation

promoting reproducibility to use this standard when introducing a new IBM. As an example we described here the recent version of the generic *TreeShotNoise* model published by Pommerening et al. (2011), Pommerening and Särkkä (2013) and Häbel et al. (2019). Instead of suggesting one or more concrete, quantitative tree characteristics we use the term "mark" here as in Chap. 4 to emphasise that the modelling focus can be on any plant size characteristic or on combinations of size characteristics.

Purpose

TreeShotNoise was developed for analysing spatio-temporal dynamics in monospecies and mixed-species forests, i.e. the temporal evolution of spatial marked point patterns in forests. The name origins from shot-noise fields, where the points are instances of time and the impulses acoustic signals (Chiu et al. 2013). Specifically the objective of the model was to understand how intraspecific interaction, growth and mortality affect the spatial structure of a forest and vice versa. The model is generic and can be parametrised for any tree species and forest ecosystem.

State Variables and Scales

The model has two hierarchical levels, individual trees and the forest, i.e. the population each tree is part of. At individual level, growth, interaction and mortality are considered. An individual tree i is described by 1. an identity number or index, 2. a location, ξ_i, of the stem centre expressed in Cartesian coordinates, 3. a mark (commonly stem diameter = diameter at breast height, measured at 1.3 m above ground in cm, but also other marks are possible) and 4. an annual absolute growth

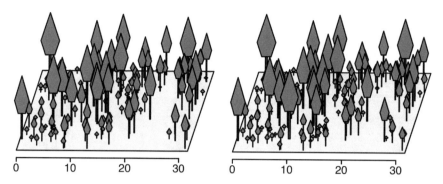

Fig. 5.18 Visualisations of the observed data (left) and of the results after 16 years of simulation (1988–2004) using the *TreeShotNoise* model (right). The visualisations relate to the interior Douglas fir (*Pseudotsuga menziesii* var *glauca* (MIRB.) FRANCO) plot 1 in the Alex Fraser Research Forest in British Columbia and were produced in R using the crown models developed by Pretzsch (2009, p. 234ff.)

rate, $\Delta m_{i,t}/\Delta t$, the latter two depending on time t given in years (Fig. 5.18). Tree interaction is spatially explicit, see the paragraph entitled *Interaction*. A rectangular observation window defines the boundaries of the forest and can be arbitrarily selected. The nine model parameters are specific to tree species.

Process Overview and Scheduling

The trees' life cycle is described by two biological sub-models operating in discrete, annual time steps. The first sub-model determines the absolute mark growth rate depending on a tree's potential mark growth rate and the interaction it faces. The second sub-model accounts for mortality simulating natural tree death depending on the mark growth during a certain reference period. The establishment of new trees has not been considered yet, since this process was not included in the data analysed so far.

At the beginning of each time step first the mortality rule is applied followed by the removal of all dead trees. Afterwards the interaction function is calculated for the residual trees, which contributes to the annual growth rates. After calculating potential interaction and mark growth it is possible to determine growth rates. Using growth rates, the tree stem diameters are now updated synchronously (Fig. 5.19).

Design Concepts

Basic principles: The growth sub-model reflects the well-known fact that the growth of some marks of trees (e.g. stem diameter, crown diameter) inside a forest is reduced compared to that of open-grown trees, which typically do not experience interaction with other trees (Newnham 1964; Botkin et al. 1972). In the *TreeShotNoise* model, as a substitute for growth data from open-grown trees growth data of the most dominant trees of the same population are used and identified through quantile regression (Cade and Noon 2003). The interaction sub-model is based on a random field for describing the interaction intensity of single trees in a forest, following Adler (1996) and Illian et al. (2008, p. 435f.). The additive superposition of interaction effects exerted by single

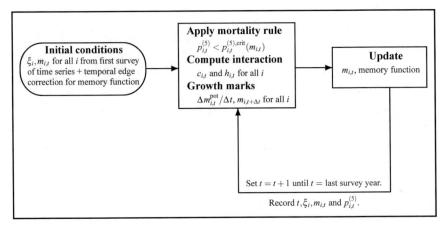

Fig. 5.19 Flowchart of a *TreeShotNoise* model simulation. Modified from Häbel et al. (2019)

trees describes the interaction intensity that a tree would face at a given location. The deterministic mortality sub-model utilises the well-known observation that trees have to maintain some level of mark growth at all times for their survival.

Emergence: *TreeShotNoise* explicitly models the life of each tree depending on growth, local interaction and mortality. Emergent system dynamics include (1) the spatial structure of the forest, (2) the distribution of tree marks and (3) self-thinning behaviour and residual tree density among other descriptive statistics.

Adaptation: Mortality enlarges the growing space available to some trees. As a consequence these trees have access to more resources, which increases the growth of tree marks.

Objectives: The objective of the aforementioned adaptive trait is to maintain or enhance individual fitness through continuous growth.

Sensing: Individual trees are assumed to be aware of their own state variables, of the model parameters related to the tree processes and of the interaction intensity at their location.

Interaction: Above-ground interaction (mostly in terms of competition for spatially distributed resources and to some degree also including neutral effects and facilitation) is modelled based on the concept of the *shot-noise field* (Illian et al. 2008). According to this approach every tree exerts a local effect, which depends on its mark and decreases with increasing distance from the tree. To derive the interaction intensity of a tree, the interaction effects of all other trees are additively aggregated. The resulting total interaction intensity is then weighted by the local effect the tree exerts at its own location. This determination of interaction intensity mainly reflects asymmetric interaction (see Sect. 2.1.1).

Stochasticity: All sub-models currently are deterministic but a stochastic variant of the mortality model is envisaged for the future, since it would more realistically reflect natural death processes.

Observation: At the end of each model run *TreeShotNoise* allows saving all state variables but also the derived variables such as the interaction intensity occurring at each tree location. In addition, summary characteristics such as the empirical mark distribution, tree density and the empirical mark variogram can be saved. The output files are in ASCII format and can easily be imported by spreadsheet and statistical software for further analysis and visualisation.

Initialisation and Input Data

TreeShotNoise is initialised with a starting configuration of trees, e.g. tree locations and tree marks (e.g. stem diameters). In past applications, we used data from original time series for this purpose. Also the length of the simulation period usually coincided with the length of the observation period of the time series. Furthermore the model is initialised with a set of nine fixed model parameters, which are read from an input file and are specific for each investigated forest. *TreeShotNoise* currently does not use input data to represent varying environmental processes, but assumes homogeneous environmental conditions throughout the observation window.

Sub-models

Tree growth: The growth process is the biological core of *TreeShotNoise* and is modelled using the potential-modifier approach (Newnham 1964; Botkin et al. 1972). In this approach, potential absolute annual growth rates are estimated, i.e. growth rates that would be observed, if the trees grew largely in absence of any interaction from other trees, as an upper quantile of the observed mark growth rates when applying quantile regression (Cade and Noon 2003). These growth rates are subsequently reduced based on inter-tree interaction.

Accordingly potential annual mark growth rate $\Delta m_{i,t}^{\text{pot}}$ is modelled for each tree i, time t and mark m through quantile regression based on the Hugershoff growth function (Hugershoff 1936; Zeide 1993, Eq. 7)

$$\frac{\Delta m_{i,t}^{\text{pot}}}{\Delta t} = k \cdot m_{i,t}^{p} \cdot e^{-q \cdot m_{i,t}}, \tag{5.29}$$

where k, p and q are model parameters. As part of the quantile regression, the *state-space* approach involves an annual updating of the mark. The updates are produced by Eq. (5.29) and as a result the growth rates correctly follow a nonlinear growth curve rather than a linear one as is often assumed when working with mean annual growth rates from periodic re-measurements (Nord-Larson 2006; Häbel et al. 2019). As the observed growth rates used in the quantile regression stem from repeated measurements in the same observational plots, the parameter estimation routines of *TreeShotNoise* account for possible within-tree correlations using the first-order autoregressive method in addition to the state-space approach as described in Nord-Larson (2006). For forest ecosystems with mixed species, function (5.29) is fitted for each species or species-trait group separately.

Finally, the interaction function $h_{i,t}$ (Eq. 5.33 below) modifies potential growth to obtain the annual absolute growth rate, $\Delta m_{i,t}$ as

$$\frac{\Delta m_{i,t}}{\Delta t} = \frac{\Delta m_{i,t}^{\text{pot}}}{\Delta t} \cdot (1 - e^{-\nu/h_{i,t}}). \tag{5.30}$$

Here ν is a further model parameter.

Tree interaction: Tree mark growth is hampered by interaction among trees. To model this impact, in each time step, first an interaction field is constructed based on the actual forest configuration given by tree locations and marks. The value of $c_{i,t}$ of this field at the location of tree i (Eq. 5.32) is considered the corresponding interaction intensity and is subsequently used to determine growth rate $\Delta m_{i,t}$ by means of Eq. (5.30).

The distance-related decrease of the local effect is modelled using a Gaussian kernel function. The local interaction effects of all trees in a forest are additively aggregated. This results in an interaction field (see also the illustration in Fig. 5.7, right), which assigns to any location ξ and time t the interaction intensity $c_t(\xi)$ as

$$c_t(\xi) = \sum_j p_{j,t}(\xi) = \sum_j m_{j,t}^{\alpha} \cdot \exp\left\{-\frac{\delta \cdot dist_j^2(\xi)}{m_{j,t}^{\beta}}\right\} \tag{5.31}$$

with positive model parameters α, β and δ; $dist_j$ is the Euclidean distance between the location of an arbitrary tree j and another location ξ in the forest.

Consequently the interaction intensity of tree i at time t can be expressed as

$$c_{i,t} = \sum_{j \neq i} p_{j,t}(\xi_i) = \sum_{j \neq i} m_{j,t}^{\alpha} \cdot \exp\left\{-\frac{\delta \cdot dist_j^2(\xi_i)}{m_{j,t}^{\beta}}\right\}. \tag{5.32}$$

The $c_{i,t}$ field values are computed with periodic boundary conditions (Illian et al. 2008) to reduce edge effects and only depend on the marks of those trees influencing tree i and on distance $dist_j(\xi_i)$ between them.

However, the impact of the interaction intensity also depends on the mark of the affected tree i. To take this into account the interaction function therefore combines the mark of tree i with its interaction intensity and is given by

$$h_{i,t} = \sum_{j \neq i} \frac{p_{j,t}(\xi_i)}{m_{i,t}^{\alpha}} = \sum_{j \neq i} \frac{m_{j,t}^{\alpha} \cdot \exp\left\{-\frac{\delta \cdot dist_j^2(\xi_i)}{m_{j,t}^{\beta}}\right\}}{m_{i,t}^{\alpha}}. \tag{5.33}$$

The term $m_{i,t}^{\alpha}$ gives the value of the interaction signal at the location ξ_i of tree i, i.e. the maximum of the local effect function of tree i. By construction, $h_{i,t}$ is scaled between 0 and 1.

Tree death: Deterministic mortality depends on a 5-year growth performance and is derived from the ratio of current and previous mark, the so-called growth multiplier $M_{i,t}$ (see Sect. 6.2.3), which can be transformed to relative growth rate (RGR). RGRs have proved to be good indicators of imminent death (Bigler and Bugmann 2003; Gillner et al. 2013). For a given tree i, a memory function (see Sect. 5.2.6) multiplicatively aggregates the growth multipliers $M_{i,t}$ of the last five years (see Eq. 6.18 in Sect. 6.2.3) according to

$$M_{i,t}^{(5)} = M_{i,t} \cdot M_{i,t-1} \cdot \ldots \cdot M_{i,t-4} \qquad (5.34)$$

and transforms them to the corresponding RGR, $p_{i,t}^{(5)}$ as

$$p_{i,t}^{(5)} = \ln M_{i,t}^{(5)}. \qquad (5.35)$$

If the simulated five-year RGR falls short of the critical value $p_{i,t}^{(5),\mathrm{crit}}$, the tree dies (see Fig. 5.15). The critical value $p_{i,t}^{(5),\mathrm{crit}}$ is given by the power function

$$p_{i,t}^{(5),\mathrm{crit}}(m_{i,t}) = a \cdot m_{i,t}^{-b} \qquad (5.36)$$

with model parameters a and b. For the first five simulation years, it is necessary to apply a temporal edge correction to the memory function (see Sect. 5.2.6), because the relative growth rates of the trees prior to the first simulation year are unknown.

TreeShotNoise and the corresponding parameter estimation routines have been implemented in R and C++. A pseudo-code detailing the model parameter estimation is included in Häbel et al. (2019).

References

Adami C, Schossau J, Hintze A (2016) Evolutionary game theory using agent-based methods. Phys Life Rev 19:1–26

Adams T, Ackland G, Marion G, Edwards C (2011) Understanding plantation transformation using a size-structured spatial population model. Forest Ecol Manag 261:799–809

Adler FR (1996) A model of self-thinning through local competition. Proc Natl Acad Sci USA 93:9980–9984

Álvarez-González JG, Zingg A, Gadow Kv (2010) Estimating growth in beech forests: a study based on long-term experiments in Switzerland. Ann Forest Sci 67:307

Baccelli F, Blaszczyszyn B (2001) On a coverage process ranging from the Boolean model to the Poisson-Voroni tesselation. Adv Appl Probab 33:293–323

Baddeley A, Rubak E, Turner R (2016) Spatial point patterns. Methodology and applications with R. CRC Press, Boca Raton, 810 p

Baptestini EM, de Aguiar MAM, Bolnick DI, Araújo MS (2009) The shape of the competition and carrying capacity kernels affects the likelihood of disruptive selection. J Theor Biol 259:5–11

Batista JLF, Maguire DA (1998) Modeling the spatial structure of tropical forests. Forest Ecol Manag 110:293–314

Bauer S, Wyszomirski T, Berger U, Hildenbrandt H, Grimm V (2004) Asymmetric competition as a natural outcome of neighbour interactions among plants: results from the field-of-neighbourhood modelling approach. Plant Ecol 170:135–145

Bäuerle H, Nothdurft A (2011) Spatial modeling of habitat trees based on line transect sampling and point pattern reconstruction. Can J Forest Res 41:715–727

Bella IE (1971) A new competition model for individual trees. Forest Sci 17:364–372

Berger U, Hildenbrandt H (2000) A new approach to spatially explicit modelling of forest dynamics: spacing, ageing and neighbourhood competition of mangrove trees. Ecol Model 132:287–302

Berger U, Hildenbrandt H, Grimm V (2002) Towards a standard for the individual-based modelling of plant populations: self-thinning and the field-of-neighbourhood approach. Nat Res Model 15:39–54

Berger U, Adams M, Grimm V, Hildenbrandt H (2006) Modelling secondary succession of neotropical mangroves: causes and consequences of growth reduction in pioneer species. Perspect Plant Ecol Evol Syst 7:243–252

Bigler C, Bugmann H (2003) Growth-dependent tree mortality models based on tree rings. Can J Forest Res 33:210–221

Botkin DB, Janak JF, Wallis JR (1972) Some ecological consequences of a computer model of forest growth. J Ecol 60:849

Boyden S, Binkley D, Shepperd W (2005) Spatial and temporal patterns in structure, regeneration, and mortality of an old-growth ponderosa pine forest in the Colorado front range. Forest Ecol Manag 219:43–55

Brown C, Law R, Illian JB, Burslem DFRP (2011) Linking ecological processes with spatial and non-spatial patterns in plant communities. J Ecol 99:1402–1414

Bugmann H (2001) A review of forest gap models. Clim Chang 51:259–305

Bugmann F, Yan A, Sykes MT, Martin P, Lindner M, Desanker PV, Cumming SG (1996) A comparison of forest gap models: model structure and behaviour. Clim Chang 34:289–313

Bullock JM, Mallada González L, Tamme R, Götzenberger L, White SM, Pärtel M, Hooftman DAP (2017) A synthesis of empirical plant dispersal kernels. J Ecol 105:6–19

Burkhart HE, Tomé M (2012) Modeling forest trees and stands. Springer, New York, 457 p

Cade BS, Noon BR (2003) A gentle introduction to quantile regression for ecologists. Front Ecol Environ 8:412–420

Canham CD, LePage PT, Coates KD (2004) A neighbourhood analysis of canopy tree competition: effects of shading versus crowding. Can J Forest Res 34:778–787

Chen BW, Gadow Kv (2002) Timber harvest planning with spatial objectives, using the method of simulated annealing. Forstwissenschaftliches Centralblatt 121:25–34

Chilès J-P, Delfiner P (1999) Geostatistics. Modeling spatial uncertainty. Wiley, New York, 695 p

Chiu SN, Stoyan D, Kendall WS, Mecke J (2013) Stochastic geometry and its applications, 3rd edn. Wiley, Chichester, 544 p

Clark PJ, Evans FC (1954) Distance to nearest neighbour as a measure of spatial relationships in populations. Ecology 35:445–453

Comas C, Mateu J (2007) Modelling forest dynamics: a perspective from point process methods. Biom J 49:176–196

Crawford J, Torquato S, Stillinger FG (2003) Aspects of correlation function realizability. J Chem Phys 118:7065–7073

Cronie O, Särkkä A (2011) Some edge-correction methods for marked spatio-temporal point process models. Comput Stat Data 55:2209–2220

Cronie O, Nyström K, Yu J (2013) Spatiotemporal modeling of Swedish Scots pine stands. Forest Sci 9:505–516

Cukier RI, Levine HB, Shuler KE (1978) Nonlinear sensitivity analysis of multiparameter model systems. J Comput Phys 26:1–42

DeAngelis DL, Grimm V (2014) Individual-based models in ecology after four decades. F1000Prime Rep 6:39

DeAngelis DL, Mooij WM (2005) Individual-based modeling of ecological and evolutionary processes. Annu Rev Ecol Evol Syst 36:147–168

Degenhardt A (1999) Description of tree distribution patterns and their development through marked Gibbs processes. Biom J 41:457–470

Degenhardt A, Pofahl U (2000) Simulation of natural evolution of stem number and tree distribution pattern in a pure pine stand. Environmetrics 11:197–208

Diggle PJ (2014) Statistical analysis of spatial and spatio-temporal point patterns, 3rd edn. CRC Press, Boca Raton, 267 p

Diggle PJ, Gates DJ, Stibbard A (1987) A nonparametric estimator for pairwise-interaction point processes. Biometrika 74:763–770

Eddelbuettel D (2013) Seamless R and C++ integration with Rcpp. Springer, New York, 220 p

Falster DF, Westoby M (2003) Plant height and evolutionary games. Trends in Ecol Evol 18:337–343

Fibich P, Lepš J (2011) Do biodiversity indices behave as expected from traits of constituent species in simulated scenarios? Ecol Model 222:2049–2058

García O (2014) A generic approach to spatial individual-based modelling and simulation of plant communities. Math Comput For Nat Res Sci 6:36–47

Gerrard DJ (1969) Competition quotient - a new measure of the competition affecting individual forest trees. Michigan State University Research Bulletin, Agricultural Experiment Station, p 20

Gillner S, Rüger N, Roloff A, Berger U (2013) Low relative growth rates predict future mortality of common beech (Fagus sylvatica L.). Forest Ecol Manag 2013:372–378

Grabarnik P, Särkkä A (2001) Interacting neighbour point processes: some models for clustering. J Stat Comput Simul 68:103–125

Grabarnik P, Särkkä A (2009) Modelling the spatial structure of forest stands by multivariate point processes with hierarchical interactions. Ecol Model 220:1232–1240

Grabarnik P, Särkkä A (2011) Modelling the spatial and space-time structure of forest stands: how to model asymmetric interaction between neighbouring trees. Procedia Environ Sci 7:62–67

Grimm V (1999) Ten years of individual-based modelling in ecology: what have we learned and what could we learn in the future? Ecol Model 115:129–148

Grimm V, Berger U (2016) Robustness analysis: deconstructing computational models for ecological theory and applications. Ecol Model 326:162–167

Grimm V, Railsback SF (2005) Individual-based modeling and ecology. Princeton University Press, Princeton, 448 p

Grimm V, Railsback SF (2012) Pattern-oriented modelling: a 'multi-scope' for predictive systems ecology. Philos Trans R Soc Lond B Biol Sci 367:298–310

Grimm V, Revilla E, Berger U, Jeltsch F, Mooij WM, Railsback SF, Thulke HH, Weiner J, Wiegand T, DeAngelis DL (2005) Pattern-oriented modeling of agent-based complex systems: lessons from ecology. Science 310:987–991

Grimm V, Berger U, Bastiansen F, Eliassen S, Ginot V, Giske J, Goss-Custard J, Grand T, Heinz SK, Huse G, Huth A, Jepsen JU, Jørgensen C, Mooij WM, Müller B, Pe'er G, Piou C, Railsback SF, Robbins AM, Robbins MM, Rossmanith E, Rüger N, Strand E, Souissi S, Stillman RA, Vabø R, Visser U, DeAngelis DL (2006) A standard protocol for describing individual-based and agent-based models. Ecol Model 198:115–126

Grimm V, Berger U, DeAngelis DL, Polhill JG, Giske J, Railsback SF (2010) The ODD protocol: a review and first update. Ecol Model 221:2760–2768

Grimm V, Augusiak J, Focks A, Frank BM, Gabsi F, Johnston ASA, Liu C, Martin BT, Meli M, Radchuk V, Thorbeck P, Railsback SF (2014) Towards better modelling and decision support: documenting model development, testing, and analysis using TRACE. Ecol Model 280:129–139

Grüters U, Seltmann T, Schmidt H, Horn H, Pranchai A, Vovides AG, Peters R, Vogt J, Dahdouh-Guebas F, Berger U (2014) The mangrove forest dynamics model mesoFON. Ecol Model 291:28–41

Häbel H, Myllymäki M, Pommerening A (2019) New insights on the behaviour of alternative types of individual-based tree models for natural forests. Ecol Model (In print)

Hasenauer H (1997) Dimensional relationships of open-grown trees in Austria. Forest Ecol Manag 96:197–206

Högmander H, Särkkä A (1999) Multitype spatial point patterns with hierarchical interactions. Biometrics 55:1051–1058

Hugershoff R (1936) Die mathematischen Hilfsmittel des Kulturingenieurs und Biologen. II. Teil: Herleitung von gesetzmäßigen Zusammenhängen [Mathematical tools for forest engineers and biologists. Part II: Deriving relationships based on natural laws]. Dresden, unpublished manuscript

Huston M, DeAngelis D, Post W (1988) New computer models unify ecological theory. BioScience 38:682–691

Illian J, Penttinen A, Stoyan H, Stoyan D (2008) Statistical analysis and modelling of spatial point patterns. Wiley, Chichester, 534 p

Kirkpatrick S, Gellat CD, Vecchi MP (1983) Optimisation by simulated annealing. Science 220:671–680

Koenker R, Park BJ (1994) An interior point algorithm for nonlinear quantile regression. J Econom 71:265–283

Law R, Dieckmann U (2000) A dynamical system for neighborhoods in plant communities. Ecology 81:2137–2148

Lenton TM, Held H, Kriegler E, Hall JW, Lucht W, Rahmstorf S, Schellnhuber HJ (2008) Tipping elements in the Earth's climate system. Proc Natl Acad Sci USA 105:1786–1793

Lewandowski A, Gadow Kv (1997) Ein heuristischer Ansatz zur Reproduktion von Waldbeständen [A method for reproducing uneven-aged forest stands]. Allgemeine Forst- und Jagdzeitung 168:170–174

Lewis PAW, Shedler GS (1979) Simulation of non-homogeneous Poisson processes by thinning. Nav Res Logist 26:403–413

Li B, Wu H, Zou G (2000) Self-thinning rule: a causal interpretation from ecological field theory. Ecol Model 132:167–173

Li Y, Ye S, Hui G, Hu Y, Zhao Z (2014) Spatial structure of timber harvested according to structure-based forest management. Forest Ecol Manag 322:106–116

Lilleleht A, Sims A, Pommerening A (2014) Spatial forest structure reconstruction as a strategy for mitigating edge-bias in circular monitoring plots. Forest Ecol Manag 316:47–53

Matérn B (1960) Spatial variation. Meddelanden fran Statens Skogsforskningsinstitut 49:1–144

Maynard Smith J (1982) Evolution and the theory of games. Cambridge University Press, Cambridge, 234 p

McNickle GG, Dybzinski R (2013) Game theory and plant ecology. Ecol Lett 16:545–555

Miina J, Pukkala T (2002) Application of ecological field theory in distance-dependent growth modelling. Forest Ecol Manag 161:101–107

Motz K, Sterba H, Pommerening A (2010) Sampling measures of tree diversity. Forest Ecol Manag 260:1985–1996

Murrell DJ, Law R (2003) Heteromyopia and the spatial coexistence of similar competitors. Ecol Lett 6:48–59

Nanos N, Larson K, Millerón M, Sjöstedt-de Luna S (2010) Inverse modelling for effective dispersal: do we need tree size to estimate fecundity? Ecol Model 221:2415–2424

Nash JF (1950) Equilibrium points in N-person games. Proc Natl Acad Sci USA 36:48–49

Neumann Jv, Morgenstern O (1944) Theory of games and economic behaviour. Princeton University Press, Princeton, 776 p

Newnham RM (1964) The development of a stand model for Douglas fir. PhD thesis, University of British Columbia, Vancouver, 201 p

Nord-Larson T (2006) Modeling individual-tree growth from data with highly irregular measurement intervals. Forest Sci 52:198–208

Nord-Larson T, Johannsen VK (2007) A state-space approach to stand growth modelling of European beech. Ann Forest Sci 64:365–374

Nothdurft A, Saborowski J, Nuske RS, Stoyan D (2010) Density estimation based on k-tree sampling and point pattern reconstruction. Can J Forest Res 40:953–967

Ogata Y, Tanemura M (1985) Estimation of interaction potentials of marked spatial point patterns through the maximum likelihood method. Biometrics 41:421–433

O'Sullivan AP, Perry JD (2013) Spatial simulation. Exploring pattern and process. Wiley-Blackwell, Chichester, 305 p

Perry DA, Oren R, Hart SC (2008) Forest ecosystems, 2nd edn. The Johns Hopkins University Press, Baltimore, 632 p

Pianosi F, Beven K, Freer J, Hall JW, Rougier J, Stephenson DB, Wagener T (2016) Sensitivity analysis of environmental models: a systematic review with practical workflow. Environ Model Softw 79:214–232

Picard N, Bar-Hen A, Mortier F, Chadaeuf J (2009) The multi-scale marked area-interaction point process: a model for the spatial pattern of trees. Scand J Stat 36:23–41

Pienaar LV, Turnbull KJ (1973) The Chapman-Richards generalization of von Bertalanffy's growth model for basal area growth and yield in even-aged stands. Forest Sci 19:2–22

Piou C, Berger U, Grimm V (2009) Proposing an information criterion for individual-based models developed in a pattern-oriented modelling framework. Ecol Model 220:1957–1967

Pommerening A (2000) Neue Methoden zur räumlichen Reproduktion von Waldbeständen und ihre Bedeutung für forstliche Inventuren und deren Fortschreibung [New methods of spatial simulation of forest structures and their implications for updating forest inventories]. Allgemeine Forst- und Jagd-Zeitung [German J Forest Res] 171:164–169

Pommerening A (2006) Evaluating structural indices by reversing forest structural analysis. Forest Ecol Manag 224:266–277

Pommerening A, Maleki K (2014) Differences between competition kernels and traditional size-ratio based competition indices used in forest ecology. Forest Ecol Manag 331:135–143

Pommerening A, Sánchez Meador AJ (2018) Tamm review: tree interactions between myth and reality. Forest Ecol Manag 428:164–176

Pommerening A, Särkkä A (2013) What mark variograms tell about spatial plant interactions. Ecol Model 251:64–72

Pommerening A, Stoyan D (2006) Edge-correction needs in estimating indices of spatial forest structure. Can J Forest Res 36:1723–1739

Pommerening A, Stoyan D (2008) Reconstructing spatial tree point patterns from nearest neighbour summary statistics measured in small subwindows. Can J Forest Res 38:1110–1122

Pommerening A, LeMay V, Stoyan D (2011) Model-based analysis of the influence of ecological processes on forest point pattern formation. Ecol Model 222:666–678

Pommerening A, Gonçalves AC, Rodríguez-Soalleiro R (2011) Species mingling and diameter differentiation as second-order characteristics. Allgemeine Forst- und Jagd-Zeitung [German J Forest Res] 182:115–129

Pommerening A, Svensson B, Zhao D, Wang H, Myllymäki M (2019) Spatial species diversity in species-rich forest ecosystems: revisiting and extending the concept of spatial species mingling. Ecol Indic (In print)

Pretzsch H (1997) Analysis and modeling of spatial stand structures. Methodological considerations based on mixed beech-larch stands in Lower Saxony. Forest Ecol Manag 97:237–253

Redenbach C, Särkkä A (2013) Parameter estimation for growth interaction processes using spatio-temporal information. Comput Stat Data Anal 57:672–683

Renshaw E, Särkkä A (2001) Gibbs point processes for studying the development of spatial-temporal stochastic processes. Comput Stat Data 36:85–105

Rice SO (1945) Mathematical analysis of random noise. Bell Syst Tech J 24:46–156

Saloranta TM, Andersen T (2007) MyLake - a multi-year lake simulation model code suitable for uncertainty and sensitivity analysis simulations. Ecol Model 207:45–60

Saltelli A, Tarantola S, Chan KP-S (1999) A quantitative model-independent method for global sensitivity analysis of model output. Technometrics 41:39–56

Saltelli A, Chan K, Scott EM (eds) (2009) Sensitivity analysis. Wiley, Chichester, 494 p

Särkkä A, Renshaw E (2006) The analysis of marked point patterns evolving through space and time. Comput Stat Data 51:1698–1718

Schmolke A, Thorbek P, DeAngelis DL, Grimm V (2010) Ecological models supporting environmental decision making: a strategy for the future. Trends Ecol Evol 25:479–486

Schneider MK, Law R, Illian JB (2006) Quantification of neighbourhood-dependent plant growth by Bayesian hierarchical modelling. J Ecol 94:310–321

Shimatani K, Kubota Y (2004) Spatial analysis for continuously changing point patterns along a gradient and its application to an Abies sachalinensis population. Ecol Model 180:359–369

Snyder RE, Chesson P (2004) How the spatial scales of dispersal, competition and environmental heterogeneity interact to affect coexistence. Am Nat 164:633–650

Stillman RA, Railsback SF, Giske J, Berger U, Grimm V (2015) Making predictions in a changing world: the benefits of individual-based ecology. BioScience 65:140–150

Stoyan D (1987) Statistical analysis of spatial point processes: a soft-core model and cross-correlations of marks. Biom J 29:971–980

Stoyan D, Penttinen A (2000) Recent applications of point process methods in forestry statistics. Stat Sci 15:61–78

Stoyan D, Stoyan H (1998) Non-homogeneous Gibbs process models for forestry - a case study. Biom J 5:521–531

Strîmbu VF, Ene LT, Næsset E (2016) Spatially consistent imputations of forest data under a semivariogram model. Can J Forest Res 46:1145–1156

Thiele JC, Grimm V (2010) NetLogo meets R: linking agent-based models with a toolbox for their analysis. Environ Model Softw 25:972–974

Tomé M, Burkhart HE (1989) Distance-dependent competition measures for predicting growth of individual trees. Forest Sci 35:816–831

Tomppo E (1986) Models and methods for analysing spatial patterns of trees. Communicationes Instituti Forestalis Fenniae, vol 138. Helsinki, 65 p

Torquato S (2002) Random heterogeneous materials. Microstructure and macroscopic properties. Springer, New York, 701 p

Tscheschel A, Stoyan D (2006) Statistical reconstruction of random point patterns. Comput Stat Data Anal 51:859–871

Vanclay JK (1994) Modelling forest growth and yield. Applications to mixed tropical forests. CABI Publishing, Wallingford, 312 p

Vogt DR, Murrell DJ, Stoll P (2010) Testing spatial theories of plant coexistence: no consistent differences in intra- and interspecific interaction distances. Am Nat 175:73–84

Weiskittel AR, Hann DW, Kerschaw JA, Vanclay JK (2011) Forest growth and yield modeling. Wiley Blackwell, Chichester, 415 p

Wenk G, Antanaitis V, Šmelko Š (1990) Waldertragslehre [Forest growth and yield science]. Deutscher Landwirtschaftsverlag, Berlin, 448 p

Wiegand T, Jeltsch F, Hanski I, Grimm V (2003) Using pattern-oriented modeling for revealing hidden information: a key for reconciling ecological theory and application. Oikos 100:209–222

Wiegand T, Moloney KA (2014) Handbook of spatial point-pattern analysis in ecology. CRC Press, Boca Raton, 538 p

Wu H, Sharpe PJH, Walker J, Penridge LK (1985) Ecological field theory: a spatial analysis of resource interference among plants. Ecol Model 29:215–243

Yeong CLY, Torquato S (1998) Reconstructing random media. Phys Rev E 57:495–506

Zeide B (1993) Analysis of growth equations. Forest Sci 39:594–616

Chapter 6
Principles of Relative Growth Analysis

Abstract The analysis of plant growth is an important interdisciplinary field of plant science and lays the foundation of individual-based research in forest ecology and management. In the past, knowledge about growth processes was a crucial prerequisite for sustainable economic planning in forestry, in this day and age, global environmental changes render growth analysis more important than ever. Marks in point process statistics (Chap. 4) can also represent growth rates for a better characterisation of tree-size dynamics and are dependent variables in individual-based modelling (Sect. 5.2). Particularly the concept of relative growth has proved to be useful in comparative studies of plant growth analysis and for growth reconstruction in dendrochronology, climate change and forest decline research. Studying relative growth rates has become a standard in plant science and is key to the concept of allometry. Relative growth rates are crucial characteristics for assessing growth performance and growth efficiency. The concept of relative growth has independently been developed and pursued in different fields of science and at different locations. In this chapter, we integrated different approaches in one consistent theoretical concept and provided many examples.

6.1 Importance of Growth and Growth Metrics

All living organisms are capable of growth in the sense of irreversible change with time, mainly in size, often in form and occasionally in number (Hunt 1982, p. 5) and growth is a universal and fundamental life process on Earth. In plants, both survival and reproduction depend on plant size and growth rate (Bigler and Bugmann 2003; Shipley 2006; Pommerening and Muszta 2015, 2016).

Growth is a common theme in biology, ecology, forestry and agriculture, yet mathematically the topic has been approached separately using different concepts and notations. Bertalanffy (1951, p. 267) described growth as an increase in size of a living system as a result of assimilation. More generally Jørgensen et al. (2000) defined growth as increase in a measurable quantity, often taken in ecology to be some form of mass or energy, such as population size or biomass. The authors distinguished between three forms of growth, i.e. growth to storage, growth to throughflow and growth to organisation.

In a forest science context, van Laar and Akça (2007, p. 201) pointed out that *growth* is the biological process whilst *increment* is the observed growth of an organism or a population during a given period of time. In production biology and forestry, yield is defined as the harvested or harvestable accumulated increment per unit area (Assmann 1970; van Laar and Akça 2007, p. 1 and p. 201, respectively). The methods presented in this chapter are general and can be applied to a wide range of organisms and biological scales, even to crystals, however, we focus on plant growth in this chapter.

The term plant growth analysis refers to quantitative methods that describe the performance of whole plant systems grown under natural, seminatural or controlled conditions. Plant growth analysis provides an explanatory, holistic and integrative approach to interpreting plant form and function. It uses observed primary data such as weights, areas, volumes and contents of plants or plant components to investigate processes involving the whole plant or a population of plants (Hunt 2003). On the same subject Wenk et al. (1990, p. 20) explained that forest growth and yield research—the corresponding counterpart in forest science—is concerned with the experimental and theoretical exploration of ecological growth patterns of individual trees and forest stands and their use for satisfying needs of human society. This suggests an intimate link between field experiments and models (Pommerening and Muszta 2016).

In the aforementioned areas of plant science, methods of plant growth analysis were developed more or less independently. Boundaries of academic subjects and unhelpful notations have so far prevented to see that many seemingly different approaches in plant growth analysis can indeed be considered as essentially one approach. In production biology, particularly in forest science, the quantification of the outcome of growth processes has been an important pre-requisite for ensuring sustainability and planning business activities. Thus the theoretical foundation of forestry activities through a mathematical description of growth processes has had a high priority. First basic population models, so-called yield tables, were already established towards the end of the 18th century and systematic experiments with a view to monitor and quantify the growth of tree populations exposed to different treatments started towards the end of the 19th century (Assmann 1970, p. 1f.). It did not take long before researchers in this area found that the possibilities for identifying strict growth laws similar to those in physics are limited and that stochastic methods from mathematical statistics are required to identify and to describe growth patterns (Assmann 1970, p. 205).

Hunt (1982, p. 1, 16) referred to the British school of plant growth analysis, which had its origin in the work of F. G. Gregory, V. H. Blackman, G. E. Briggs, R. A. Fisher and colleagues. A detailed history of this school can be found in Evans (1972, p. 190ff.). The methods of this school amount to quantifying the growth of whole plants and populations by means of mathematical-statistical methods and provided a useful framework for ecological, genetical, physiological and agricultural studies. Together with his colleagues F. Fiedler, Do. Gerold, De. Gerold, A. Nicke, K. Preußner, K. Römisch, H. Wätzig and R. Zimmermann at Tharandt/Dresden Technical University in Germany, G. Wenk founded a quantitative plant science school in forestry, starting in the 1970s approximately at the same time as the British school formed at Sheffield and Aberystwyth Universities. The Tharandt school characterised the growth of trees by using the concept of relative plant growth and here particularly the approach of analysing growth functions. Eventually this school developed the population model BEM and the size class model VESO for predicting the growth of trees (Wenk et al. 1990; Wenk 1994). There is also evidence of empirical work on relative tree growth by Soviet researchers (Antanaitis and Zagreev 1969) at the same time, however, a theoretical treatment of the subject seems to be lacking. Another parallel and detailed work on relative tree growth has been carried out in Finland by Kangas (1968), but with fairly limited uptake by the international research community. The work of these research schools is unique, as the concept of relative growth has so far found only few scientific applications in forest science, much in contrast to general plant science.

Studying relative growth rates has found many applications in ecology. Schnute (1981), for example, used the concept for modelling the growth of fish. Bentil et al. (2007) used RGRs for modelling the growth of invasive species and Grime and Hunt (1975) for explaining the adaptivity of local flora. Larocque and Marshall (1993) studied competition effects in trees using relative growth rates.

Modelling growth processes to confirm the results of the analysis and to project future ecological growth patterns has been an important concern of researchers in this field. The mathematical-statistical analysis and modelling of plant growth has started in the middle of the 19th century parallel to the first advances in plant physiology. It was at that time that the first functions describing logistic plant growth were developed and published. One of the oldest growth functions is that by Gompertz (1825), though originally designed for a different purpose. Since then many more functions describing plant growth have been published. For good overviews of growth functions see Hunt (1982), Zeide (1993) and Bolker (2008).

Like other parts of quantitative plant science, the concept of relative plant growth, involving the analysis and modelling of plant growth rate relative to plant size, has been developed independently at different locations more or less at the same time. It has provided valuable insights into the growth patterns of plants and has extensively been used in plant physiology and ecology (Grime and Hunt 1975; Ingestad 1982; Hunt and Cornelissen 1997; Shipley 2006; Houghton et al. 2013). The concept is also closely related to plant mortality and is a pre-requisite for quantifying and modelling allometric relationships in plants. Numerous studies using methods of relative plant growth have been and are still being published and they have also been applied in animal science, for an overview see Shimojo et al. (2002). A particular benefit of studying relative plant growth is the avoidance, as far as possible, of the inherent differences in scale between contrasting organisms so that their performances may be compared on an equitable basis (Hunt 1990, p. 6). As such relative growth rate is

a standardised measure of productive capacity of a plant and allows the comparison
of plants that differ in initial size, age or environmental conditions (Larocque and
Marshall 1993; Pommerening and Muszta 2016).

6.2   Concept of Relative Growth

6.2.1   Definition of Growth Processes

Let $y(t)$ denote the state of a plant characteristic at time t, e.g. the weight, area,
volume or biomass of a plant. This is modelled by a strictly increasing continuously
differentiable real-valued function, $F(t)$ (Eq. 6.1), defined on the interval $[0, \infty)$.
This function has at least one inflection point and possesses an upper horizontal
asymptote:

$$y = F(t) \text{ with } 0 \le t < \infty \tag{6.1}$$

Function $F(t)$ represents cumulative growth, e.g. the total biomass attained by a
plant at any particular age (Assmann 1970, p. 41), see Fig. 6.1.

The first derivative of growth function $F(t)$ is referred to as instantaneous absolute growth (AGR) or—to draw an analogy to mechanics—*growth velocity* (Wenk
1978; Hunt 1982, p. 16). In forest science, this is often referred to as *current annual
increment, CAI*:

$$y'(t) \equiv \frac{dy}{dt} = f(t) \tag{6.2}$$

Since function $f(t)$ is the derivative of function $F(t)$, it is positive and continuous.
Positivity follows from the fact that the growth function $F(t)$ is strictly increasing
(see Fig. 6.1), and $f(t)$ is continuous because growth function $F(t)$ is continuously
differentiable. Growth function $F(t)$ is selected so that its rate of growth, $f(t)$,
displays a sharp increase, followed by a rapid decrease and eventually there is a
slow tapering-off. As a result $f(t)$ has an asymmetric shape. The maximum value
of function $f(t)$ corresponds to the inflection point of function $F(t)$. The value of
$f(t)$ is close to zero, when t is a very small or a very large number, corresponding
to the horizontal asymptotes of $F(t)$ (Pommerening and Muszta 2016).

Absolute growth rate depends on the current state of the plant size characteristic
and is therefore not helpful to growth analysts when comparing plants of different
sizes (Causton and Venus 1981, p. 17). In such situations, relative growth, p, is often
studied in addition to absolute growth.

Relative growth velocity or instantaneous relative growth rate (RGR; in forest
science termed relative increment) is also a function of time and is defined
as the increase in size relative to the growth characteristic (Pommerening and
Muszta 2016).

Fig. 6.1 Relationship between a cumulative growth, an absolute instantaneous and a relative growth rate function. The symbol t_I denotes the time when the inflection point of the growth curve occurs. The symbol t_{max} corresponds with the upper asymptote denoted y_{max}. Modified from Pommerening and Muszta (2016)

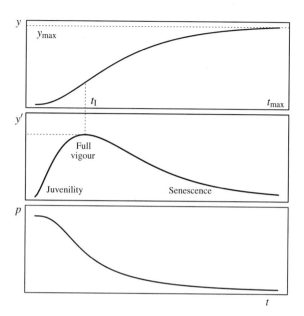

Using the chain rule for differentiation of a complex function, the sequence of equations below shows that relative growth rate is equal to the derivative of log $y(t)$ with respect to time t, see also Fisher (1921), Causton (1977, p. 213) and Kangas (1968, p. 28):

$$\frac{d}{dt} \log y(t) = \frac{d \log y}{dy} \cdot \frac{dy(t)}{dt} = \frac{1}{y(t)} \cdot \frac{dy(t)}{dt} = \frac{y'(t)}{y(t)} = \frac{f(t)}{F(t)} = p(t) \quad (6.3)$$

Studying the relative growth of $y(t)$ is therefore equivalent to studying the absolute growth of $\log y(t)$. The relationship between relative growth and logarithmic size characteristics is an important consideration, which is particularly relevant to allometry as discussed in Sect. 6.2.4.

Instantaneous relative growth rate can initially exhibit very large values or values around 1 (if early growth before the inflection point is exponential) and typically decreases with increasing time. The curve of relative growth rate declines throughout growth in a "reverse sigmoid" manner (Causton 1977, p. 207): In the first years function p decreases slowly, then more rapidly followed by a slow decrease towards senescence (see Fig. 6.1). Shortly before death, RGR is close to zero, which makes this characteristic interesting for mortality studies (see Sect. 5.2.6). For causing this decrease a combination of factors have been suggested, including an accumulation of non-photosynthetic biomass in the form of stems and roots, self-shading of leaves and decreases in local concentrations of soil nutrients (Paine et al. 2012; Philipson et al. 2012).

Hunt (1982, p. 16) motivated relative growth by an example of two plants that achieved the same absolute growth rate but had different initial sizes. In this example, he concluded that a measure of growth is needed, which takes this original difference in size into account. In a similar way, Murphy and Pommerening (2010) explained that modelling relative growth rate is an analysis where the influence of the growth variable is excluded. Wenk et al. (1990, p. 78) also stated that relative growth is an expression of "growth energy" and Causton (1977, p. 197) asserted that relative growth rate is a measure of the efficiency of plant material to produce new material and that it is a crucial physiological characteristic. Since RGR varies widely between species, Houghton et al. (2013) concluded that relative growth rate is a useful metric for separating species into functional groups and in ecological theory. As such RGR has become a central parameter determining a species' growth strategy (Grime 1977). The authors also provided a meta-analysis on the common finding that herbaceous plants have higher relative growth rates than woody plants.

We can continue the analogy to mechanics by defining *growth acceleration*, i.e. the rate of change of the rate of change, as the second derivative of the growth function $F(t)$ (Schnute 1981; Shimojo et al. 2002):

$$y''(t) = f'(t) = \frac{d^2 y}{dt^2} \tag{6.4}$$

Similar to mechanics, growth acceleration is the change in growth velocity or growth rate divided by time taken. The concept of *relative growth acceleration* can then be defined as in Eq. (6.5), see also Schnute (1981) and Zeide (1993):

$$z(t) = \frac{y''(t)}{y'(t)} = \frac{d^2 y}{dt^2} \frac{1}{y'(t)} \tag{6.5}$$

Shimojo et al. (2002) could also show that the following relations hold linking relative growth acceleration, $z(t)$, relative growth rate (RGR), $f(t)/F(t)$, absolute growth rate (AGR), $f(t)$, and absolute growth, $F(t)$:

$$\frac{f(t)}{F(t)} = \frac{y''(t)}{y'(t)} = z(t) = p(t) \tag{6.6}$$

However, according to our calculations Eq. (6.5) is only satisfied, if $F(t)$ is an exponential function, see Pommerening and Muszta (2016, Appendix 2). In later work, Shimojo (2006) even went a step further and defined the concept of *growth jerk*, i.e. the derivative of growth acceleration with respect to time.

Growth velocity and growth acceleration are of theoretical importance and not measurable. In a practical research context, plants are measured at discrete points in time. In this context, Hunt (1982, 1990, p. 10f. and p. 8, respectively) distinguished between functional and classical approaches of plant growth analysis drawing on previous work by Causton. In the analysis based on growth functions, time-series or any kind of repeated surveys provide data for curve fitting: Characteristics like instantaneous growth rates are then calculated from the fitted functions and not directly from the observed data (Hunt 1982, p. 15). In the classical approach, time-series data including a number of survey periods are analysed using *mean growth rates* (or *mean periodic increments* in forest science) as introduced in the next section. Differences in sample size between the two analysis approaches may apply but otherwise they are not mutually exclusive (Pommerening and Muszta 2016).

6.2.2 Absolute Growth Rate

As instantaneous growth rates cannot be measured in practice, the difference between growth characteristics of interest is usually studied at discrete points in time, $t_1, t_2, \ldots, t_n$, which for example are scheduled survey years. In this context the period between two discrete points in time is denoted $\Delta t = t_k - t_{k-1}$ with $k = 2, \ldots, n$. For ease of notation in the remainder of this section we set $y(t_k) = y_k$ and $p(t_k) = p_k$ etc. and assume equidistant time periods. However, the notation can also be modified to accommodate unequal time periods.

> *Mean periodic increment* or *mean absolute growth rate*, in the context of discrete growth data, is the difference in the value of a particular plant characteristic y at different times t_k and t_{k-1} divided by Δt.

This can be written as

$$\bar{i}_k = \frac{y_k - y_{k-1}}{t_k - t_{k-1}} = \left(\frac{\Delta y}{\Delta t} \right)_k . \tag{6.7}$$

Since growth function $F(t)$ is differentiable, this difference quotient is proportional to derivative $F'(t)$. Indeed, $\bar{i}_k = F'(s)$ where s denotes a point in time located somewhere between times t_k and $t_k - 1$. The exact location of s is unknown, but as the difference in time, Δt, grows smaller, point s will be close to t_k and the continuity of $F'(t)$ implies that $F'(s)$ will be close to $F'(t_k)$. Thus considering a short time period, the mean absolute growth rate, $\bar{i}_k$, is approximately equal to the instantaneous growth rate $F'(t_k)$.

When the mean absolute growth rate is positive, this indicates that during the short time period Δt the plant size characteristic grows. When $\bar{i}_k = 0$, this is an indication that the plant size characteristic does not change during the short time period. Also, when $\bar{i}_k < 0$ the plant size characteristic appears to shrink or even decays in that period (Pommerening and Muszta 2016).

In the remainder of this chapter, for ease of reading and understanding equations we consider absolute growth rate with reference to annual time steps where $t_k -$

$t_{k-1} = 1$. Thus, absolute growth rate, $\bar{i}_k$, simplifies to

$$i_k = y_k - y_{k-1}. \tag{6.8}$$

However, should $t_k - t_{k-1} \neq 1$, it is important to give the time difference due consideration. Absolute growth rates of trees have been studied much in forest science, see for example Assmann (1970) and Pretzsch (2009).

6.2.3 Relative Growth Rate

According to Blackman (1919), Fisher (1921), Whitehead and Myerscough (1962) and Hunt (1982, 1990), *mean periodic relative increment* or *mean relative growth rate*, $\overline{p}_k$, is the difference of the logarithms of y_k and y_{k-1} divided by Δt, see also Causton (1977, p. 213):

$$\overline{p}_k = \frac{\log\ y_k - \log\ y_{k-1}}{t_k - t_{k-1}} = \frac{\log(y_k/y_{k-1})}{\Delta t} \tag{6.9}$$

The R listing below demonstrates how Eqs. (6.7) and (6.9) can be implemented using tree stem diameter of one tree as an example:

```
> AGR <- NA
> for (i in 2 : length(dbh)) {
+ AGR <- (dbh[i] - dbh[i - 1]) / (surveyYear[i] -
+ surveyYear[i - 1])
+ RGR <- (log(dbh[i]) - log(dbh[i - 1])) / (surveyYear[i] -
+ surveyYear[i - 1])
+ }
```

Since it is recommended to avoid `for` loops in R, the same results can be achieved with the `diff()` function:

```
> AGR <- diff(dbh, lag = 1, differences = 1) /
+ diff(surveyYear, lag = 1, differences = 1)
> RGR <- diff(log(dbh), lag = 1, differences = 1) /
+ diff(surveyYear, lag = 1, differences = 1)
```

The setting `lag = 1` tells function `diff()` that we are interested in successive differences and `differences = 1` ensures that the function is only executed once.

Fisher (1921) defined mean relative growth rate as amount of change per unit area of material per unit area of time. Blackman (1919) originally referred to Eq. (6.9) as "efficiency index" and "specific growth rate", see also Causton and Venus (1981, p. 37). From the last term in Eq. (6.9) we can see that mean RGR can be interpreted as the logarithm of the ratio of successive size measurements divided by the corresponding time interval. Mean growth rate is thought to reflect systematic variation

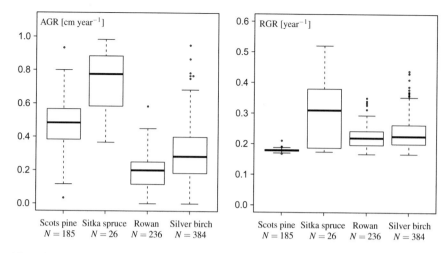

Fig. 6.2 A comparison of absolute and relative growth rates of four species in a mixed-species woodland at Pen yr Allt Ganol in Gwydyr Forest (North Wales, UK). Modified from Pommerening and Muszta (2016)

in physiology, allocation and leaf construction (Houghton et al. 2013). Quantifying RGR is a method for measuring and comparing plant growth potential reflecting intrinsic growth physiology (Turnbull et al. 2008) and $\overline{p}_k$ is the most common RGR characteristic used in the literature.

Pommerening and Muszta (2016) analysed absolute growth rates (AGR) and relative growth rates (RGR) in a mixed-species woodland in North Wales. This is a very common and traditional application of the concept of relative plant growth (Fig. 6.2). The growth rates in this example are based on surveys made in 2002 and 2007. Scots pine (*Pinus sylvestris* L.) and Sitka spruce (*Picea sitchensis* (BONG.) CARR.) were dominant species that form the main forest canopy, whilst rowan (*Sorbus aucuparia* L.) and silver birch (*Betula pendula* ROTH.) were species of understorey regeneration. Sitka spruce was also partly present in the understorey. The non-native Scots pine and Sitka spruce trees were originally planted on the site in 1931 and the two native broadleaved species colonised naturally. A growth analysis is interesting here for anticipating the future species composition in this woodland.

Over- and understorey species understandably showed very different tree sizes, which suggest the use of RGR for better comparison. As expected the two main-canopy species Scots pine and Sitka spruce have markedly higher absolute growth rates than the understorey species (Fig. 6.2, left). This confirms Causton's and Venus' (1981, p. 17) statement that absolute growth rate is often roughly proportional to plant size. Relative growth rate, however, gives a different impression and reveals that Sitka spruce had the highest mean relative growth rate of all species followed by rowan and silver birch. Scots pine—although a dominant main-canopy species—apparently had the lowest relative growth rate. It is therefore likely that the next forest generation at

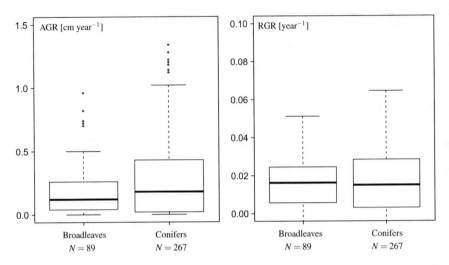

Fig. 6.3 Absolute and relative growth rates of broadleaves and conifers in a mixed-species wood-land at Coed y Brenin (plot 7) in North Wales (UK), see Fig. 4.37. The broadleaves include birch (*Betula spp.*), oak (*Quercus spp.*), rowan (*Sorbus aucuparia* L.), sycamore (*Acer pseudoplatanus* L.) and willow *Salix spp.* The conifers are Douglas fir (*Pseudotsuga menziesii* (MIRB.) FRANCO), Japanese larch (*Larix kaempferi* (LAMB.) CARR.), Scots pine (*Pinus sylvestris* L.) and Sitka spruce (*Picea sitchensis* (BONG.) CARR.)

Pen yr Allt Ganol will include a mix of Sitka spruce and native broadleaves, if left undisturbed by man.

It is also interesting to note that the variation of species-specific growth rates was quite different for AGR and RGR. Growth rate variation was much more variable with RGR and more homogeneous for AGR.

In a similar way, we carried out a growth rate analysis at Coed y Brenin (plot 7). Here the growth rates related to the period 2006–2011 and we were interested in differences between the species/trait groups broadleaves and conifers (Fig. 6.3). Douglas fir (*Pseudotsuga menziesii* (MIRB.) FRANCO) was originally planted in 1985, but struggled and other species subsequently colonised the site. Also here we consid-ered that comparing growth rates may give hints about a possible, future dominance of one group over the other.

All species occurring at Coed y Brenin (plot 7) were approximately of the same age. In contrast to the results in Fig. 6.2 the growth analysis at Coed y Brenin (plot 7) did not reveal any major differences in the distribution of growth rates between the two species/trait groups. Considering median growth rates, conifers had a slightly higher AGR than broadleaves whilst the latter showed slightly higher RGR compared to the former, but these differences were marginal. The growth rates of the conifers varied more than those of the broadleaves in this woodland. However, it appears that both species/trait groups had equal chances as far as their growth rates were concerned.

Larocque and Marshall (1993) reviewed and investigated the relationship between RGR and competition in red pine (*Pinus resinosa* AIT.) stands in Canada. In this study, RGR decreased with increasing tree size before the onset of competition and when competition was not severe. Under severe competitive stress RGR increased with tree size. They concluded that small trees were more efficient than large trees at producing new biomass before the onset of competition. Competition reduced the efficiency of small trees relative to large trees.

Again, for ease of reading and understanding equations we consider annual growth rates only where $\Delta t = 1$ in the remainder of this section. Thus, relative growth rate, $\overline{p}_k$, simplifies to

$$p_k = \log y_k - \log y_{k-1} = \log(y_k/y_{k-1}). \tag{6.10}$$

Also here it should be emphasised that cases of $\Delta t \neq 1$ (in whatever unit time is measured in a given study) need to be given full consideration, e.g. by computing mean annual RGR as in Eq. (6.9).

Independently of Blackman and Hunt, Wenk (1978) and other authors from forest science defined relative growth rate more directly and intuitively as absolute growth rate divided by the plant size characteristic. Apparently this approach has a long tradition in forest science, going back to authors like Hartig, Koenig, Schneider, Pressler and Breymann in the 18th and 19th centuries (Prodan 1965, p. 433). Since we consider discrete points in time, the plant size characteristic in the denominator can now refer to the beginning, y_{k-1}, or to the end, y_k, of the survey period leading to upper (+) and lower (−) bounds. Equation (6.10) elegantly avoids this problem and relates to an unknown point in time between k and $k-1$ (Pommerening and Muszta 2016). This unknown point in time is near the centre between k and $k-1$, as a comparison with Pressler's increment formula reveals (see Fig. 6.4). In forest science, Pressler (1865) simply assuming a linear increase of y suggested the formula

$$p_k^0 = 2\frac{y_k - y_{k-1}}{y_k + y_{k-1}}, \tag{6.11}$$

thus dividing AGR by the mean of y_k and y_{k-1}, which was also proposed by Fisher (1921) without reference to Pressler (1865). Müller (1915) also mentioned the use of the geometric mean in the denominator and there are even more variants of calculating relative growth rates, however, all of them differ from p_k. Using upper and lower bounds leads to equations

$$p_k^+ = \frac{y_k - y_{k-1}}{y_{k-1}} \quad \text{and} \tag{6.12}$$

$$p_k^- = \frac{y_k - y_{k-1}}{y_k}. \tag{6.13}$$

Wenk et al. (1990, p. 78) argued for the use of Eq. (6.13) in the research work of his school, as y_{k-1} can take very small values near zero. Also, experimentally only past growth can be measured and the current size characteristic y_k is naturally always related to the end of that growth period. Other authors familiar with growth rates in economics preferred Eq. (6.13) and in fact p_k, p_k^+ and p_k^- can be easily converted to one another according to Eq. (6.14):

$$p_k^+ = \frac{p_k^-}{1 - p_k^-}; \quad p_k^- = \frac{p_k^+}{1 + p_k^+}; \quad p_k^+ = e^{p_k} - 1; \quad p_k^- = 1 - \frac{1}{e^{p_k}} \qquad (6.14)$$

Other important relationships following from Eq. (6.14) include $p_k = \log(1 + p_k^+)$ and $p_k = -\log(1 - p_k^-)$.

In the context of production biology such as forestry, it is important to note that p_k^+ multiplied by age is equal to 1, when the mean annual increment (MAI) culminates. MAI is the temporal mean of a growth function, i.e. $y(t)/t$. In the point where $p(t)$ multiplied by t (where t is age) is equal to 1, (CAI) is equal to MAI. If $p(t) < 1/t$ then MAI has already culminated, if $p(t) > 1/t$ MAI has not yet culminated (Prodan 1965, p. 434f.).

Pommerening and Muszta (2016) illustrated the relationships between p_k, p_k^0, p_k^+ and p_k^- using stem analysis data (Fig. 6.4). For small values of relative growth rate all three definitions lead to almost the same results whilst increasingly larger deviations from p_k can be observed with increasing relative growth rate, whereby p_k^+ and p_k^- form the upper and lower bounds as previously discussed. Since the underlying growth function $F(t)$ is increasing, $y_{k-1} < 0.5(y_k + y_{k-1}) < y_k$ implies $p_k^- < p_k < p_k^+$, which is confirmed in Fig. 6.4. Pressler's relative growth rate apparently is an acceptable approximation of p_k for small RGR.

Absolute growth rate can be calculated from RGR as the product of plant characteristic and relative growth rate:

$$i_k = y_{k-1}e^{p_k} - y_{k-1} = y_{k-1}p_k^+ = y_k p_k^- \qquad (6.15)$$

For projecting growth the concept of the *growth multiplier*, also referred to as *growth factor* and *growth coefficient*, has proved useful (Wenk 1972; Kangas 1968; Evans 1972; Hunt 1982). The idea of the growth multiplier is to calculate a current size characteristic from a past size characteristic in a multiplicative way:

$$y_k = y_{k-1}\frac{y_k}{y_{k-1}} = y_{k-1}M_k, \qquad (6.16)$$

where factor M_k is the growth multiplier.

The growth multiplier is a function of relative growth rate and defined as the ratio of a particular plant size characteristic at different times (Wenk 1972).

Fig. 6.4 A comparison of the relative growth rates p_k, p_k^0, p_k^+ and p_k^- using the annual stem analysis data (volume growth) of Sitka spruce (*Picea sitchensis* (BONG.) CARR.) tree no. 4000 at Cefn Du (plot 1), Clocaenog Forest (North Wales, UK). Modified from Pommerening and Muszta (2016)

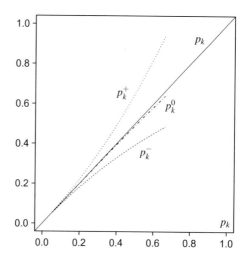

Naturally Eq. (6.16) implies that the growth multiplier also allows backcasting growth, i.e. calculating the value of a previous growth characteristic from its present value through $y_{k-1} = y_k/M_k$.

The use of M_k leads to an integrated form of the relative growth rate (West et al. 1920; Wenk 1978). Growth multipliers therefore offer an alternative to integrating functions of relative growth rate (Wenk 1972). Part of the importance of M_k stems from the fact that the growth multiplier plays a crucial role in predicting future growth based on relative growth rates through a recursive use of $y_k = y_{k-1}M_k$ (Pommerening and Muszta 2015).

Circumstances where $M_k > 1$ indicate growth, the condition $M_k = 1$ occurs where there is no growth and with $M_k < 1$ the corresponding plant size characteristic shrinks or even decays.

Depending on how relative growth rate is defined, M_k can be calculated in one of the following ways:

$$M_k = e^{p_k} = 1 + p_k^+ = \frac{1}{1 - p_k^-} \tag{6.17}$$

Note that M_k always remains the same metric regardless of the RGR definition used. From Eq. (6.17) follow the important relationships $p_k = \log M_k$, $p_k^+ = M_k - 1$ and $p_k^- = 1 - 1/M_k$.

Evans (1972, p. 197) and Hunt (1982, p. 17) referred to the growth multiplier as Backmans efficiency index, which is supposed "to represent the efficiency of the plant as a producer of new material, and to give a measure of the plant's economy in working". Obviously growth multipliers as functions of relative growth rate offer another possibility of relating different approaches to quantifying relative growth to one another.

Relative growth rates can be multiplicatively aggregated over several years or otherwise defined growth periods. The aggregation is achieved by multiplying the growth multipliers of the n observed growth periods. Wenk et al. (1990, p. 100) referred to this cumulative measure as the *generalised growth multiplier* $M^{(n)}$. The calculation of the generalised growth multiplier from relative growth rates again depends on the definition of RGR:

$$M^{(n)} = e^{p_1 + p_2 + \cdots + p_n} = e^{\sum_{k=1}^{n} p_k} \tag{6.18}$$

$$M^{(n)} = (1 + p_1^+) \cdot (1 + p_2^+) \cdot \ldots \cdot (1 + p_n^+) = \prod_{k=1}^{n} (1 + p_k^+) \tag{6.19}$$

$$M^{(n)} = \frac{1}{(1 - p_1^-) \cdot (1 - p_2^-) \cdot \ldots \cdot (1 - p_n^-)} = \frac{1}{\prod_{k=1}^{n} (1 - p_k^-)} \tag{6.20}$$

As with M_k note that $M^{(n)}$ are identical in all three equations. Average relative growth rates from empirical time series data over a number of growth periods can be obtained by applying the *geometric* rather than the arithmetic mean to generalised growth multipliers based on the relationships in Eq. (6.17):

$$\widetilde{p}_k = \log(\sqrt[n]{M^{(n)}}) \tag{6.21}$$

$$\widetilde{p}_k^+ = \sqrt[n]{M^{(n)}} - 1 \tag{6.22}$$

$$\widetilde{p}_k^- = 1 - \frac{1}{\sqrt[n]{M^{(n)}}} \tag{6.23}$$

Finally, in analogy to relative growth rate, growth acceleration can be calculated from empirical data in the following ways:

$$z_k^+ = \frac{\Delta p}{p_{k-1}^{\cdot\cdot}}; \quad z_k^- = \frac{\Delta p}{p_k^{\cdot\cdot}}; \quad z_k = \log p_k^{\cdot\cdot} - \log p_{k-1}^{\cdot\cdot}, \tag{6.24}$$

where the upper index ".." can denote either "+", "−" or " ".

6.2.4 Multiple RGR and the Concept of Allometry

Often more than one RGR of the same plant is measured. In that case it is interesting to study the relationship between two RGR of the same organism. To illustrate the problem, Sloboda (pers. comm., Fig. 6.5) for example suggested defining a matrix for projecting the growth of total tree height (h) and stem diameter (d) in a single equation. The matrix includes the growth multipliers relating to both size variables, i.e.

$$\begin{bmatrix} h_k \\ d_k \end{bmatrix} = \begin{bmatrix} M_{h,k} & 0 \\ 0 & M_{d,k} \end{bmatrix} \begin{bmatrix} h_{k-1} \\ d_{k-1} \end{bmatrix} = \begin{bmatrix} M_{h,k}\, h_{k-1} \\ M_{d,k}\, d_{t-1} \end{bmatrix}. \tag{6.25}$$

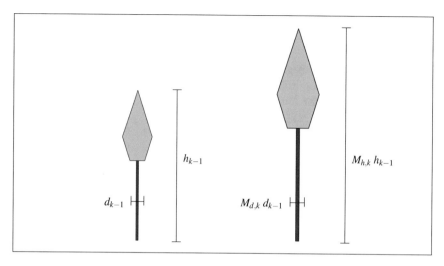

Fig. 6.5 Illustration of the principle of the Sloboda matrix in Eq. (6.25)

As we know from Eq. (6.17), the growth multipliers $M_{h,k}$ and $M_{d,k}$ are only different forms of RGR. In the matrix approach of Eq. (6.25), the two RGR for total height and stem diameter are thus used separately for projecting height and diameter from $k - 1$ to k through matrix multiplication.

It is now instructive to take a closer look at the relationship between the two RGRs, which in the above example were expressed as $M_{h,k}$ and $M_{d,k}$. This relationship can be quantified through the concept of *allometry*, also referred to as *biological scaling* or *allometric scaling*. Allometry originally described the scaling relationships between body size and metabolic rates. The concept has been expanded to include morphological (e.g. lifespan, heart rate and body length, body mass), physiological (e.g. metabolic rates, growth rates and body size) and ecological traits (e.g. growth rates of plants and seed size, animal territories and body size) (Mosimann 1970; West and Brown 2005).

As a biological concept allometry is part of the field of relative growth (Gayon 2000). In any organism, there are relationships between different size characteristics of an organism and also between one of these dimensional elements and the whole organism.

According to Huxley (1932) and Teissier (1934) an allometric relationship between two plant size characteristics, say $x(t)$ and $y(t)$, can be expressed in the form

$$\frac{dy}{dt}\frac{1}{y(t)} = \left(\frac{dx}{dt}\frac{1}{x(t)}\right)m(t). \tag{6.26}$$

This equation relates changes in $\log y(t)$ to changes in $\log x(t)$. Specifically it states that $\log y(t)$ changes proportionally with $\log x(t)$ over short time periods, assuming that $m(t)$ is constant. The function $m(t)$ mediating the changes is often referred to as the *allometric coefficient* (or *exponent*).

Allometric coefficients are key biological characteristics that describe the way in which resources are allocated to different parts of a plant (Gayon 2000): An increase of $x(t)$ by 1% corresponds to an increase by $m(t)$ percent in $y(t)$. Allometric coefficients can be interpreted as compounded growth rates, i.e. as rates of change involving more than one plant size characteristic (Hunt 1990, p. 15). The better known integrated representation of the allometric equation is

$$y(t) = b\, x(t)^{m(t)}, \tag{6.27}$$

where b is a model parameter. Note that Eq. (6.27) is a consequence of Eq. 6.26 only, if the allometric coefficient is constant for all times t. Empirical research has provided evidence that $m(t)$, however, is rarely constant. In that case the model parameter b turns into a complicated function $b(t)$. Gayon (2000) provided an extensive discussion of the biological meaning of model parameter b.

The condition $m(t) = 1$ indicates *isometric* growth, i.e. both tree characteristics change at the same rate and as a consequence the original properties between two size characteristics $x(t)$ and $y(t)$ remain unchanged. If $m(t) > 1$, there is a *positive* or *progressive* allometric relationship implying that $y(t)$ changes faster than $x(t)$, which leads to a change of proportions between $x(t)$ and $y(t)$. If $m(t) < 1$, there is a *negative* or *degressive* allometric relationship, i.e. $x(t)$ changes faster than $y(t)$. Abruptly changing trends of allometric relationships often point to environmental conditions that have changed, where as a consequence a tree suddenly allocated more biomass to one part of its organism at the expense of another. Therefore studying allometric relationships is of particular interest in the context of plant interaction (Pommerening and Muszta 2016).

Based on Eqs. (6.14) and (6.17) the relative growth rates of size characteristics x and y in the case of discrete points in time are related as

$$m_k = \frac{p_{x,k}}{p_{y,k}} = \frac{\log(1 + p_{x,k}^+)}{\log(1 + p_{y,k}^+)} = \frac{\log(1 - p_{x,k}^-)}{\log(1 - p_{y,k}^-)}. \tag{6.28}$$

Here m_k is an approximation of $m(t)$. Equation (6.28) shows that the use of p_k (Eq. 6.9) leads to a simpler expression of the allometric relationship based on relative growth rates. Also, the interpretation of m_k is made easier by the ratio $p_{x,k}/p_{y,k}$: Values of $m_k < 1$ imply $p_{y,k} > p_{x,k}$ while $m_k > 1$ is caused by $p_{x,k} > p_{y,k}$ whatever size variables are used for x and y.

In the following listing, RGR is calculated from stem-analysis data with annual measurements relating to only one tree separately for stem diameter (lines 3–7) and total height (lines 9–13) using Eq. (6.28). The allometric coefficient m_k is calculated in lines 15–17, here the results for m, mplus and mminus should be the same.

```
1  > for (i in 2 : length(myData$age)) {
2  +   # Stem diameter dbh
3  +   myData$pd[i] <- (log(myData$d[i]) - log(myData$d[i - 1]))
4  +   myData$pdplus[i] <- (myData$d[i] - myData$d[i - 1]) /
5  +     myData$d[i - 1]
6  +   myData$pdminus[i] <- (myData$d[i] - myData$d[i - 1]) /
7  +     myData$d[i]
8  +   # Total height
9  +   myData$ph[i] <- (log(myData$h[i]) - log(myData$h[i - 1]))
10 +   myData$phplus[i] <- (myData$h[i] - myData$h[i - 1]) /
11 +     myData$h[i - 1]
12 +   myData$phminus[i] <- (myData$h[i] - myData$h[i - 1]) /
13 +     myData$h[i]
14 + }
15 >  m <- myData$pd / myData$ph
16 >  mplus <- log(1 + myData$pdplus) / log(1 + myData$phplus)
17 >  mminus <- log(1 - myData$pdminus) / log(1 - myData$phminus)
```

Using function diff() the three different RGR measures can alternatively be computed as:

```
> myData$pd <- diff(log(myData$pd), lag = 1, differences = 1)
>
> myData$pdplus <- diff(myData$dbh, lag = 1,
+ differences = 1) / myData$dbh[1 : (length(myData$dbh) - 1)]
>
> myData$pdminus <- diff(myData$dbh, lag = 1,
+ differences = 1) / myData$dbh[2 : length(myData$dbh)]
```

The relationships in Eq. (6.28) allow the modelling of an unknown RGR, $p_{y,k}$, of a plant size characteristic based on the knowledge of RGR, $p_{x,k}$, of another characteristic of the same plant and known m_k, e.g. $p_{y,k} = p_{x,k}/m_k$. Analysing the change of allometric coefficient over time gives valuable clues for understanding changing environmental conditions of a tree during its life time (Fig. 6.6, left).

For example the trend curve of the allometric coefficient in Fig. 6.6 reveals a global minimum at approximately 25 years and a global maximum to be expected at around 70 years. Between 15 and 40 years there is a trend of negative allometry between total tree height and stem diameter, i.e. height developed faster than diameter. Diameter growth, however, finally caught up with height growth at an age of approximately 40 years. After 25 years of age (the point of fastest height growth), diameter growth gained over height growth and gradually changed the relationship back to positive allometry.

The trend of increasing positive allometry and thus strong stem-diameter growth continued in a sigmoid fashion until the end of the lifetime of tree no. 486. Allometric patterns can markedly vary even among trees of the same forest stand and depend on genetic and environmental factors as well as on competition.

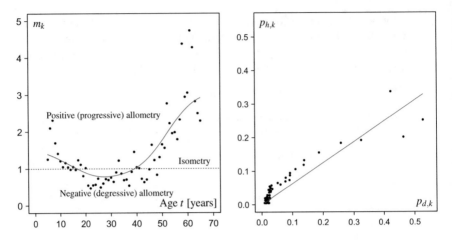

Fig. 6.6 Left: Annual allometric coefficient, m_k, in terms of height (y) and diameter (x) of Sitka spruce (*Picea sitchensis* (BONG.) CARR.) tree no. 486 in Gwydyr Forest (Pen yr Allt Ganol) over age. For the trend curve non-parametric regression involving a Gaussian kernel and a bandwidth $h = 20$ years was used. Right: RGR of total tree height ($p_{h,k}$) over RGR of stem diameter ($p_{d,k}$) for the same tree based on Eq. (6.10) for estimating the mean allometric coefficient. The intercept was set to zero

The R listing below explains how to compute the non-parametric trend curve in lines 1f. and how to add it to the scatterplot in lines 7f. The index value of -1 in line 1 excludes the first observation where no growth is available. m[] denotes the allometric coefficient as in Eq. 6.28.

```
1  > trend <- ksmooth(tdata$age[-1], m[-1], kernel = "normal",
2  + bandwidth = 20)
3  > par(mar = c(2, 2, 0.5, 0.5))
4  > plot(tdata$age[-1], m[-1], las = 1, ylab = "", xlab = "",
5  + cex = .9, col = "black", pch = 19, axes = FALSE,
6  + ylim = c(0, 5), xlim = c(0, 70))
7  > lines(trend, xlab = "", ylab = "", main = "", las = 1,
8  + lty = 1, lwd = 2, col = "red")
9  > abline(h = 1, lty = 2)
10 > axis(1, lwd = 2, cex.axis = 1.8)
11 > axis(2, las = 1, lwd = 2, cex.axis = 1.8)
12 > box(lwd = 2)
```

In many applications it may also be useful to estimate a mean allometric coefficient as a summary characteristic for the whole life or observation time of a tree. One way to achieve this is by linear regression (Fig. 6.6, right).

We return to example using tree no. 486 and the allometric relationship between height and diameter growth is again assumed to be of interest. The corresponding RGRs are used and setting the intercept to zero yields a slope parameter that gives a conservative estimate of the mean allometric coefficient (see the code listing below). In this case $m_k = 0.62$, which is close to $2/3$, the theoretical allometric coefficient for the relationship between tree total height and stem diameter (Pretzsch 2010; Niklas and Spatz 2012):

```
lm.1 <- lm(ph ~ 0 + pd, data = tdata)
Call:
lm(formula = ph ~ 0 + pd, data = tdata)

Residuals:
Min 1Q Median 3Q Max
-0.087672594590 -0.001094961227 0.010882742638 0.025379870218
    0.073967664858

Coefficients:
Estimate Std. Error t value Pr(>|t|)
pd 0.621647731810 0.026704611179 23.27867 < 2.22e-16 ***
---
Signif. codes: 0 '***' 0.001 '**' 0.01 '*' 0.05 '.' 0.1 ' ' 1

Residual standard error: 0.026590317603 on 60 degrees of
    freedom
(1 observation deleted due to missingness)
Multiple R-squared: 0.90031505491, Adjusted R-squared:
    0.89865363916
F-statistic: 541.89630384 on 1 and 60 DF, p-value: <
    2.22044605e-16
```

By contrast, the arithmetic mean is $\overline{m}_k = 1.44$ and the geometric mean is $\widetilde{m}_k = 1.21$. From a theoretical point of view, again the geometric mean should be more appropriate than the arithmetic mean. For example volume RGR of trees, $p_{v,k}^+$, can be estimated from diameter and height growth multipliers using the term $M_{h,k}\, M_{d,k}^{\widetilde{m}_k} - 1$ (Sloboda, pers. comm.). According to Eq. (6.14) $p_{v,k}^+$ can then be transformed to $p_{v,k} = \log(1 + p_{v,k}^+)$.

The *allometric partitioning theory* assumes general, invariant allometric relationships between tree characteristics (Enquist and Niklas 2001) whilst the *optimal partitioning theory* suggests that plants allocate biomass to the organ that acquires the most limiting resource (McCarthy and Enquist 2007). The latter implies that, for example, tree crowns may laterally expand in an attempt to catch more light when light is scarce. Both theories are supported by much empirical evidence. Pretzsch (2010) pointed out that the two theories do not contradict each other but that under conditions of optimal resource availability allometric coefficients as per the allometric partitioning theory can be expected. However, when environmental conditions are not optimal, the allometric coefficient may differ within a certain allometric corridor.

Combining models of relative growth and allometrics is a natural, alternative choice for modelling plant growth, as these two concepts are closely related. This was clearly in Huxley's mind when he entitled his book about allometry "Problems of relative growth" (Huxley 1932). Following this tradition Wenk et al. (1990) and Wenk (1994) have shown how several characteristics of individual plants and of plant populations can be simultaneously modelled by a combination of relative growth function and allometric coefficients (Pommerening and Muszta 2016).

6.2.5   Functions of Relative Growth Rate

In the analysis of functions, as previously mentioned, observed data are not directly analysed but used for model fitting. Summary characteristics are then calculated from the models. Mean absolute growth rate can for example be simply calculated from a growth function as

$$\frac{F(t) - F(t - \Delta t)}{\Delta t}. \tag{6.29}$$

In analogy, mean relative growth rate in an analysis using growth functions is given by the ratio

$$\frac{F(t) - F(t - \Delta t)}{F(t)\,\Delta t}. \tag{6.30}$$

Hunt (1982) dedicated a whole book to this research strategy and explained that it is a branch of mathematical modelling. The rationale is that a mathematical expression or group of expressions behaves in some way like a real system and can then be referred to as a mathematical model of that system (Hunt 1982, p. 47). In the same way Wenk's research school as documented in his book (Wenk et al. 1990) modelled relative plant growth not only for predicting future yields from stands of trees but also for interpreting the model parameters like statistical characteristics to achieve a deeper understanding of tree growth. This is considered as a model-based plant growth analysis.

Attempts to directly analyse growth observations can sometimes result in a scattered and distorted picture of reality. A mathematical function fitted to those observations may regain much of the clarity with which the reality is perceived by the experimenter (Hunt 1982, p. 53). The fitted function can often be of greater value to the experimenter than the data from which it was derived. Also functional methods give relative growth rates with smaller variances than those yielded by the classical method (Causton and Venus 1981, p. 59). On the other hand, every mathematical model comes with underlying assumptions, which need to be verified when applying the model.

Modelling relative growth rates serves two purposes, 1. an improved analysis of growth performance and efficiency and 2. the prediction/reconstruction of future or past growth rates.

It is always good advice to use mechanistic or semi-mechanistic growth functions where possible. This is particularly important when temporal extrapolations are intended. Polynomials are for example generally a poor choice and lack theoretical foundation (Vanclay 1994, p. 9f.). Growth functions with few model parameters that have a biological meaning and thus can be interpreted are also useful for making quick plausibility checks.

Hunt (1982), Wenk et al. (1990, p. 79) and Zeide (1993) gave a number of plant growth functions and provided detailed discussions. They are often combinations of power functions and exponential functions (Zeide 1989) and are special cases of a general form (Pommerening and Muszta 2016).

Table 6.1 Frequently used growth functions and functions of absolute and relative growth rate with model parameters a, b and c, where t denotes time or age. Modified from Pommerening and Muszta (2015)

Function name	Growth function	Absolute growth rate	Relative growth rate
Chapman-Richards	$a(1-e^{-bt})^c$	$abce^{-bt}(1-e^{-bt})^{c-1}$	$bc(1-e^{-bt})^{-1}$
Gompertz	$ae^{-be^{-ct}}$	$abce^{-ct}e^{-be^{-ct}}$	bce^{-ct}
Korf	$ae^{-bt^{-c}}$	$abct^{-c-1}e^{-bt^{-c}}$	$bct^{-(1+c)}$
Logistic	$a(1+ce^{-bt})^{-1}$	$abce^{-bt}(1+ce^{-bt})^{-2}$	$bc(c+e^{bt})^{-1}$
Monomolecular	$a(1-ce^{-bt})$	$abce^{-bt}$	$bc(e^{bt}-c)^{-1}$
Weibull	$a(1-e^{-bt^c})$	$abct^{c-1}e^{-bt^c}$	$bct^{c-1}(e^{bt^c}-1)^{-1}$

An overview of functions of relative growth rate and of asymptotic relative growth rate are given in Table 6.1.

The Chapman-Richards function is a very flexible and accurate growth function published by Richards (1959). It can be interpreted as a generalisation of the Bertalanffy (1957) growth function for animal growth and has frequently been used to model tree and tree population growth (Pienaar and Turnbull 1973).

Gompertz (1825) originally proposed his function for describing age distribution in human populations. Only a century later it was applied as a growth model by Winsor (1932). Interestingly, the corresponding function of relative growth rate is an elementary function of age. It has therefore also been referred to as function of exponential decay (Laird et al. 1965). The Gompertz function is often used in biological studies and Wenk (1969) successfully extended the Gompertz function for modelling relative growth of ten-year survey periods:

$$p^{10}(t) = e^{-c_1 \cdot t'\left(1-e^{-c_2 \cdot t'\left(1-e^{-c_3 \cdot t'}\right)}\right)} \tag{6.31}$$

In function $p^{10}(t)$, the main parameter, c_1, also referred to as *growth parameter*, accounts for the overall shape of the growth curve and has been linked to individual tree vigour and to site quality. The growth parameter largely corresponds to parameter c of the Gompertz function in Table 6.1, particularly in the function's simplified version $p(t) = e^{-c \cdot t}$ (Wenk et al. 1990, p. 80). Murphy and Pommerening (2010) could re-confirm that model parameter c_2 is also related to environmental factors, particularly to latitude, soil moisture and soil nutrient regime. Function $p^{10}(t)$ can be considered to be a mathematical expression of the "growth energy" of a tree and is interpreted as a summary characteristic. At stand level, and in the absence of systematic changes in environmental conditions, the growth parameter has proved to be constant through time for many tree species and in such situations c_1 equals stem volume RGR at the time of culmination of the current annual increment (Wenk 1978). The growth parameter is negatively correlated with stem volume RGR and for individual trees, on any given site, it has been shown that small values of c_1 imply

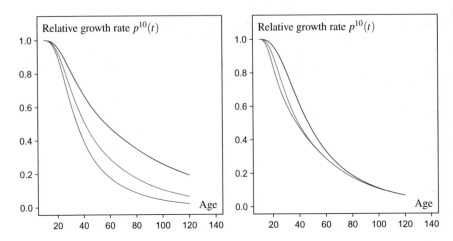

Fig. 6.7   RGR over age based of the modified Gompertz function $p^{10}(t)$ (Wenk 1969, Eq. 6.31). The model parameters used were: Left: $c_1 = 0.15$ (black), $c_1 = 0.25$ (red), $c_1 = 0.35$ (blue), $c_2 = 1.0$. Right: $c_1 = 0.25$, $c_2 = 0.5$ (black), $c_2 = 1.5$ (red), $c_2 = 3.5$ (blue). Model parameter c_3 was set to $c_3 = 0.40$ for all curves. Age was recorded in years

increased tree vigour. Smaller, more suppressed trees have lower RGR and therefore higher c_1 values (Wenk et al. 1990, see Fig. 6.7, left). Light demanding and fast growing species tend to have larger c_1 values than shade tolerant and slow growing species. The effect of the growth parameter is modified in the early years of growth by parameters c_2 and c_3. Large values of c_2 indicate stagnating juvenile growth. With most European tree species this effect lasts only for 40–60 years depending on parameter values (Murphy and Pommerening 2010, see Fig. 6.7, right). For trees beyond that age function $p^{10}(t)$ converges towards $e^{-c_1 \cdot t'}$. Parameters c_1, c_2 and c_3 are always positive and based on empirical studies the latter can, in the majority of cases, be set to a constant value of 0.4 for a wide range of intermediate to shade tolerant species and to a constant value of 1.0 for light demanding species. Absolute age of the tree or stand is transformed according to $t' = (\text{age} - 10)/10$ (Wenk et al. 1990), whilst for tropical species values of 2 and 3 have been suggested instead of 10. The function is extremely flexible whilst remaining relatively parameter parsimonious and therefore ensures good statistical fit and extrapolation capabilities (Wenk et al. 1990, see Fig. 6.7). Gerold and Römisch (1977) proposed a method for converting ten-year RGR, as estimated by function $p^{10}(t)$, to annual RGR, which is required when fitting the function, see Murphy and Pommerening (2010) for details. For Sitka spruce (*Picea sitchensis* (BONG.) CARR.) in Wales (UK) Murphy and Pommerening (2010) found c_1 values between 0.15 and 0.35 and c_2 values between 0.50 and 3.5 based on stem analyses.

Korf proposed his growth function in 1939 and it has been rediscovered by Lundqvist (1957). The Korf function has been applied to the growth of various tree characteristics (Zeide 1993) and Zeide (1989) referred to this function as a power decline function because asymptotic relative growth can be presented as an elementary power function.

The logistic growth function (Verhulst 1838), according to Causton (1977, p. 198) and Hunt (1982, p. 126) also known as autocatalytic function, has been a famous model in ecology. Unfortunately it lacks both theoretical foundation and accuracy (Zeide 1993), but still is often in use.

Originally developed in physical chemistry, the monomolecular growth function is also known as Mitscherlich function after a German agronomist who used it at the beginning of last century. Zeide (1993) also referred to an early use by Weber (1891). The monomolecular function is one of the simplest of asymptotic functions and has no inflection point; hence its biological plausibility is rather limited.

Although originally intended to describe a probability distribution, the Weibull function has turned out to be a very reliable empirical model for tree growth (Zeide 1993).

Kangas (1968, p. 69) independently suggested the function $p(t) = ae^{bt^{-c}}$ for modelling the growth multiplier of Eq. (6.16) and referred to it as the *growth coefficient function* (Pommerening and Muszta 2015).

Zeide (1993) and Pommerening and Muszta (2016) pointed out that all growth functions in Table 6.1 have a common element. It is interesting to note that the functions of relative growth rate share even more similarities than the growth functions. The functions of relative growth rate also have fewer model parameters than the growth functions and the functions of absolute growth. The relative growth rate function terms are also simpler and it is therefore possible to argue that using the concept of relative growth rate helps to standardise growth functions. The reduction of model parameters is another desirable property.

Figure 6.8 and Table 6.2 give an impression of how the functions of relative growth rate can be fitted to observed relative tree volume data. Naturally stem diameter, biomass or leaf-area-index growth data can alternatively be used. Judging by the statistics in Table 6.2 and the curves in relation to the observed data in Fig. 6.8, the Chapman-Richards function is the best choice in this case, whereby the algebraic difference form (Eq. 6.32) even leads to further improvement. The fitted function can now be used to carry out plant growth analyses based on relative growth.

Table 6.2 Model parameters, *Bias* and *RMSE* relating to the Chapman-Richards, the Gompertz and the Korf model of relative growth rate (Table 6.1) applied to the data of the Sitka spruce tree no. 486 in Gwydyr Forest (Pen yr Allt Ganol, North Wales, UK). See also Fig. 6.8. Modified from Pommerening and Muszta (2016)

Function name	b	c	*Bias*	*RMSE*
Chapman-Richards	−0.03967	5.28045	0.00014	0.05376
Chapman-Richards (Eq. 6.32)	0.02963	4.01008	−0.00147	0.02961
Gompertz	13.32683	0.10821	0.01604	0.05499
Korf	28.35671	0.26424	−0.00819	0.05865

Whilst most growth projection models in forest science and ecology are based on AGR (Larocque and Marshall 1993), the fitted function of relative growth can be inserted in Eq. (6.16) to obtain a growth multiplier, so that the growth multiplier thus acts as a wrapper of any growth function. Depending on environmental factors and competition the model parameters may even change over time for one individual or population and produce different relative growth rates. The relative growth rates of other characteristics of the same plant are estimated through allometric relationships and simultaneous regression techniques. Wenk et al. (1990) and Wenk (1994) showed how population growth models can thus be based on the concept of relative growth. Pommerening and Muszta (2015) explored this further by demonstrating that individual plant and population models using RGR are based on similar principles. Also Dyer (1997, p. 102ff.) developed a basal area growth disaggregation model for loblolly pine (*Pinus taeda* L.) plantations in the southern US based on growth multipliers.

In this context, it is worth noting that the algebraic difference form of growth functions (see Burkhart and Tomé 2012, p. 145ff.) as originally suggested by Bailey and Clutter (1974) is also a way of modelling growth multipliers. Equation (6.32) for example shows the algebraic difference form of the Chapman-Richards growth function:

$$y(t) = y(t - \Delta t) \left[\frac{1 - e^{bt}}{1 - e^{b(t - \Delta t)}} \right]^c \tag{6.32}$$

In Eq. (6.32), the second term in square brackets essentially constitutes the growth multiplier as defined in Eq. (6.16). Using this growth multiplier the current value of y, $y(t)$, is calculated from the previous value at time $t - \Delta t$ (Wenk et al. 1990, p. 204f.). Any function of Table 6.1 can be expressed in the algebraic difference form. The multiplier can then be turned to RGR using one of the relationships in Eq. (6.17), see Fig. 6.8 (right). The advantage of this approach is that it is possible to use the original, perhaps more familiar AGR versions of growth functions directly.

6.2.5.1 Modelling Individual Plant Growth

The strategy of modelling individual plant growth is straightforward: 1. A suitable function of relative growth rate is selected (either from Table 6.1 or from other publications). 2. A primary plant size characteristic is identified, e.g. tree volume. 3. Other plant size characteristics, e.g. tree height and tree diameter, are linked to the function of relative growth rate of the primary plant size characteristic through allometric coefficients. 4. The 2–3 model parameters of the function of relative growth rate and the two allometric coefficients are estimated simultaneously through nonlinear regression. Jones et al. (2009, p. 219f.) described how such more complex types of nonlinear regression can be calculated in R using the function `optim()` and we provided a listing towards the end of this section.

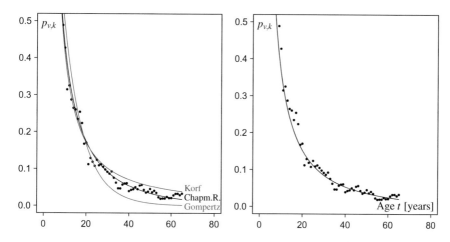

Fig. 6.8 Left: The three best functions of Table 6.1 fitted to the relative annual volume growth rate, $p_{v,k}$ of Sitka spruce tree no. 486 in Gwydyr Forest (Pen yr Allt Ganol, North Wales, UK). For model statistics see Table 6.3. Right: The algebraic difference form of the Chapman-Richards growth function (Eq. 6.32) applied to the same data. Modified from Pommerening and Muszta (2016)

Wenk et al. (1990, p. 174ff.) selected primary and other plant size characteristics in such a way that error propagation was effectively reduced: They identified tree volume as a three-dimensional size characteristic to be the primary characteristic and one-dimensional total tree height and stem diameter as other characteristics. However, there is, of course, no need to strictly follow this recommendation and tree volume can also be replaced by weight or biomass.

To illustrate this methodology we have used stem-analysis data of a Sitka spruce (*Picea sitchensis* (BONG.) CARR.) and of a sweet chestnut tree (*Castanea sativa* MILL.) from North Wales (UK, Fig. 6.9). Stem-analysis data typically include annual trees size characteristics such as for example stem volume, total tree height and stem diameter at 1.3 m above ground level. As function of relative growth we selected the well-known and frequently used Chapman-Richards function, but any of the other functions in Table 6.1 would perform reasonably similar (Pommerening and Muszta 2015).

For presenting observed data and models efficiently, we used the reciprocal of the growth multiplier, i.e. $1/e^{p_k}$, here, which can be easily calculated both for observed and estimated RGR. Like the growth multiplier, also its reciprocal is a function of RGR and has low values at early age that rapidly increase and approach 1 towards maturity and senescence. The relative growth rates and corresponding curves relating to total tree height and stem diameter are closer than any of them is to relative volume growth, which represents a different size dimension. Conifers and particular spruce are typically easier to model than broadleaves, as we can see by comparing the results in the two graphs of Fig. 6.9.

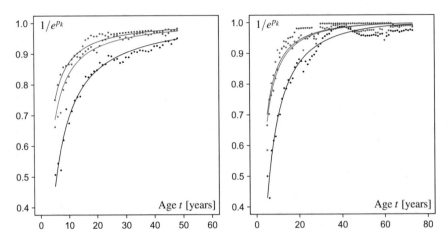

Fig. 6.9 Reciprocal of the growth multiplier based on p_k for (left) Sitka spruce (*Picea sitchensis* (BONG.) CARR.) tree no. 5000 in Clocaenog Forest (North Wales, UK) at Cefn Du (plot 1) and (right) for sweet chestnut (*Castanea sativa* MILL.) tree no. 1513 at Gwydyr Forest (Artist's Wood) over age. Black: p_k related to stem volume, blue: p_k related to total height, red: p_k related to stem diameter

The special point of interest in this modelling approach is that only $p_{v,k}$ is explicitly modelled using the Chapman-Richards function of relative growth. $p_{h,k}$ (height-based RGR) and $p_{d,k}$ (diameter-based RGR) are estimated from $p_{v,k}$ and $p_{h,k}$, respectively, through two constant allometric coefficients, m_h and m_d, which act both as model parameters and interpretable summary characteristics.

Through recursive use of Eq. (6.16) it is possible to describe the observed, integrated function $y(t)$ of volume, total height and stem diameter. Since it is challenging to model three related tree growth rates by using two constant allometric coefficients, we restricted the modelling to a tree age starting with ten years. Volume over time is estimated using the first observed volume measurement at age 10. Before that age tree RGR can be very varied. Then the growth multiplier based on $\hat{p}_{v,k}$ estimated from the Chapman-Richards function is repeatedly applied to that value until the final value of age. Following this $\hat{p}_{h,k}$ is calculated from $\hat{p}_{v,k}$ and the allometric coefficient m_h. Then the growth multiplier based on $\hat{p}_{h,k}$ is repeatedly applied to that value until the final value of age. Finally $\hat{p}_{d,k}$ is calculated from $\hat{p}_{h,k}$, the allometric coefficient m_d and again stem diameter over time is computed from the corresponding growth multiplier.

The fit for Sitka spruce tree no. 5000 is obviously quite satisfying (Fig. 6.10, left). The modelling of the sweet chestnut tree no. 1513 proved much more challenging (Fig. 6.10, right). This can also be understood from the *RMSE* values in Table 6.3. Particularly the assumption of constant allometric coefficients does not hold for this tree: Apparently there were several times during the life of this tree when height growth markedly changed, i.e. at age 20, 30 and 65. Likewise diameter growth abruptly changed over time, particularly at age 45. The comparison of model

Table 6.3 Model parameters and *RMSE* relating to the Chapman-Richards of relative growth rate applied (Table 6.1) to the data of the Sitka spruce tree no. 5000 in Clocaenog Forest (Cefn Du, plot 1) and sweet chestnut tree no. 1513 in Gwydyr Forest (Artist's Wood) both from North Wales (UK). Model parameters and *RMSE* relate to RGR of stem volume, total height and stem diameter. See also Figs. 6.9 and 6.10

Tree no.	Stem volume (m^3)			Total height (m)		Stem diameter (cm)	
	b	c	RMSE	m_h	RMSE	m_d	RMSE
5000	−0.00935	3.72599	0.01255	2.47648	0.01130	1.16644	0.01258
1513	−0.03406	4.26270	0.02166	3.93540	0.01251	0.69008	0.01604

curve and observed growth characteristic highlights such trends that were caused by abruptly changing environmental conditions. In this particular case the sweet-chestnut tree in question was several times browsed and bark-stripped by introduced American grey squirrels (*Sciurus carolinensis* GMELIN) that especially targeted the tree's crown.

From Fig. 6.10 (left) it is also clear that tree no. 5000 showed a continued growth of all three size variables at advanced age, whilst total height of tree no. 1513 started to level off at an age between 30 and 40 years. The allometric coefficients m_h of both trees tell us that on average volume RGR was considerably larger than height RGR, particular in the sweet chestnut tree. For tree no. 5000, height RGR was on average slightly larger than diameter RGR ($m_h \approx 1.2$). However, in tree no. 1513, stem diameter grew on average faster than height ($m_d < 1$).

Obviously this is only an example and the analyst is completely free to select any other three growth characteristic, should they be of interest and available.

The following coding is a good summary of the modelling procedure discussed in this section. In lines 3–10, RGR of volume, total height and stem diameter are calculated from the observed data of a stem analysis with annual measurements. The following lines 12–38 all relate to the nonlinear regression. They include a function (lines 12–20) simulating volume RGR from a relative growth function (lines 13f.) and height and stem-diameter RGR by using estimated allometric coefficients. Function `calcAllRelativeGrowthRates()` is then used in a loss function (lines 22–27), where the squared differences between observed and estimated RGR are summed as part of the least squares procedure. The weights `wV`, `wH` and `wD` can be used to assign relative importance to the three size variables and are set in lines 31–33. Finally, based on the function `optim()` the nonlinear regression is coded in lines 36–38 with start parameters set in line 35. Note that the loss function and the arguments of the loss function are listed as arguments at the beginning of the interface of function `optim()`. Once the regression finished, the function `calcAllRelativeGrowthRates()` can be employed again to estimate the relative growth rates (line 40). `abdn.L2$par` is a vector that includes the estimated model parameters. The vector with estimated tree volume is initialised with the first value of observed volume in line 42. Following this any subsequent volume is estimated using the growth multiplier coded as `exp(dn$pvx[i])`. Total height and stem diameter are estimated in analogy.

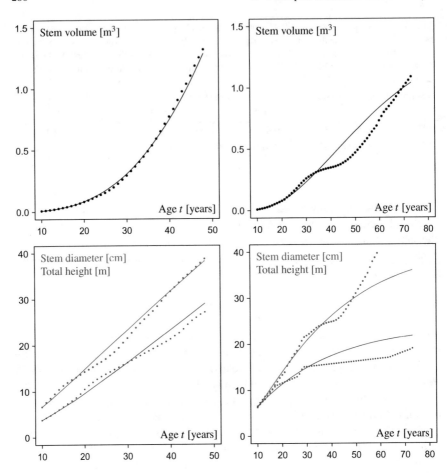

Fig. 6.10 Stem volume, total height and stem diameter development over time of (left) Sitka spruce (*Picea sitchensis* (BONG.) CARR.) tree no. 5000 in Clocaenog Forest (North Wales, UK) at Cefn Du (plot 1) and (right) sweet chestnut (*Castanea sativa* MILL.) tree no. 1513 at Gwydyr Forest (Artist's Wood)

```
 1  > # Calculate observed relative volume, height and diameter
 2  + growth rates.
 3  > myData$pv <- NA
 4  > myData$ph <- NA
 5  > myData$pd <- NA
 6  > for (i in 2 : length(myData$age)) {
 7  + myData$pv[i] <- (log(myData$v[i]) - log(myData$v[i - 1]))
 8  + myData$ph[i] <- (log(myData$h[i]) - log(myData$h[i - 1]))
 9  + myData$pd[i] <- (log(myData$d[i]) - log(myData$d[i - 1]))
10  + }
11  >
12  > calcAllRelativeGrowthRates <- function(xdata, abdn) {
13  +   # Chapman Richards
```

```
14  +   xdata$pvx <- abdn[1] * abdn[2] / (1 - exp(-abdn[1] *
15  +   xdata$age))
16  +   # Allometric relationships
17  +   xdata$phx <- xdata$pvx / abdn[3]
18  +   xdata$pdx <- xdata$phx / abdn[4]
19  +   return(xdata)
20  + }
21  >
22  > loss.L2 <- function(abdn, xdata, wV, wH, wD) {
23  +   xdata <- calcAllRelativeGrowthRates(xdata, abdn)
24  +   xdev <- wV * (xdata$pv - xdata$pvx)^2 + wH * (xdata$ph -
25  +   xdata$phx)^2 + wD *(xdata$pd - xdata$pdx)^2
26  +   return(sum(xdev, na.rm = TRUE))
27  + }
28  >
29  > # Regression b, c, m1 and m2 (allometric coefficients) for
30  + volume, height and diameter
31  > weight.v <- 0.33
32  > weight.h <- 0.33
33  > weight.d <- 0.33
34
35  > abdn0 <- c(-0.67, -0.068, 0.5, 2.56)
36  > abdn.L2 <- optim(abdn0, loss.L2, xdata = myData,
37  + wV = weight.v, wH = weight.h, wD = weight.d, control = list(
38  + maxit = 30000, temp = 2000, trace = TRUE, REPORT = 500))
39
40  > dn <- calcAllRelativeGrowthRates(myData, abdn.L2$par)
41  > myData$v.est <- NA
42  > myData$v.est[1] <- myData$v[1]
43  > for (i in 2 : length(myData$age))
44  +   myData$v.est[i] <- myData$v.est[i - 1] * exp(dn$pvx[i])
```

6.2.5.2 Modelling the Growth of Plant Cohorts and Populations

In the same way as it is possible to model individual plants one can also model groups or cohorts of a plant population or whole plant populations (Pommerening and Muszta 2015). In this case, the growth rates are calculated from population summary characteristics. Since modelling populations as a whole is not the focus of this book, we will only cover this topic briefly. Details of this approach are also documented in Wenk and Nicke (1985) and in Wenk (1994).

Drawing an analogy to the example used in the previous section we can, for example, model volume per hectare, top height and quadratic mean diameter of a forest stand. Let us denote the corresponding relative growth rates as $p_{V,k}$, $p_{H,k}$, and $p_{D,k}$ using capital letters for population volume (V), height (H) and diameters (D) in the subscripts.

Ignoring recruitment of saplings the methodology is almost exactly the same as for individual trees with the exception that there is a need to account for trees leaving the forest stand. These losses can be due to forest management or to natural mortality

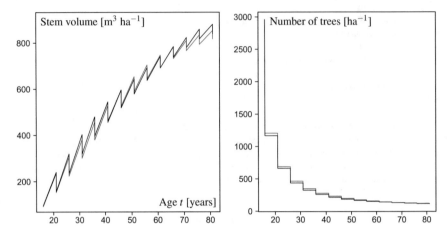

Fig. 6.11   Stand volume (left) and number of trees per hectare (right) development over time of the British Douglas fir (*Pseudotsuga menziesii* (MIRB.) FRANCO) yield class model for yield class 24, initial spacing 1.7 × 1.7 m and crown thinning (Edwards and Christie 1981). Black: Yield table curves. Red: Model curves

or can be a combination of both. For simplicity we introduce just one additional function that we simply refer to as loss function here, $l_{V,k}$, to collectively take care of death events as a result of disturbances (Wenk et al. 1990, p. 159):

$$l_{V,k} = 1 - \frac{Q}{M_{V,k}}, \qquad (6.33)$$

where Q is the ratio of V_k^{res}/V_{k-1}^{res} i.e. the ratio of successive residual stand volumes (superscript "res" denotes "residual" here). The ratio Q defines the loss of trees and must not exceed the volume growth multiplier, as negative values of stand volume are not defined. With $Q = 1$, $p_{V,k} = l_{V,k}$ and the forest stand does not grow.

The loss function is therefore a ratio of two multipliers subtracted from one and can also be estimated with the Chapman-Richards relative growth rate function (Pommerening and Muszta 2015). Forest stand volume is then calculated and projected in the following way (considering that the superscripts "prior" define the forest state before disturbance, "lost" the part of the tree population lost and "res" the state of the residual forest after disturbance):

$$V_{k-1}^{lost} = V_{k-1}^{prior} \times l_{V,k-1} \qquad (6.34)$$
$$V_{k-1}^{res} = V_{k-1}^{prior} - V_{k-1}^{lost}$$
$$V_k^{prior} = V_{k-1}^{res} \times M_{V,k}$$

In a first step, the volume per hectare of dead trees, i.e. the absolute loss in terms of volume, is calculated as the product of the volume of the forest stand before the disturbance, V_{k-1}^{prior}, and the volume loss rate, $l_{V,k-1}$. Then residual stand volume, V_{k-1}^{res}, constitutes the difference between stand volume before disturbance, V_{k-1}^{prior}, and the absolute volume loss, V_{k-1}^{lost}. Finally the volume of the forest stand before disturbance for the next time step, V_k^{prior} is calculated as the product of the residual stand volume of the previous time step, V_{k-1}^{res}, and the volume growth multiplier of the next time step, $M_{V,k}$.

In analogy to volume projection, the development of a density measure such as trees per hectare can be modelled. Stand height is also modelled in a similar way as outlined in the last line of Eq. (6.35) following the concept of projecting individual-tree heights.

Finally, the quadratic mean diameter, dg_k^{prior}, of the forest stand before disturbance is calculated from stand basal area before disturbance, G_k^{prior}, and the number of trees per hectare before disturbance, N_k^{prior}, using the following two equations:

$$G_k^{\text{prior}} = \frac{V_k^{\text{prior}}}{f_H} \tag{6.35}$$

$$dg_k^{\text{prior}} = 100 \times \sqrt{\frac{4 \times G_k^{\text{prior}}}{\pi \times N_k^{\text{prior}}}}$$

f_H is a static form height function. Such form height relationships are available for many species and countries. The equations of this section can be included in a regression routine, for example in the `optim()` function of R as demonstrated in the last section (Jones et al. 2009, p. 219f.). As a function of relative growth rate we again selected the Chapman-Richards function (see Table 6.1), but any of the other functions is suitable, too.

To illustrate this method we have used Douglas fir (*Pseudotsuga menziesii* (MIRB.) FRANCO) data from British yield tables (Edwards and Christie 1981), specifically those relating to yield class 24, initial spacing 1.7 × 1.7 m and crown thinning. Yield tables can be interpreted as tabular summary characteristics of forest stands, whereby the yield classes represent different environmental conditions resulting in a larger or smaller carrying capacity. Naturally any other aggregated plant population data can be selected for this purpose (Pommerening and Muszta 2015).

The yield table data are provided for five-year intervals and as a consequence relative growth rates and growth multipliers also relate to five-year periods.

In addition to the yield table data, we have used the UK form height function for Douglas fir suggested by (Matthews and Mackie 2006, p. 325):

$$f_H = -0.509255 + 0.426679 \times H, \tag{6.36}$$

where H is stand top height in metres.

The temporal development of the actual population size characteristics volume per hectare, top height and quadratic mean diameter (not shown) were calculated from relative growth rates as explained in Eqs. (6.34) and (6.35), see Fig. 6.11.

The obvious similarity between individual-tree and population modelling of relative growth rates suggests a link between these two modelling levels (see for example Cao 2014). The idea of this approach is to combine the advantages of different modelling resolutions, particularly to employ information of population models (that are mathematically more tractable and statistically more stable) for improving individual-tree models. This strategy is often referred to as *disaggregation*.

6.2.6 Sampling and Growth Rate Combinations

The possibilities for applying growth rates and functions discussed in the previous sections to arbitrary growth characteristics to $y(t)$ are unlimited. The applications can range from dry weight, biomass to leaf area, stem volume, basal area and stem diameters. Often measurements are destructive, e.g. for biomass and dry weight, and such destructive measurements are then referred to as "harvests" in the plant science literature, see for example Evans (1972, p. 44f.). This often implies that for establishing growth rates, the measurements of different plants or the averages of several plants have to be used (Evans 1972, p. 247). In this context, Hoffmann and Poorter (2002) provided useful advice on unbiased estimators of mean relative growth rates.

If, however, many non-destructive measures are made on the same individuals, as this is common practice in long-term monitoring in forest science (longitudinal studies), then the error structure of the model fit must take this into account and mixed-effect models for repeated-measures data can be used (Paine et al. 2012; Philipson et al. 2012; Zhao et al. 2014).

Naturally, it is possible to study the growth of individual plants, of groups of plants and of whole plant populations. Evidently RGR is the result of complex processes determined by physiology, morphology and biomass (Shipley 2006). This characteristic is also simultaneously affected by genetic, ontogenetic and environmental factors (Grime and Hunt 1975). Therefore much effort has been put into partitioning relative growth rates (e.g. Hunt 1982; Hunt and Cornelissen 1997; Shipley 2006; Rees et al. 2010). An example of a widely quoted partitioning approach is

$$RGR = NAR \times SLA \times LMR, \qquad (6.37)$$

where NAR = net assimilation rate, SLA = specific leaf area and LMR = leaf mass ratio. In a meta-analysis, Shipley (2006) found that NAR generally was the best predictor of RGR, but that as light intensity decreased the importance of SLA increased on the expense of NAR. The relationship between LMR and RGR is apparently inconsistent (Houghton et al. 2013). There are many such interrelations and Hunt

(1990, p. 83ff.) provided a good summary. In addition, Ingestad (1982) summarised studies proving that nutrient uptake rates are closely related to relative growth rates. Combinations of growth rates were referred to as *compounded growth rates* by Hunt (1990, p. 15). They involve more than one plant characteristic, such as the whole plant's rate of dry weight increase per unit of its leaf area. One of the characteristics may not be a plant characteristic, as in the rate of dry matter production per unit area of land or in the unit leaf rate (Hughes and Freeman 1967).

To account for the continuous accumulation of non-productive tissues in perennial plants, Brand et al. (1987) suggested the *relative production rate*, i.e. the logarithmic ratio of current AGR and the AGR of the previous year or period. A related measure was introduced in dendrochronological research by Nowacki and Abrams (1997) as the *percentage of relative growth change*. Interestingly Ramseier and Weiner (2006) found that the unweighted size of plant neighbours was an important determinant of a target plant's RGR regardless of its own size (Pommerening and Muszta 2016).

6.3   Size-Dependent Relative Growth Rates

As relative growth rate continuously decreases with increasing time and size, criticism has frequently been noted when, for example, comparisons between species with different initial sizes were carried out. As a rationale to explain the decline of RGR with size it is often put forward that through self-shading and tissue ageing plants become increasingly inefficient as they get larger leading to systematic changes in physiology, morphology and allocation (Rees et al. 2010). The effect of declining RGR with size is referred to as *ontogenetic drift* (see Evans 1972, p. 16). The size dependency of RGR implies that mean RGR as defined in the literature and in this chapter is, at least partly, an artefact of initial size and could potentially mask important relationships (Turnbull et al. 2008; Paul-Victor et al. 2010; Paine et al. 2012; Philipson et al. 2012). When comparing individuals at a given point in time, RGR cannot distinguish between individuals that grow slowly because they are large, and individuals that grow slowly because they are pursuing a slow growth strategy (Rose et al. 2009). Using methods of *size correction* or *size standardisation*, Turnbull et al. (2008) could, for example, demonstrate that small-seeded species are not necessarily physiologically better adapted for rapid growth than large-seeded species. Since relative growth rate is already a standardised measure, discussions are still ongoing in which context size correction/standardisation is required. A common method of size standardisation is to fit a suitable growth curve to RGR data from multiple sampling and then to calculate RGR for all species at a common reference size, see for example Rees et al. (2010). This method essentially means replacing time-dependent RGR by size-dependent RGR, which is an allometric relationship, see Sect. 6.2.4. Already Larocque and Marshall (1993) and Dyer (1997) reported relationships between RGR and tree size.

In order to address this problem, several authors have devised what they referred to as size correction. The general principle of this approach involves 1. fitting a growth curve to observed data including size and time, where size depends on time, i.e. $y(t)$ or $y'(t)/y(t)$. 2. Then the RGR function of the same model needs to be fitted to the RGR data. 3. Next the growth function is solved for t to yield a relationship where time depends on size, i.e. $t(y)$ or $t(y'/y)$. 4. Finally age in the RGR function is substituted for size using the inverted growth function. The sequential use of steps 1–4 is a way of obtaining the relationship between y'/y and y (Rose et al. 2009; Paul-Victor et al. 2010; Rees et al. 2010; Pommerening and Muszta 2015).

For example inverting the Chapman-Richards growth function for t provides a possibility to convert a size characteristic to time/age:

$$t = \frac{\ln\left(1 - e^{\frac{\ln y/a}{c}}\right)}{b} = -\frac{1}{b}\ln\left(1 - \left(\frac{y}{a}\right)^{\frac{1}{c}}\right) \tag{6.38}$$

Analysing three tree stems sampled for stem analysis in the usual time-dependent way (Fig. 6.12, left) shows hardly any differences in their relative growth rates. The growth rates here relate to stem diameter. Particularly the RGRs of tree no. 1 and 3 are very similar and the respective model curves almost run in parallel. Tree no. 4 instead has markedly larger relative growth rates than the other two trees up to the age of 20.

Now the described size-correction method was applied relating the relative growth rates to stem diameter. The results change our interpretation (Fig. 6.12, right): Looking at the growth patterns from the point of view of size (stem diameter in cm) tells us that the RGR patterns of tree no. 3 and 4 are in fact closer and that the growth pattern of tree no. 1 is rather different. We also learn that initial and final tree sizes were

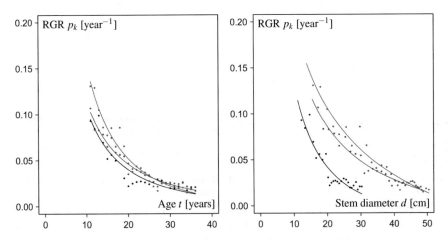

Fig. 6.12 Three stem-analysis trees from the same Sitka spruce (*Picea sitchensis* (BONG.) CARR.) plantation site Clocaenog 10 in North Wales (UK). Tree no. 1 (black), tree no. 3 (blue) and tree no. 4 (red). The Chapman-Richards RGR growth model (see Table 6.1) was used for defining the trend lines in the left graph and the size correction of Eq. (6.38) in the right graph

quite different. Size correction helped to differentiate between the growth rate patterns more clearly and to recognise the relationships between the RGRs of the three trees. In a comparable situation, Rose et al. (2009) and Rees et al. (2010) argued that Fig. 6.12 (right) represents a fairer comparison, since size has a stronger influence on relative growth rates than time.

In Fig. 6.12 (right), observed RGR values were directly plotted over size. This raises the question why we need to invert growth functions and to go through the 4-step procedure outlined above instead of modelling size-dependent RGR in the first place. Clearly the general trend of declining RGR with size is not very different from that for RGR and time.

A size-dependent analysis of RGR is also supported by the fact that trees in natural and selection forests can persist to remain small for hundred years and more and then emerge to become fully-grown trees once an opportunity arises as a consequence of a disturbance (Schütz 2001b). Such trees then in terms of growth behave like juvenile trees suggesting that size matters more than age. Weiner et al. (2001) argued that the so-called age-related decline in forest productivity of tree populations as well as of individual trees is primarily a size-related decline. For example, the well-documented pattern that declines in forest productivity occur earlier on more fertile sites (Ryan et al. 1997) may be interpreted as a simple outcome of size-dependent growth: Under better conditions trees reach the size at which growth begins to decline sooner. In tree and forest modelling, the modelling of size-dependent absolute growth rates is quite common, as individual-tree age is not always available and size-dependent growth functions help to generalise tree models.

RGR can therefore primarily be regarded as a function of size, i.e. $p(y(t))$ rather than $p(t, y)$. It is assumed that RGR has a kind of "nested" or indirect dependency on time and size is used as a proxy for time in this modelling approach. In general plant science, direct size-dependent modelling of relative growth rates has only been attempted on rare occasions.

For modelling size-dependent RGR directly it is possible to start with a simple power function that approaches zero for large plant sizes and corresponds with the allometric equation (Eq. 6.27), i.e.

$$\overline{p}_k = a_0 \, y^{-b_0}. \tag{6.39}$$

Here $\overline{p}_k$ is the mean relative growth rate (RGR, Eq. 6.9). In the case of stem analyses with annual measurements, $\overline{p}_k$ simplifies to p_k (Eq. 6.10). In Eq. (6.39), a_0 is a location parameter and b_0 a shape parameter. A comparison of the two graphs in Fig. 6.13 emphasises that RGR size correction clearly implies a size-dependent analysis of relative growth rates. The trend curves in both graphs are almost identical. An alternative to Eq. (6.39) is the exponential function

$$\overline{p}_k = a_1 \, e^{-b_1 \, y}, \tag{6.40}$$

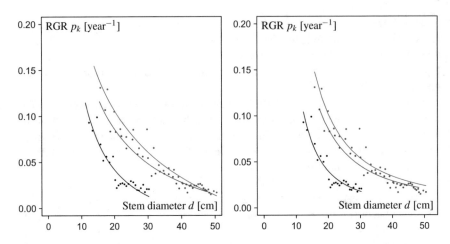

Fig. 6.13 Three stem-analysis trees from the same Sitka spruce (*Picea sitchensis* (BONG.) CARR.) plantation site Clocaenog 10 in North Wales (UK). Tree no. 1 (black), tree no. 3 (blue) and tree no. 4 (red). The Chapman-Richards RGR growth model (see Table 6.1) in combination with the size correction of Eq. (6.38) was used for defining the trend lines in the left graph and a simple power function (Eq. 6.39) in the right graph

where model parameters a_1 and b_1 play a role similar to a_0 and b_0. Another alternative is the relative growth function based on the Hugershoff function of Eq. (5.30) in Chap. 5:

$$\overline{p}_k = k \ y^{a_2-1} \ e^{-b_2 \, y} \qquad (6.41)$$

Growth data collected in general plant science are often of a different nature than in forest science. In the former, it is very typical to use data stemming from snapshot harvests, i.e. data collected at one point in time only. In such a case the RGR data cloud often suggests a model shape that is very different from what we see in Fig. 6.13. As a result quite different model types have been suggested. In fact the relationship between RGR and plant size varies considerably and Larocque and Marshall (1993, Fig. 3) illustrated the changes in this relationship in tree plantations and found that they depend on the stage of development.

Regression for size-dependent RGR is carried out similar to the regression technique we used for time-dependent RGR. As in the previous listing, first the observed relative growth rates need to be calculated. Following that function `calcGrowth-Function()` is defined (lines 1–9). This function wraps the model describing the size-dependent RGR trend and the three options of Eqs. (6.39), (6.40) and (6.41) are given. Currently activated is Eq. (6.39). Again the loss function `loss.L2()` uses function `calcGrowthFunction()` to calculate estimated RGR and finally the sum of squared differences between observed and estimated RGR, which serves as optimisation criterion in function `optim()`. The actual regression is coded in lines 19f. using start parameters set in line 18.

```
 1  > calcGrowthFunction <- function(size, abdn) {
 2  + # Power decline equation
 3  + px <- abdn[1] * size^abdn[2]
 4  + # Negative exponential distribution
 5  + # px <- abdn[1] * exp(-abdn[2] * size)
 6  + # Modified from Zeide (1993, p. 609, Eq. 7)
 7  + # px <- abdn[1] * size^(abdn[2] - 1) * exp(-abdn[3] * size)
 8  + return(px)
 9  + }
10  >
11  > loss.L2 <- function(abdn, xdata) {
12  + pxs <- calcGrowthFunction(xdata$size, abdn)
13  + xdev <- (xdata$p - pxs)^2
14  + return(sum(xdev, na.rm = TRUE))
15  + }
16
17  > # Regression
18  > abdn0 <- c(-0.67, 0.068)
19  > abdn.L2 <- optim(abdn0, loss.L2, xdata = myData, control =
20  + list(maxit = 30000, temp = 200, trace = TRUE, REPORT = 500))
```

In the literature, often a linear relationship between RGR and size is assumed. Iida et al. (2014), for example, related size-dependent growth and mortality with architectural traits of 145 tropical tree species using the linear relationship of Eq. (5) in Table 6.4. Dyer (1997, p. 63) modelled the linear relationship between relative growth rate and relative size (tree stem diameter divided by median stem diameter, Eq. (4) in Table 6.4) of trees. The author was particularly interested in the slope parameters of this model and used them to identify changes in this relationship over time and across densities. An example of the approach described in Eq. (2) of Table 6.4 is given in Sect. 7.2.8.

In natural forests, the patterns of RGR are, however, different. Using, for example, the time series of interior Douglas fir (*Pseudotsuga menziesii* var *glauca* (MIRB.) FRANCO) in the Alex Fraser Research Forest (BC, Canada, LeMay et al. 2009) reveals the same declining trend as for the stem analyses of individual trees in Fig. 6.13. The colours representing relative growth rates of different survey years do not show any

Table 6.4 Linear relationships between RGR and size used in the literature. y_m is the median of y

Reference	Model	Eq.
Wenk (1996, pers. comm.)	$M_k = a + b \cdot y$	(1)
Wenk (2003, pers. comm.)	$i_k = a + b \cdot y$[1]	(2)
Ramseier and Weiner (2006)	$\overline{p}_k = a + b \cdot y$	(3)
Dyer (1997)	$\overline{p}_k = a + b \cdot \frac{y}{y_m}$	(4)
Ryan et al. (1997)	$\overline{p}_k = a + b \cdot \log y$	(5)
Houghton et al. (2013)	$\log \overline{p}_k = a + b \cdot \log y$	(6)

[1] This equation models AGR and eventually yields $\overline{p}_k$ through transformation: $i_k/y = a/y + b \Leftrightarrow \overline{p}_k^+ = a/y + b \rightarrow \overline{p}_k = \log(p_k^+ + 1)$

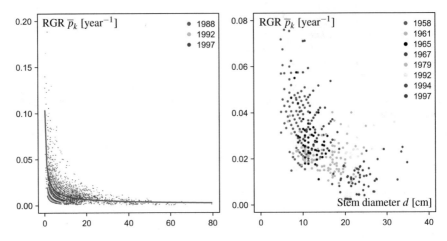

Fig. 6.14 Left: The declining trend of size-dependent relative growth rates of trees in a semi-natural woodland of interior Douglas fir (*Pseudotsuga menziesii* var *glauca* (MIRB.) FRANCO) in the Alex Fraser Research Forest (BC, Canada). The red trend curve was modelled using Eq. (6.39). Right: RGR data from a birch (*Betula pendula* ROTH.) time series at Bedgebury (Kent, UK) analysed as part of the Tyfiant Coed project (Bangor University, UK). The years indicate the beginning of the survey period used for calculating mean relative growth rates

obvious trend, i.e. the observed relative growth rates can be found throughout the survey years, which is typical of uneven-aged natural woodlands (Fig. 6.14, left).

From these results we can conclude that the trends of size-dependent relative growth rates are quite similar in stem analysis data and in time series involving uneven-aged woodlands. For modelling such RGR patterns we can use Eqs. (6.39)–(6.41).

However, when analysing data from even-aged plantations we found quite different trends. Figure 6.14 (right), for example, shows size-dependent RGR in a British birch time series. The data were collected in a forest grown as even-aged, mono-species plantation. The reason for the difference in trends is that in plant populations, where all plants were planted and are of the same age, the range of sizes is limited and as a consequence so is RGR.

Following the patterns of the coloured point clouds, we can clearly see in Fig. 6.14 (right) that every survey year contributes a small, distinctive point cloud, which by itself does not follow the trend of a declining power function. All point clouds pulled together do conform with the trend known from stem analyses and uneven-aged forests (Fig. 6.15). The point clouds of individual survey years, however, have an elliptic shape suggesting a linear relationship (like those reviewed in Table 6.4). Such linear relationships are also known from other plant-growth science studies (Larocque and Marshall 1993; Turnbull et al. 2008; Houghton et al. 2013).

At the beginning of a time series observing plants of the same age, at a stage of early forest stand development, the point-cloud ellipses are almost vertical with only a small tilt to the right or left. With progressing forest development and increasing

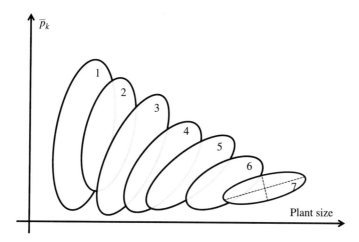

Fig. 6.15 Schematic temporal progression of the RGR point clouds in even-aged plant populations. The numbers refer to different forest development stages corresponding to discrete census years. The dashed lines in ellipse no. 7 represent the semi-major and semi-minor ellipse axes. (The arbitrary numbers of seven point clouds has been chosen for convenience and clarity.)

tree size the tilt increases and there is some overlap between point clouds. The tilting is a consequence of increasing variance of size and decreasing RGR variance in subsequent surveys. These two simultaneous effects initially increase but then gradually decrease the strength of the linear relationship. Another possibly complementary explanation for the trends in Fig. 6.15 is that individual trees with large RGR values move faster on declining trajectories of relative growth than trees with small initial RGR values that also tend to end up with smaller absolute sizes. Often tree growth, however, moves on non-parallel trajectories that intersect during the observation time.

Given an initial, elliptic point cloud with an almost vertical main axis, these growth effects lead to a situation where the ellipses of all subsequent data clouds are increasingly tilted, because trees with larger RGR values tend to develop larger tree sizes faster. This also implies that we can draw conclusions about the physiological age and the development stage of a sampled plantation when analysing the data ellipsis: The flatter the data ellipse and the smaller the positive slope of the semi-major axis, the older and more advanced the stage of succession or woodland development.

For example the comparatively young conifer cohort at Coed y Brenin (plot 7) was associated with a fairly upright RGR-size data ellipse in 2011, whilst the much older Sitka spruce cohort at Clocaenog (plot 1) had a much flatter, almost horizontal ellipse (see Fig. 6.16) in 2007.

Also trees with initially larger RGR values can sometimes have a smaller final size than others from the same site whilst all other conditions were the same. Still the abovementioned explanation is a good theory that helps to conciliate the seemingly odd RGR data from even-aged monocultures with the point cloud shapes known from stem analyses and natural forests.

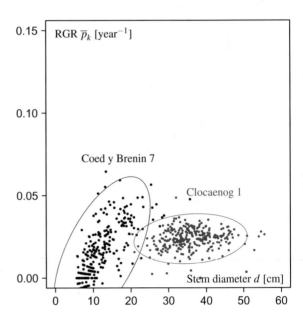

Fig. 6.16 RGR-size 95%-confidence ellipses of the conifers in Coed y Brenin (plot 7) and of Sitka spruce at Clocaenog (plot 1) both from even-aged plantations in North Wales (UK). The former tree cohort was planted in 1985 and the latter in 1951

Data from even-aged plantations typically find a parallel in data from plant trials reported in general plant science. Also here all plants of a given trial have the same age and are planted and harvested at the same time. Therefore we consider the pattern sketched in Fig. 6.15 an important, general problem.

As a first step in modelling this phenomenon it is possible to consider the confidence ellipses of the bivariate normal distribution. Each point cloud representing a specific survey year in Fig. 6.14 (right) can be described by such confidence ellipses (Muszta, 2017, pers. comm.). The orientation of any ellipsis is determined by the semi-major or main axis.

The linear models of Table 6.4 should ideally match the semi-major axis of each data ellipse as closely as possible. Identifying the parameters of the semi-major axes of a whole system of ellipses as indicated in Fig. 6.15 is a major contribution to describing the growth processes involved and eventually to modelling them.

Standardised major axis (SMA) regression techniques help to approximate the semi-major axes of data ellipses. They are related to principal component analysis, a multivariate approach (Legendre and Legendre 2012; Warton et al. 2012).

The purpose of line fitting here is not to predict but to summarise the relationship between two variables. In the spirit of data or dimension reduction the resulting line is a summary in the sense that a single variable is used to describe two-dimensional data (Warton et al. 2006). For carrying out SMA regressions we used the smatr R package (Warton et al. 2012) and the data ellipses were visualised with the car package.

The R listing below shows how to apply the packages car and smatr for visualising the confidence ellipses and calculating a regression line that is close to the semi-major axes of the ellipses. After selecting a survey year in line 4 the confidence ellipse is estimated in lines 5f. The standardised major axis regression is coded in lines 7f. A summary of the results can be produced with the command in line 9. The coef() function of the smatr allows extracting the slope parameter (line 10).

```
1  > library(car)
2  > library(smatr)
3  >
4  > singleSurvey <- myData[myData$year == 1958, ]
5  > ellipse <- dataEllipse(cbind(singleSurvey$dbh,
6  + singleSurvey$RGR), levels = 0.95, draw = FALSE)
7  > sma.lm <- sma(RGR ~ dbh, data = singleSurvey,
8  + method = "SMA")
9  > summary(sma.lm)
10 > slope <- coef(sma.lm)[[2]]
11 >
12 > plot(singleSurvey$dbh, singleSurvey$RGR, axes = FALSE,
13 + ylab = "", xlab = "", main = "", pch = 16, cex = 1.0,
14 + ylim = c(0, 0.08), xlim = c(0, 40), col = "red")
15 > lines(ellipse, col = "red")
16 > curve(coef(sma.lm)[[2]] * x + coef(sma.lm)[[1]],
17 + from = min(singleSurvey$dbh), to = max(singleSurvey$dbh),
18 + col = "red", add = T)
19 > axis(side = 1, lwd = 2, las = 1, cex.axis = 1.7)
20 > axis(side = 2, lwd = 2, las = 1, cex.axis = 1.7)
21 > box(lwd = 2)
```

The data, the confidence ellipse and the SMA regression line can be visualised using the code in lines 12–21. The confidence ellipse is plotted in line 15 using the lines() function and the SMA regression line is plotted in lines 16–18. Here again the function coef() of the smatr package provides the model parameters, i.e. intercept and slope.

The visualisation of data ellipses and SMA regression lines show that the latter are close to the semi-major axes of the ellipses (Fig. 6.17, left). The slope coefficients of the SMA regression lines can then be plotted over mean size (Fig. 6.17, right) to show the progression of the data ellipses with increasing size. The general trend is that of negative slopes at the beginning which become positive with a certain mean size (here approximately 17 cm). Some curves also start with large positive values. The slope coefficients reach a maximum and then gradually approach zero. This trend has also been observed in other work (Dyer 1997).

It is now possible to compare the slope trend lines of different time series (Fig. 6.18). Among the four Sitka spruce (*Picea sitchensis* (BONG.) CARR.) time series studied in the Tyfiant Coed project (Bangor University) only Glasfynydd 2068 has one observation with a negative slope. There were some clear differences between the four sites. It is interesting to see that the most fertile site (Glasfynydd 2068) with the greatest carrying capacity had the lowest trend line (the data ellipses tended to be quite flat indicating weak relationships between size and RGR), while the poorest site (Coed y Brenin 2021) showed the highest trend line, i.e. the relationship between tree size and corresponding RGR was particularly strong here.

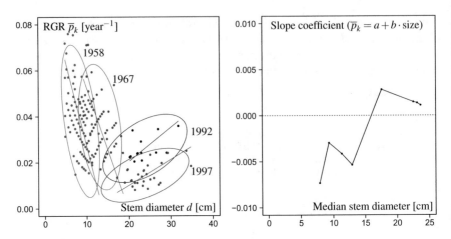

Fig. 6.17 Left: Selection of 95%-confidence ellipses and SMA regression lines relating to the birch time series at Bedgebury, see Fig. 6.14. Right: The slope coefficients of the SMA regression lines over median stem diameter

These interesting results merit further research using a wide range of data sources. The context and the special conditions of the linear relationship between RGR and size often assumed in the literature have now become much clearer. This relationship can only be found in data where all plants are of the same age and it is part of a larger pattern across several discrete survey periods that eventually shows the well-known trend of RGR decline.

Fig. 6.18 The slope coefficients of the SMA regression lines over median stem diameter of four Welsh Sitka spruce (*Picea sitchensis* (BONG.) CARR.) time series analysed as part of the Tyfiant Coed project (Bangor University, UK)

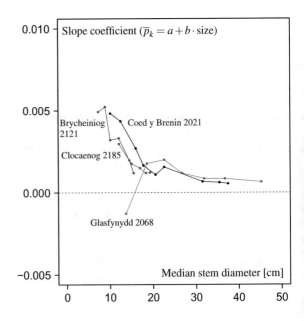

Fig. 6.19 Relative growth rates at Artist's Wood, a managed selection forest dominated by Douglas fir (*Pseudotsuga menziesii* (MIRB.) FRANCO) and originally planted in 1921 (see Schütz and Pommerening 2013). The two surveys included the growth periods 2002–2007 and 2007–2011. The model curves are based on Eq. (6.39)

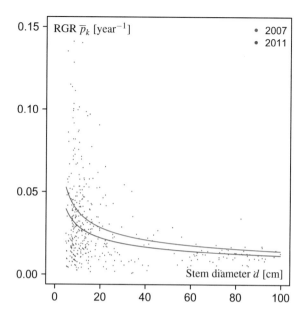

In uneven-aged forest stands, however, the situation is different, see Fig. 6.19. Here RGR is not limited to a particular size range in each survey, but the observations occur throughout the stem-diameter range as in Fig. 6.14 (left). This is also true for managed woodlands, as we can see in Fig. 6.19. Here it is even difficult to separate the RGR observations from 2007 to 2011.

The power function of Eq. (6.39) fitted separately to the data from the two survey years suggests two curves that almost run in parallel, where the curve describing the 2007 data is located above the 2011 curve. This may imply that the average relative growth rates of trees of the same size have dropped between 2007 and 2011.

One could imagine this as the average small tree (at the beginning of the size range) "travelling" on a lower trajectory towards maturity and senescence. However, previous analyses by the authors have shown that such curves of different surveys can also occasionally intersect or coincide.

6.4 Growth Rates as Marks in Point Process Statistics

Growth rates can also be considered as interesting marks in the analysis of marked point patterns. This is an intriguing extension of spatially explicit growth analysis. However, so far this possibility has not been used much.

Biondi et al. (1994) analysed stem diameter and AGR based on tree basal area from a 10-year growth period using the mark variogram (see Sect. 4.4.7.2). The authors found very little dependence of AGR on tree locations, whereas stem-diameter showed a clear spatial dependence in their study.

To illustrate the potential of spatially explicit growth analysis, we have selected plot 2 of the Alex Fraser Research Forest (BC, Canada) that was already introduced in Chap. 4, see Figs. 4.34 and 7.26.

The growth rates were calculated as means according to Eqs. (6.7) and (6.9) relating to the growth period 1997–2004, whilst the stem-diameter marks were taken from 2004 (Fig. 6.20). Although exactly the same tree locations were used in all three maps and the scaling of marks was visually adjusted for better comparison, the three maps differ markedly. It is important to note that seemingly missing trees may have very small or zero growth rates. Particularly large are the differences of the maps using stem diameters (left) and RGR (right) as marks: As expected large marks on the left corresponded to small marks on the right and vice versa. The coefficient of mark variation was largest for RGR (1.04), followed by stem diameter (1.00) and AGR (0.73). The differences in variation are clearly not as large as one might expect from studying the maps in Fig. 6.20.

Next we applied two mark correlation functions to the three different marks as discussed in Sect. 4.4.7.2, the mark correlation function $k_{mm}(r)$ and the mark variogram $\gamma_m(r)$. For the ease of comparison the 95% pointwise envelopes (Sect. 4.4.9) were omitted and the mark variograms were normalised.

The corresponding R coding uses the spatstat package and follows the pattern of spatial computations of Chap. 4. The spatstat object is created in lines 1f. Here it is important to change the definition of marks in line 2 depending on the size and growth variable intended to study. The range of distances r and the discrete evaluation points are set in line 3.

```
1  > myDataP <- ppp(myData$x, myData$y, window = xwindow,
2  + marks = myData$dbh) # myData$AGR, myData$RGR
3  > myR <- seq(0, 20, 0.25)
4  >
5  > kmm <- markcorr(myDataP, function(m1, m2) {m1 * m2},
6  + r = myR, correction = "translate", method = "density",
7  + kernel = "epanechnikov", bw = 0.8)
8  >
9  > mv <- markvario(myDataP, r = myR, correction = "translate",
10 + method = "density", kernel = "epanechnikov", bw = 1.3,
11 + normalise = TRUE)
```

Then the mark correlation function $\hat{k}_{mm}(r)$ is estimated in lines 5–7 and the mark variogram $\hat{\gamma}_m(r)$ in lines 9–11. For details on the settings see Chap. 4.

For stem diameters the mark correlation function indicated that up to 5 m there are small trees of similar size (Fig. 6.21, left). At distances $r \approx 10$ m and $r \approx 14$ m larger trees of similar size occur. Since AGR is proportional to size, the red $\hat{k}_{mm}(r)$ curve follows an overall trend similar to the black, however, the minima and maxima are not as pronounced as with stem diameter. This result seems to support the findings by Biondi et al. (1994). Very different are the outcomes for RGR marks: On first sight it appears as if maxima and minima are swapped for the curves related to

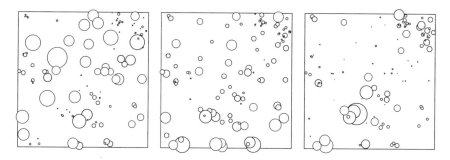

Fig. 6.20 Plot 2 of the Alex Fraser Research Forest (BC, Canada) in a mostly pure stand of interior Douglas fir (*Pseudotsuga menziesii* var *glauca* (MIRB.) FRANCO) in 2004. Plot size is 31.62 m × 31.62 m. Marks used were stem diameter (left), stem-diameter based AGR (centre) and stem-diameter based RGR (right)

stem diameter and RGR as marks. The blue $\hat{k}_{mm}(r)$ curve starts with large values to decrease towards a minimum where the black curve has its first maximum at around 5 m. Then the blue curve briefly runs in parallel with the black curve until $r \approx 10$ m followed by a sudden drop. At $r \approx 14$ m the RGR related blue $\hat{k}_{mm}(r)$ curve forms a large minimum which is almost a perfect reflection of the maximum of the stem-diameter $\hat{k}_{mm}(r)$ curve. This somewhat contrary behaviour of the RGR curve is surely related to the fact that large-sized trees typically have small relative growth rates. Spatially this means that at short distances there are many small, productive trees with large RGR values. At around 14 m distance large trees occur that in relative

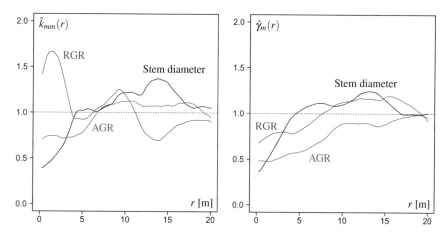

Fig. 6.21 Spatial characteristics estimated for plot 2 of the Alex Fraser Research Forest (BC, Canada) in a mostly pure stand of interior Douglas fir (*Pseudotsuga menziesii* var *glauca* (MIRB.) FRANCO) in 2004. Left: Mark correlation function $\hat{k}_{mm}(r)$ with bandwidth $h = 0.8$ m. Right: The corresponding mark variograms $\hat{\gamma}_m(r)$ with bandwidth $h = 1.3$ m. In both cases the Epanechnikov kernel (Eq. 4.28) and three different marks were used

terms are much less productive and therefore have very small relative growth rates. Apparently the test function of the mark correlation function is very suitable for diagnosing the relationship between size and growth marks. We obtained a different impression from using the mark variogram as a diagnostic tool (Fig. 6.21, right). This characteristic differentiates less between two growth rates than the mark correlation function.

The stem-diameter related, black $\hat{\gamma}_m(r)$ curve indicates trees of similar size up to 5 m. Thereafter there is an increasing trend of unequal size marks, i.e. trees at short distances are of similar size while pairs of trees at large distances are increasingly different as this is often the case in woodlands. For AGR also the mark variogram trend is similar to that of stem diameter, which again supports the findings of Biondi et al. (1994). However, throughout the distance range considered the AGR values of pairs of trees remain to be similar. Although the blue RGR curve of $\hat{\gamma}_m(r)$ appears to run almost in parallel to that of AGR, we note positive association with similar mark values until $r \approx 7$ m and beyond this point negative association with dissimilar RGR values until $r = 20$ m. Due to the different test function the mark variogram obviously emphasises other aspects of the size/growth relationship. In all cases the correlation range is around 20 m. The combined use of different size/growth marks and mark correlation functions has been particularly helpful in this analysis.

References

Antanaitis V, Zagreev V (1969) Prirost Lesa [Forest increment]. Izdatel'stvo lesnaja promyšlennost', Moscow, 240 p

Assmann E (1970) The principles of forest yield study. Studies in the organic production, structure, increment and yield of forest stands. Pergamon Press, Oxford, 506 p

Bailey RL, Clutter JL (1974) Base-age invariant polymorphic site curves. For Sci 20:155–159

Bentil DE, Osei BM, Ellingwood CD, Hoffmann JP (2007) Analysis of a Schnute postulate-based unified growth mode for model selection in evolutionary computations. BioSystems 90:467–474

Bigler C, Bugmann H (2003) Growth-dependent tree mortality models based on tree rings. Can J For Res 33:210–221

Biondi F, Myers DE, Avery CC (1994) Geostatistically modeling stem size and increment in an old-growth forest. Can J For Res 24:1354–1368

Blackman VH (1919) The compound interest law and plant growth. Ann Bot 33:353–360

Bolker BM (2008) Ecological models and data in R. Princeton University Press, Princeton, 396 p

Brand DG, Weetman GF, Rehsler P (1987) Growth analysis of perennial plants: the relative production rate and its yield components. Ann Bot 59:45–53

Burkhart HE, Tomé M (2012) Modeling forest trees and stands. Springer, New York, 457 p

Cao QV (2014) Linking individual-tree and whole-stand models for forest growth and yield prediction. For Ecosyst 1:1–8

Causton DR (1977) A biologist's mathematics. Edward Arnold, London, 326 p

Causton DR, Venus JC (1981) The biometry of plant growth. Edward Arnold, London, 307 p

Dyer ME (1997) Dominance/suppression competitive relationships in loblolly pine (Pinus taeda L.) plantations. PhD dissertation, Virginia Tech, Blacksburg, Virginia, USA, 155 p

Edwards PN, Christie JM (1981) Yield models for forest management. Forestry Commission Booklet, vol 48. Forestry Commission, Edinburgh, 32 p

Enquist BJ, Niklas KJ (2001) Invariant scaling relations across tree-dominated communities. Nature 410:655–741

Evans GC (1972) The quantitative analysis of plant growth. Blackwell Scientific Publications, Oxford, 734 p

Fisher RA (1921) Some remarks on the methods formulated in a recent article on "The quantitative analysis of plant growth". Ann Appl Biol 7:367–372

Gayon J (2000) History of the concept of allometry. Am Zool 40:748–758

Gerold D, Römisch K (1977) Eine Möglichkeit zur Ableitung jährlicher Zuwachsprozente aus 10-jährigen Prozenten [A method for deriving annual relative increment from 10-year values]. Wissenschaftliche Zeitschrift der Technischen Universität Dresden 26:945–946

Gompertz B (1825) On the nature of the function expressive of the law of human mortality, and on a new mode of determining the value of life contingencies. Philos Trans R Soc 115:513–585

Grime JP (1977) Evidence for the existence of three primary strategies in plants and its relevance to ecological and evolutionary theory. Am Nat 111:1169–1194

Grime JP, Hunt R (1975) Relative growth rate: it's range and adaptive significance in a local flora. J Ecol 63:393–422

Hoffmann WA, Poorter H (2002) Avoiding bias in calculations of relative growth rate. Ann Bot 80:37–42

Houghton J, Thompson K, Rees M (2013) Does seed mass drive the differences in relative growth rate between growth forms? Proc R Soc B 280:20130921

Hughes AP, Freeman PR (1967) Growth analysis using frequent small harvests. J Appl Ecol 4:553–560

Hunt R (1982) Plant growth curves: the functional approach to plant growth analysis. Cambridge University Press, Cambridge, 248 p

Hunt R (1990) Basic growth analysis: plant growth analysis for beginners. Unwin Hyman, London, 112 p

Hunt R (2003) Growth analysis, individual plants. In: Thomas B, Murphy DJ, Murray D (eds) Encyclopaedia of applied plant sciences. Academic Press, London, pp 588–596

Hunt R, Cornelissen JHC (1997) Components of relative growth rate and their interrelations in 59 temperate plant species. New Phytol 135:395–417

Huxley JS (1932) Problems of relative growth. Lincoln Mac Veagh Dial - The Dial Press, New York, 276 p

Iida Y, Poorter L, Sterck F, Rahman Kassim A, Potts MD, Kubo T, Kohyama TS (2014) Linking size-dependent growth and mortality with architectural traits across 145 co-occuring tropical tree species. Ecology 95:353–363

Ingestad T (1982) Relative addition rate and external concentration; driving variables used in plant nutrition research. Plant Cell Environ 91:443–453

Jones O, Maillardet R, Robinson A (2009) Introduction to scientific programming and simulation using R. Chapman & Hall/CRC, Boca Raton, 453 p

Jørgensen SE, Patten BC, Straškraba M (2000) Ecosystems emerging: 4. growth. Ecol Model 126:249–284

Kangas Y (1968) Beschreibung des Wachstums der Bäume als Funktion ihres Alters [Describing the growth of trees as a function of age]. Acta Forestalia Fennica 90:136 (Helsinki)

Laird AK, Tyler SA, Barton AD (1965) Dynamics of normal growth. Growth 29:233–248

Larocque GR, Marshall PL (1993) Evaluating the impact of competition using relative growth rate in red pine (Pinus resinosa Ait.) stands. For Ecol Manag 58:65–83

Legendre P, Legendre L (2012) Numerical ecology, 3rd edn. Elsevier. Oxford, 990 p

LeMay V, Pommerening A, Marshall P (2009) Spatio-temporal structure of multi-storied, multi-aged interior Douglas fir (Pseudotsuga menziesii var. glauca) stands. J Ecol 97:1062–1074

Lundqvist B (1957) On the height growth in cultivated stands of pine and spruce in Northern Sweden. Meddelande fran Statens Skogsforsk 47:64

Matthews RW, Mackie ED (2006) Forest mensuration: a handbook for practitioners. Forestry Commission, Edinburgh, 330 p

McCarthy MC, Enquist BJ (2007) Consistency between an allometric approach and optimal partitioning theory in global patterns of plant biomass allocation. Funct Ecol 21:713–720

Mosimann JE (1970) Size allometry: size and shape variables with characterizations of the lognor-
mal and generalized gamma distributions. J Am Stat Assoc 65:930–945

Müller U (1915) Lehrbuch der Holzmeßkunde [Forest mensuration], 2nd edn. Verlagsbuchhandlung
Paul Parey, Berlin, 398 p

Murphy ST, Pommerening A (2010) Modelling the growth of Sitka spruce (Picea sitchensis (Bong.)
Carr.) in Wales using Wenk's model approach. Allg Forst Und Jagdztg 181:35–43

Niklas KJ, Spatz H-Ch (2012) Plant physics. The University of Chicago Press, Chicago, 426 p

Nowacki GJ, Abrams MD (1997) Radial-growth averaging criteria for reconstructing disturbance
histories from presettlement-origin oaks. Ecol Monogr 67:225–249

Paine CE, Marthews TR, Vogt DR, Purves D, Rees M, Hector A, Turnbull LA (2012) How to fit
nonlinear plant growth models and calculate growth rates: an update for ecologists. Methods Ecol
Evol 3:245–256

Paul-Victor C, Züst T, Rees M, Kliebenstein DJ, Turnbull LA (2010) A new method for measuring
relative growth rate can uncover the costs of defensive compounds in Arabidopsis thaliana. New
Phytol 187:1102–1111

Philipson CD, Saner P, Marthews TR, Nilus R, Reynolds G, Turnbull LA, Hector A (2012) Light-
based regeneration niches: evidence from 21 dipterocarp species using size-specific RGRs.
Biotropica 44:627–636

Pienaar LV, Turnbull KJ (1973) The Chapman-Richards generalization of von Bertalanffy's growth
model for basal area growth and yield in even-aged stands. For Sci 19:2–22

Pommerening A, Muszta A (2015) Methods of modelling relative plant growth rate. For Ecosyst
2:5

Pommerening A, Muszta A (2016) Relative plant growth revisited: towards a mathematical standardisation of separate approaches. Ecol Model 320:383–392

Pressler M (1865) Das Gesetz der Stammbildung [The law of stem formation]. Verlag Arnold,
Leipzig, 153 p

Pretzsch H (2009) Forest dynamics, growth and yield: from measurement to model. Springer,
Heidelberg, 664 p

Pretzsch H (2010) Re-evaluation of allometry: state-of-the-art and perspective regarding individuals
and stands of woody plants. In: Lüttge U, Beyschlag W, Nüdel B, Francis D (eds) Progress in
Botany, vol 71. Springer, Heidelberg, pp 339–369

Prodan M (1965) Holzmesslehre [Forest mensuration]. J. D. Sauerländer's Verlag, Frankfurt, 644 p

Ramseier J, Weiner A (2006) Competitive effect is a linear function of neighbour biomass in
experimental populations of Kochia scoparia. J Ecol 94:305–309

Rees M, Osborne CP, Woodward FI, Hulme SP, Turnbull LA, Taylor SH (2010) Partitioning the
components of relative growth rate: how important is plant size variation. Am Nat 176:E152–E161

Richards FJ (1959) A flexible growth function for empirical use. J Exp Bot 10:290–300

Rose KE, Atkinson RL, Turnbull LA, Rees M (2009) The costs and benefits of fast living. Ecol Lett
12:1379–1384

Ryan MG, Binkley D, Fowness JH (1997) Age-related decline in forest productivity: pattern and
process. Adv Ecol Res 27:213–262

Schnute J (1981) A versatile growth model with statistically stable parameters. Can J Fish Aquat
Sci 38:1128–1140

Schütz JP (2001) Der Plenterwald und weitere Formen strukturierter und gemischter Wälder [The
selection forest and other types os structured and mixed species forests]. Parey Buchverlag, Berlin,
207 p

Schütz JP, Pommerening A (2013) Can Douglas fir (Pseudotsuga menziesii (Mirb.) Franco) sustainably grow in complex forest structures? For Ecol Manag 303:175–183

Shimojo M, Asano Y, Ikeda K, Ishiwaka R, Shao T, Sato H, Matsufuji Y, Ohba N, Tobisa M, Yano
Y, Masuda Y (2002) Basic growth analysis and symmetric properties of exponential function
with base e. J Fac Agric Kyushu Univ 47:55–60

Shimojo, M (2006) Introducing viewpoints of mechanics into basic growth analysis-(II) relative growth rate compared with energy in wave function. J Fac Agric Kyushu Univ 51:289–291

Shipley B (2006) Net assimilation rate, specific leaf area and leaf mass ratio: which is most closely correlated with relative growth rate? A meta-analysis. Funct Ecol 20:565–574

Teissier G (1934) Dysharmonies et discontinuités dans la croissance [Disharmonies and discontinuities in growth]. Acta Science et Industrie, vol 95. Hermann, Paris, 620 p

Turnbull LA, Paul-Victor C, Schmid B, Purves DW (2008) Growth rates, seed size and physiology: do small-seeded species really grow faster? Ecology 89:1352–1363

van Laar A, Akça A (2007) Forest mensuration. Managing forest ecosystems, vol 13. Springer, Dordrecht, 383 p

Vanclay JK (1994) Modelling forest growth and yield: applications to mixed tropical forests. CABI Publishing, Wallingford, 312 p

Verhulst P-F (1838) Notice sur la loi que la population pursuit dans son accroissement [A note on population growth]. Correspondence Mathematiques et Physiques 10:113–121

von Bertalanffy L (1951) Theoretische biologie (Theoretical biology), vol 2. Zürich, 418 p

von Bertalanffy L (1957) Quantitative laws in metabolism and growth. Q Rev Biol 32:217–231

Warton DI, Wright IJ, Falster DS, Westoby M (2006) Bivariate line-fitting methods for allometry. Biol Rev 81:259–291

Warton DI, Duursma RA, Falster DS, Taskinen S (2012) Smatr 3 - an R package for estimation and inference about allometric lines. Methods Ecol Evol 3:257–259

Weber R (1891) Lehrbuch der Forsteinrichtung [Textbook of forest planning]. Springer, Berlin, 468 p

Weiner J, Stoll P, Muller-Landau H, Jasentuliyana A (2001) The effects of density, spatial pattern, and competitive symmetry on size variation in simulated plant populations. Am Nat 158:438–450

Wenk G (1969) Eine neue Wachstumsgleichung und ihr praktischer Nutzen zur Herleitung von Volumenzuwachsprozenten [A new growth equation and its practical use to derive volume increment]. Archiv für Forstwesen 18:1085–1094

Wenk G (1972) Zuwachsprognosen, Vorratsfortschreibung und Aufstellung bestandesindividueller Ertragstafeln mit Hilfe von Wachstumsmultiplikatoren [Increment prognoses, projection of stand volume and stand-specific yield tables on the basis of growth multipliers]. Wissenschaftliche Zeitschrift der Technischen Universität Dresden 21:1247–1249

Wenk G (1978) Mathematische Formulierung von Wachstumsprozessen in der Forstwirtschaft [Mathematical formulation of growth processes in forestry]. Beiträge für die Forstwirtschaft, vol 1, pp 25–30

Wenk G (1994) A yield prediction model for pure and mixed stands. For Ecol Manag 69:259–268

Wenk G, Antanaitis V, Šmelko Š (1990) Waldertragslehre [Forest growth and yield science]. Deutscher Landwirtschaftsverlag, Berlin, 448 p

Wenk G, Nicke A (1985) Zur Prognose der Bestandesentwicklung [Projecting stand development]. Beiträge für die Forstwirtschaft 173–176

West GB, Brown JH (2005) The origin of allometric scaling laws in biology from genomes to ecosystems: towards a quantitative unifying theory of biological structure and organization. J Exp Biol 208:1575–1592

West C, Briggs GE, Kidd F (1920) Methods and significant relations in the quantitative analysis of plant growth. New Phytol 19:200–207

Whitehead FH, Myerscough PJ (1962) Growth analysis of plants. The ratio of mean relative growth rate to mean relative rate of leaf area increase. New Phytol 61:314–321

Winsor CP (1932) The Gompertz curve as a growth curve. Proc Natl Acad Sci 18:1–8

Zeide B (1989) Accuracy of equations describing diameter growth. Can J For Res 19:1283–1286

Zeide B (1993) Analysis of growth equations. For Sci 39:594–616

Zhao X, Corral-Rivas J, Temesgen H, von Gadow K (2014) Forest observational studies - an essential infrastructure for sustainable use of natural resources. For Ecosyst 1:8

Chapter 7
Human Disturbances and Tree Selection Behaviour

Abstract Natural disturbances and disturbances caused by humans are common and frequent features in forest ecosystems and there are also interactions between these two types of disturbances. Some specialised ecosystems even owe their existence and structure to the regular occurrence of disturbances. Given the comparatively long lifetime of managed and natural forests, disturbances are inevitable and, given the global environmental and societal changes of our age, are likely to increase. Studying natural disturbances has a fairly long tradition in forest ecology, however, anthropogenic disturbances such as those caused by accidental human activities and by professional forest management have so far received comparatively little attention. Yet they often influence forest structures much more than natural disturbances and other processes. A new type of experiment, the *marteloscope*, has emerged and was designed to carry out research on human decision making and marking behaviour in forests. It complements existing types of experiments and can also be combined with computer experiments that extend traditional field experiments and allow time-lapse analyses.

7.1 Impacts and Disturbances

Impacts and disturbances are related concepts. *Impact* is usually understood as a high force or shock, a collision, i.e. the action of one object coming forcibly into contact with another, an effect or influence. This includes the striking of one body against another, the force or impetus transmitted by a collision and the (powerful) effect or the impression of one thing, person or action on another (Hornby 2010, p. 778). Helms (1998, p. 93) noted that impact is a spatial or temporal change in the environment caused by human activity. Newton (2007, p. 213) pointed out that *impact assessment* "is designed to assess the impact of human activities (such as timber harvesting or deforestation) by comparing results of models with and without the human activity". In research, for example, it is possible to quantify the impact of scientific journals in various research communities and this is known as *impact factor*.

© Springer Nature Switzerland AG 2019
A. Pommerening and P. Grabarnik, *Individual-based Methods*
in Forest Ecology and Management, https://doi.org/10.1007/978-3-030-24528-3_7

A common thought associated with the term impact and cause to much anxiety is the possible collision of meteorites with our planet Earth. However, impact analysis is also a common term outside natural sciences in regulatory/jurisdictional and in economic fields where the likely consequences of new measures are anticipated and conflicts with other measures are identified before they are introduced. In fact, this rationale is also the basis of impact analysis in forest management and of the marteloscope experiment described in this chapter. Incidentally, in Britain and Ireland, variants of continuous cover forestry are referred to as low impact silviculture and low impact silvicultural systems (LISS) (Pommerening and Murphy 2004, see Sect. 3.4).

In ecology, the impacts of *disturbances* can only be analysed *retrospectively*, i.e. after they have happened. Puettmann et al. (2009, p. 150), Helms (1998, p. 49), Kimmins (2004, p. 520) and Newton (2007, p. 148) have suggested elements of the following definition of disturbance:

> Any sudden, temporary, discrete and relatively rare event that causes a profound change and disruption in the dynamic, functions and/or structure of an ecosystem, a community or a population and change the availability of resources or the physical environment. Typical natural ecological disturbances are fires, flooding, windstorm and insect outbreak. Typical anthropogenic disturbances include thinning and harvesting.

Impacts and disturbances cause major disruptions but also provide opportunities for new directions in the development of forest ecosystems and they trigger successional processes (Röhrig et al. 2006, p. 33). They have a profound effect on forest development, since they kill vegetation and thus release growing space, making it available to other plants to occupy and are major determinants of forest structures (Oliver and Larson 1996, p. 89ff.). Disturbances have traditionally been divided into *exogenous*, i.e. those originating outside the ecosystem (e.g. fire, wind, pollutants, introduced animals or pathogens, humans etc.) and *endogenous*, i.e. those originating from within the system (e.g. epidemics of native insects and pathogens, herbivory etc.). In practice, it is quite difficult to separate the two due to their interrelatedness (Perry et al. 2008, p. 86).

Risk is a term referring to the flip side of disturbances and express, particularly in terms of wind and fire, the anxiety associated with human thinking about loss of trees and capital. For a long time until almost recently this way of thinking was predominant in forestry. For a long time disturbances were considered only a bad thing to be avoided and prevented. From a conservation point of view there has been the attitude that human disturbances irrevocably damage a forest stand (Oliver and Larson 1996, p. 91). Interestingly, some ecologists view human interventions that limit natural disturbances as the real disturbance agents (Peter Attiwill, pers. comm. cited in Puettmann et al. 2009, p. 89).

Otto (1994, p. 322ff.) referred to disturbances as "break downs in forests", which can be characterised by sudden drops in basal area or biomass of live trees. In his opinion, disturbances are the most important drivers of forest dynamics and completely new directions of forest development are possible. Often setbacks to earlier phases of stand development or succession occur. Puettmann et al. (2009, p. 143ff.) have advocated that forest managers should view disturbances and associated impacts on ecosystems in a similar manner to insurance companies, i.e. by considering overall disturbance probabilities and by accepting a wider range of possible outcomes for individual forest stands. According to this view, undisturbed forests are no longer regarded as the norm and the stochastic nature as well as the uncertainty of ecological processes are fully taken into account. This view opens up opportunities providing flexibility for forest managers and planners to use a wider range of treatments and to work with natural processes. As a consequence forest stands are allowed to develop within an envelope or *realisation space* of possible conditions and multiple development trajectories are acceptable.

Consider, for example, a concept where the maximum basal area development, i.e. the natural basal area development, which represents the carrying capacity of a given site, defines the upper envelope of the realisation space (Fig. 7.1).

The dashed green curve corresponds to 80% of maximum basal area development. A possible and plausible convention is that thinnings are triggered whenever the current basal area reaches or exceeds the dashed curve. The dotted dark blue and the solid light blue curves represent two possible development paths within a time window defined by t_0 and t_1 that eventually lead to two different final states (Gadow 2005, p. 265). Obviously basal area can be replaced by biomass and other suitable measures including a combination of variables.

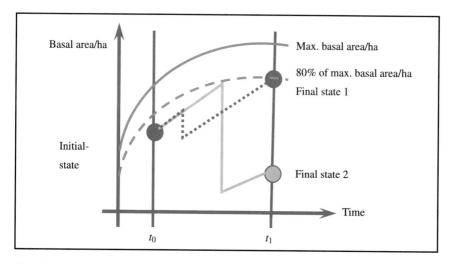

Fig. 7.1 Realisation space limited by the maximum basal area development over time and two possible development trajectories (modified from Gadow 2005, p. 265)

In this context, Kimmins (2004, p. 602ff.) coined the term *ecological rotation* (ER) in analogy to rotations in forestry and defined it as

> Period required for a given site to return to the predisturbance ecological condition or to some other desired stage.

The definition clearly stresses the similarity between natural and anthropogenic disturbances. Kimmins (2004, p. 605) also stated that the length of an ecological rotation is determined by three variables, namely

- the degree to which the ecosystem condition has been altered by disturbance,
- the rate at which the ecosystem condition recovers from disturbance and
- the frequency with which disturbance is repeated.

Two of these variables are strikingly similar to two forest management parameters of thinnings, i.e. thinning intensity and thinning cycle, see Sect. 3.6. Disturbances can last for a short time in the case of fires or windstorms or much longer periods, such as during a glacier's advance and retreat (Oliver and Larson 1996, p. 89). Gibson (2002) and Newton (2007, p. 148) maintained that disturbance regimes should be described using the following characteristics:

Extent   and spatial pattern of the disturbed area,

Intensity   or the strength of the disturbance (e.g. fire temperature or wind speed),

Severity   or the amount of damage that occurred to the forest (e.g. the number of individual trees killed or damaged),

Timing   including the frequency (the number of disturbances per unit time), the turnover rate or rotation period (the mean time taken for the entire forest area to be disturbed) and the turnover time or return interval (the mean time between disturbances),

Interactions between different types of disturbance (e.g. drought increases fire intensity).

For each of these characteristics mean, mode or median as well as variation should be calculated and presented together with frequency distributions in order to fully characterise a disturbance regime (Gibson 2002; Newton 2007, p. 148).

Impact events and disturbances typically lead to a loss of trees/reduction of tree density and to a modification of forest structure. As a consequence the microclimate, patterns of ground vegetation, nutrient cycles and tree growth change among others. The significance of disturbances is the creation of available growing space by elimination of plants previously occupying the growing space (Oliver and Larson 1996, p. 89).

After humans and fire, wind is probably the most common disturbance to forests with scales of damage that range from single tree to many hectares (Perry et al. 2008, p. 108). Other natural disturbances include floodings, snow/ice, frost and drought events, pathogens and invasive species.

The assessment of the impact of human activities on forests is of fundamental importance for conservation planning and management. Often, a key objective is to determine whether a given forest is able to withstand or tolerate a particular anthropogenic disturbance regime. Such analyses lie at the heart of defining approaches to sustainable forest management and depend not only on characterising the disturbance regime, but on understanding how the forest responds to different types and patterns of disturbance (Newton 2007; Kimmins 2004, p. 149 and p. 516ff., respectively).

Kramer (1988, p. 201f.) provided interesting examples of interactions between natural and anthropogenic disturbance regimes. As it has been a long-standing desire in forest management to mitigate negative effects of disturbances on forests, particularly wind and snow, this interaction has been studied comparatively well. The fact that for example thinnings in Norway spruce (*Picea abies* (L.) KARST.) plantations have caused windthrow immediately after the event and with increasing top height has given rise to successful thinning regimes that address this problem with adaptive thinning regimes. Forest cutting, burning, land clearing and other human disturbances partly mask and minimise the effects of natural disturbance. In managed forests, human disturbances are generally more frequent than natural ones (Oliver and Larson 1996, p. 93).

Gadow (1996) reflecting on changes in forests stated that modifications of forest structure caused by management are not always taken very seriously in the scientific literature although they often have a far greater effect on forest development than

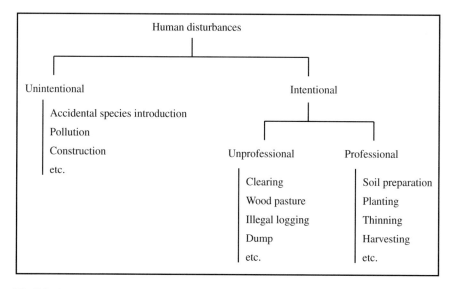

Fig. 7.2 Overview of human disturbances in forest ecosystems

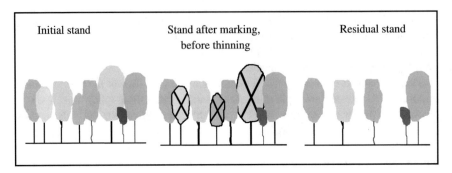

Fig. 7.3 The principle of the thinning-event analysis: Human marking behaviour is analysed immediately after marking a forest stand and before trees are felled. This provides the opportunity of
revising the decision making. The initial forest stand, the stand after marking but before thinning
and the residual stand are analysed simultaneously. Adapted from Gadow (2005, p. 56)

natural growth. Human disturbances can be *unintentional* and *intentional, unpro-
fessional* and *professional* (see Fig. 7.2). They generally have similar basic effects
on forests, i.e. trees cease to live and forest structure is modified. However, there
are a number of special properties associated with anthropogenic disturbances. The
intentional professional ones are usually planned, i.e. the associated objectives and
the time, when the event is scheduled for, are known. This allows an impact analysis
before the actual intervention is carried out and at least theoretically corrections,
if necessary, can be made prior to implementation, i.e. prior to actually cutting the
trees, see Fig. 7.3. This situation is reminiscent of the idea of a dependent permanent
sample, i.e. two different forest states are measured at the same time and at the same
location thus reducing the sampling error by the possibility of subtracting twice the
covariance (Mandallaz 2008, p. 185ff., see Sect. 1.4).

7.2 Human Tree Selection and Marking Behaviour

In the preface of his textbook "Planning in a Forest Enterprise" from 1972, Gerhard
Speidel wrote that the environment we currently live in owes much to the decisions
of human beings. He concluded that "decision making is among the most fascinating
and most responsible activities in this world". At the most basic level decision making
in forest management often relates to the selection of individual trees in a thinning
or harvesting context, e.g. which trees to leave in a forest stand and which to remove.
What factors influence the decision making and to what degree do decisions differ
between different persons? Do different decisions matter at all?

    If adopting a wide perspective, the idea of analysing intentional professional
human disturbances and producing outcome summaries has a long tradition in forest
growth and yield. Since the end of the 19th century systematic trials have been carried
out with the objective to study the interaction between natural processes, i.e. mainly
growth, birth and death processes, on one hand and goal-oriented human disturbances
on the other (Pretzsch 2009, p. 101ff.).

The first meaningful results of these experiments have been available since the 1950s (Sterba 2010) and the book publications by Assmann (1970) and Kramer (1988) provided good summaries of this research. All the experiments reported in these books have in common that human disturbances were carried out as ideal or textbook treatments to identify the best course of action for a given objective.

In the past, it was often assumed that humans marking trees for thinnings or as habitat trees, do this more or less precisely according to textbook opinions, forest plans or other instructions. However in practical forest management, thinnings and other forest operations are not always carried out according to plan or according to textbooks. The selection of supposedly "desirable", "undesirable" or indifferent trees for a given purpose, may that be timber production or conservation, is a challenging task for any human being and a serious limitation on the potential for continuous cover forestry in some countries (Pommerening et al. 2015). Often decision making in the field is delegated to staff that have not enjoyed a university education in ecology and forest management or have little experience in marking trees. Even given the same management objectives the marking behaviour of several experienced foresters or machine operators can be very different. Naturally, no matter how detailed instructions are, there is likely to be some variation between the decision making of different individuals. This can be referred to as *variability between people*. On the other hand even one and the same experienced forest manager can make different decisions concerning which trees to select for thinnings or other purposes when asked at different times during the course of a year. As any human behaviour, also tree marking behaviour depends on weather, general mood and starting point in the forest to name but a few factors. This can be considered as *variability within people*.

Idealised textbook forest management is also often assumed in tree growth models that allow the forest manager to project the current forest state into the future. Such models are an essential tool for identifying the best course of action in long-term sustainable forest management. However, how many of these projections are really helpful, if they do not account for the uncertainty introduced by human decision making in these calculations?

Human tree selection behaviour also goes far beyond the question of tree selection for thinnings. The same basic research questions arise when selecting habitat trees for conservation, when people choose trees for their burial in forest cemeteries or visitors decide, which tree to have their picnic under, and when selecting Christmas trees in a Christmas tree plantation. All this is about decision making on individual trees in forests, the behaviour of humans in the environment and about interactions between humans and trees. However, the same questions and methodology can also be applied to the selection of trees by deers and squirrels for bark stripping or browsing and to similar tree selections by animals. Considering the two main factors, humans and trees, the decision process is influenced by both of them, i.e. partly by human predisposition and preferences and partly by the trees that attract different humans in different ways.

There are a number of fundamental research questions. First, it is useful to establish how much agreement there is actually among test persons. After quantifying the general agreement, clusters of similar behaviour and outliers must be identified, in order to uncover those individuals that made the largest contribution to the lack of agreement. Covariates such as tree size, timber quality, habitat value but also personal background information can then help to explain the individual behaviour. Finally the question must be addressed, if the lack of agreement matters or whether there is a sufficiently common pattern in the selection behaviour that is compatible with the corresponding forest management objectives. Specific research questions include

- Can different tree selection behaviour be attributed to, for example, gender, age or occupation?
- Do forestry staff educated in different institutions select trees differently?
- Is there any geographic relationship?
- How do individuals respond to training and are they willing to change their behaviour?
- What effect do tree species composition and structure have on tree selection?

Gadow (2005) referred to the analysis of human disturbances as a method of silvicultural controlling, as a preventive sustainability control and as truly adaptive management, since the decisions made can be revised before final implementation (see Fig. 7.3). In addition, forest impact analysis leads to transparency of decision making in forest management and thus to professional credibility. It also provides useful information for modelling person-specific thinning and harvesting strategies to be incorporated in tree and forest simulators. The analysis of human disturbances helps to predict the consequences of interventions and keeps data up to date. Research in human tree selection behaviour has only begun and constitutes basic research with a large potential to bridge natural sciences and psychology. In an ideal way it combines basic research with science that is highly relevant to the forest industry at the same time. It is an inspiring, novel research direction at the interface between natural sciences, social sciences, psychology and ecology using strictly interdisciplinary approaches by combining statistical and other methods from outside forest science with forestry knowledge. This research is of strategic interest to forest companies, forest administrations and conservation agencies. Since marteloscopes are increasingly used in forestry related training and education, the research methods introduced in this chapter can also be used for assessing the quality of training programmes and the training needs of different parts of society. Marking exercises and training sessions clearly improve forestry education and training and contribute to life-long learning and continuing professional development. Thus forestry staff can re-confirm skills and knowledge in regular sessions similar to hunters and stalkers who have to train the command of their weapons on a regular basis and acquire new skills. This is particular important in times of global changes and helps to adopt adaptive management in situations where known relationships rapidly invalidate (Pommerening et al. 2015). There is also great potential for *citizen science* (Hecker et al. 2018): Pommerening et al. (2018), for example, analysed the data from 36 forestry training events in Great Britain that were provided by the Ae Training Centre of the GB Forestry Commission and published them jointly. Considerable added value can be created by training organisations joining forces with specialised analysts who can then help to analyse global trends in thinning behaviour and to assess training quality. Finally, even as part of open-day events at universities and colleges marking exercises and experiments can be organised to motivate prospective students. In the same way other groups of people outside forestry with a very different professional background can carry out tree markings as team-building events.

7.2.1 Problem and Origins

Many problems in medicine, politics and psychology are related to situations where a certain number of individuals select subjects or items from a range of choices (Stoyan et al. 2018b). For example pathologists may independently consider histological samples and judge on absence or presence of carcinoma (Stoyan et al. 2018a). In elections, usually a large number of voters vote for their parties and political representatives of choice (Brams and Fishburn 1978) and this method is studied in political science with a view to understand the election process and the behaviour of voters has been termed *approval voting*. In the statistical literature, test persons are referred to as raters (see for example Fleiss et al. 2003). Using this term we can describe the general problem as follows:

There is a group of r raters or voters and n subjects, items or candidates. Every rater evaluates every item by marking approvals by "1" and disapprovals by "0", i.e. the classification is binary. The array of $r \times n$ marks "0" and "1" is considered as data and analysed in various ways by well-known statistical methods. In the application of tree selection behaviour, r is relatively small and n comparatively large, i.e. a relatively small number of raters rates a large number of items (Stoyan et al. 2018b).

This definition shows that the selection of items and the behaviour of humans performing this selection is in fact a very common problem that is also studied in other research fields. It is not specific to forest science and has entered this domain only comparatively late. In the mid 1990s, Prof. Klaus von Gadow initiated a research group at Göttingen University in Germany investigating the tree selection behaviour of forest managers and machine operators in different forest ecosystems. The group designed a special survey method for data gathering which went by the names *thinning-event inventory* and *harvesting-event inventory*. The key idea of this survey method was to schedule the data gathering at the time of tree marking prior to the actual tree removal. In contrast to traditional forest inventory methods, the thinning-event inventory captured both the initial forest stand conditions and the residual stand at the same time. The changes in forest structure could then be analysed and decisions could be revised if necessary (see Fig. 7.3).

Towards the end of the 1990s a group at AgroParisTech-ENGREF at Nancy
(France) around Max Bruciamacchie realised the potential of this research idea for
training and education in forest management. The group at Nancy offered field-based
training courses to forestry professionals and students. In these courses, the participants were then asked to mark trees for thinnings on a sheet of paper similar to a
questionnaire. Their choices were analysed using specialised software or MS Excel
macros. Personalised result and feedback sheets were handed out to every participant at the end of the training session. In order to attach a new brand to this type
of research plot, the group at Nancy coined the name marteloscope (from French
martelage—marking) for these training sites. From these beginnings the idea of
marteloscopes spread through the networks of ProSilva, AFI (Association Futaie
Irrégulière) and other professional forestry organisations in France, Switzerland,
Britain and Ireland.

In the first decade of this century, the first author and his Tyfiant Coed project team
at Bangor University used the marteloscope idea in a training project in North Wales.
Poore (2011), Susse et al. (2011) and Soucy et al. (2016) described the application
of marteloscopes for education and training:

> The marteloscope is a didactic tool and a permanent plot within the forest
> in which tree measurements and associated software are linked to provide a
> framework for in-forest training in selection and as part of integrated training
> in silviculture.

The popularity of marteloscopes is currently on the increase, however, its original
research purpose has only been pursued at few institutions.

Early studies have already cast doubt on the assumption that forestry staff select
trees in good agreement (Zucchini and Gadow 1995; Füldner et al. 1996; Daume
et al. 1997). The authors of these studies have found only little agreement in the
marking behaviour among forestry professionals.

Spinelli et al. (2016) studied the silvicultural results (in terms of basal area and
trees per hectare) performed by a number of test persons with different professional
backgrounds in mixed continuous-cover-forestry woodlands in Northern Italy. They
found no significant difference in the marking behaviour of test persons from different
professional groups, however, they also identified a substantial lack of agreement in
terms of the selection of individual trees. The authors speculated that different practical experience in tree marking is a possible explanation for the lack of agreement.

Vítková et al. (2016) could demonstrate that education and subsequent training can
profile people's choices in terms of tree selection behaviour. The authors reported tree
marking experiments involving test persons with different experience and education.
They required the test persons to perform the marking twice in the same experimental
forest, once before and once after training in crown thinning methods. Experts were
reluctant to adopt the new thinning method and the training led to confusion and
decreasing agreement in this group. In contrast, novices, i.e. test persons without

previous experience, responded well to the training and the agreement in this group was significantly higher than among the experts.

Pommerening et al. (2018) also found little agreement in tree marking when analysing 36 marteloscope experiments from all over Britain, where two different thinning types were applied, i.e. crown and low thinning. Overall agreement was low but particularly so in crown-thinning experiments. As the latter is an important method of continuous cover forestry (see Sect. 3.4) and British forestry is increasingly adopting this forest management type, the authors' results suggested that there is a need to provide more training related to crown thinnings. Interestingly there was no correlation between measures of forest structure and Fleiss' kappa or other agreement characteristics. The authors also found that more complex forest structure appears to facilitate the decision process.

7.2.2 Marteloscope Experiments

A marteloscope is typically set up as a research plot with rectangular boundaries (see also Appendix B). 100×100 m is often a suitable size for long-term plots, where the number of trees to be included should ideally be between 150 and 500 trees. A marteloscope of this size takes a test person approximately three hours to complete. In general, the area should be sufficiently large so that the test persons do not influence each other's decision making. In a commercial forestry context, it can also be recommended to select an area where thinnings have not occurred during the last ten years, so that the thinning urgency is high. Otherwise the test persons may struggle to find sufficient options for decisions. For practical and statistical reasons it is good practice to consider setting up two marteloscope plots in the same forest type at close proximity (twin plots). As time goes by the two plots are thinned in turns by the local forest owner (as part of routine forest management) so that one twin can be used for marteloscope research or training at all times whilst the twin—i.e. the plot that has most recently been thinned—is used for demonstration purposes.

Every tree typically has a unique identity number, which is painted on the stem surface with waterproof paint as clearly as possible and should be visible from afar. If feasible one can consider painting tree numbers twice on each tree from opposite directions for better identification. A minimum of tree measurements should include stem diameters (with a lower threshold of 5–7 cm). In some countries, lower diameter thresholds of 17 cm are recommended. This, however, leads to heavily censored data that influence the test persons decisions (i.e. small trees cannot be selected) and ultimately to biased results.

Apart from stem diameter, surveying should ideally also include tree locations, total heights (at least on a sample basis), volume/biomass, habitat value and timber quality. Marteloscopes are not very different from research plots commonly used in silviculture and growth & yield research. In fact, plots from the latter two research fields can often be re-used as marteloscopes which offers the benefit of having past growth rates at the experimenter's disposal. In marteloscope experiments, however,

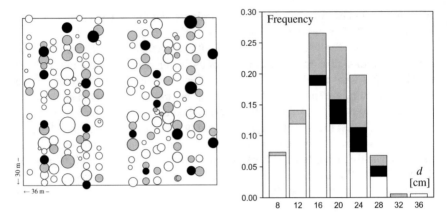

Fig. 7.4 Map and proportions of the frame (black) and competitor trees (grey) marked by one participant as part of a small temporary marteloscope experiment at Clocaenog Forest in North Wales (UK) in 2006. The proportions of the remaining trees are shown in white. Stem diameter is denoted by d

the research focus is primarily on humans and their behaviour. Part of this human behaviour naturally is the interaction with trees.

Mapping the stem centre locations of trees is useful for logistic and practical reasons, since maps can be produced (see Fig. 7.4, left). These help to maintain the experiment but can also serve as aids for orientation when handed out to test persons, particularly when the marteloscope area is large. The map can also be used to visualise the choice of a particular test person, as this is the case in Fig. 7.4 (left). The corresponding stacked empirical diameter distribution is an example of simple descriptive statistics (Fig. 7.4, right). In this case, an extraction rack runs through the centre of this Sitka-spruce *Picea sitchensis* (BONG.) CARR. marteloscope a curious feature, since the selection of trees near roads and rides has additional implications, e.g. the potential damage to live trees when extracting felled stems.

Table 7.1 gives an example of a simple marking sheet. The design of the marking sheet may vary considerably depending on the purpose of the training session or experiment and can also be implemented in a software application for tablet computers. The design of the marking sheet surely has an influence on the marking behaviour. It is therefore advisable to consider the design carefully and to be resourceful in order to achieve an unbiased outcome of the experiment. For example it is possible to leave the marking sheet completely blank and to ask the test persons to note only those trees that they want to select. Statistically speaking the marking sheet constitutes a questionnaire and handing out an empty sheet of paper to the test persons would probably reduce the influence of the marking sheet on the selection behaviour to a minimum.

In the data processing, the marking sheets are digitalised unless the data were already entered with a computer tablet during the marking process. A cross or tick

Table 7.1 Design of a typical, basic tree marking sheet for use in marteloscope research and training. DBH is stem diameter at breast height and measured in centimetres. "Frame" is short for frame tree and a mark in column "Thin" implies that a tree is selected for removal. Modified from Pommerening et al. (2015)

Tree No.	Species	DBH	Frame	Thin
1	Birch	55.4		×
2	Scots pine	60.6	×	
3	Scots pine	61.5		×
4	Birch	33.5		
5	Birch	42.1		
6	Scots pine	52.3		
7	Birch	15.6		
8	Birch	53.7		×
9	Scots pine	64.3	×	
10	Birch	24.2		
...	...	...		
...	...	...		
...	...	...		

indicating tree selection is converted to a '1'. No selection results in '0', so that a typical test-person data column consists of a sequence of 0's and 1's.

Prior to the experiment 10–20 test persons need to be recruited. The recruitment should support the purpose of the experiment, e.g. test persons could be recruited to achieve a balance in gender, geography of a given country, years of experience in forest management, education etc. It is, however, also possible to use existing or scheduled marteloscope training events for analysing the behaviour of trainees. In that situation, the analysis can provide valuable feedback to the training organisers and also help to evaluate the training quality.

Each marteloscope experiment must have clear objectives and depending on these more or less detailed instructions, example marking or even training is given to the test persons prior to the experiment. This is often accompanied by a brief qualitative and quantitative description of the forest stand (see Appendix A). Instructions should give the test persons an idea of the type(s) of trees to select and of the approximate number of trees and/or basal area to be marked. Vítková et al. (2016), for example, were interested in the test persons' ability to mark for crown thinnings (see Chap. 3) in Ireland and carried out one experiment each before and after delivering a training workshop on crown thinning with the same test persons. There must be a clear, measurable definition of the marking strategy the test persons are asked to adopt. However, it is also possible not to give any instructions at all in order to measure the intuitive behaviour of the test persons or their current state of knowledge/experience. This would be a very viable strategy for understanding traditional management practices of, for example, first nations. It is also an option to carry out one experiment without instructions and another one that gives clear instructions prior to the marking in order to understand how the test persons respond to them. Instructions become even more useful when supported by practical marking demonstrations in an adjacent woodland. An example instruction in a crown-thinning context is:

- Identify 80–120 frame trees per hectare, using timber quality as the main selection criterion.
- Thin to release frame trees, removing 1–3 competitors each as part of a crown thinning.
- Retain at least 18 m^2 ha^{-1} basal area.
- Place a tick next to trees you select for removal in the appropriate column of the marking sheet.

It is also good practice to record the test person's names, gender, work affiliation, professional and geographic backgrounds. Any additional information can potentially turn out as useful covariates or for post-stratification and aid the interpretation of the results. To this end specific forms requesting this information and perhaps also individual marking strategies can be of great value.

During the experiment the test persons should mark the trees on their marking sheets independently. This can be facilitated by sending them into the marteloscope at staggered times and from spatially different starting points. Should the experimental design include group work it is obviously important to note the group affiliations.

To avoid "strategic behaviour" the organiser should repeatedly assure the test persons that their results and any other personal data will be treated anonymously.

It is always a good idea to get the local forest manager on board and to secure her or his enthusiasm and support. S/he may even help to make a nearby cabin or small office available that can be used for analysing and printing the results on site, which is particularly useful in a training context. Then every test person should receive an individual result sheet for personal feedback. If requested the organiser should be prepared to walk the test persons through the marteloscope after the completion of the marking to discuss individual questions or interesting trees. It is a good idea to provide pencils and hot drinks in cold weather to pleasantly predispose test persons.

Pommerening et al. (2018) suggested subsetting trees of a given marteloscope in the analysis: In their research, the authors found evidence that differences in behaviour of different test persons can potentially be better elaborated when focussing on trees that are difficult to rate, since it is psychologically easier for humans to agree on obvious negative cases (Matonis et al. 2016). In practical terms, a group of experimenters could pre-select a subset of trees in a marteloscope that they collectively perceive as difficult to judge on. This subset is not revealed to the test persons. In the analysis, the experimenters then analyse the markings once for all trees and once for the subset only. This will allow to understand how trees that are difficult to judge on influence the outcome of the experiment.

7.2.3 Reference Marking

A key question often asked is what reference can be used to compare human decisions with. There is, of course, the possibility to compare with the marking of an established expert. However, also experts can make mistakes or have a certain agenda and there is always the danger that an expert marking is subjective. By contrast, basal area or volume growth rate is an objective criterion that can be used as a reference based on the idea of sustainability, i.e. that under normal circumstances not more should be removed than will re-grow until the next intervention is due, see Sect. 7.2.8. Under certain circumstances equilibrium models describing ideal sustainable size structures can also act as references (Schütz and Pommerening 2013; Brzeziecki et al. 2016). Another reference can, for example, be the dispersion of frame trees and yet other characteristics have a kind of internal reference like many spatial characteristics, see Chap. 4.

Spatial Simulation

For local thinning regimes (Chap. 3), the selection and permanent marking of frame trees is usually the first step in stand management. These frame trees are commonly the most vigorous trees in a given forest. They should also have an optimal spacing, e.g. either fairly regular (with maximum distances) or clustered (with minimum distances) pattern. In terms of the point process modelling approaches introduced in Chap. 5, this corresponds to the problem of modelling a spatial subprocess based on an existing point pattern that cannot be modified.

A simple example of how a computer simulation can provide an objective solution of this problem has been suggested by Pommerening and Särkkä (2013). The method guarantees a pattern of large-diameter frame trees that is as regular as possible similar to the idea of a Matérn hard-core process (Illian et al. 2008, p. 388f., Chap. 5), which is often a silvicultural requirement: At the beginning of a simulation n_f frame trees are selected. First, all trees are sorted by diameter in descending order (line 4 in the code below). Then the $1/3$ largest trees are appointed as candidate frame trees, ncand, (line 5). Now the number of candidate frame trees is reduced to n_f, the number of final frame trees, that form the most regular pattern among the largest trees of the forest. For this purpose each candidate frame tree i is marked by $\min(dist_j)$, the distance to the nearest candidate frame tree j (lines 8–16). Finally the frame tree candidate with the smaller stem diameter from the pair of trees with the smallest value of $\min(dist_j)$ is discarded and $\min(dist_j)$ is recomputed for the remaining frame tree candidates. This procedure is repeated until the specified number of final frame trees, n_f, is achieved (lines 18–44).

```
1  > selectFrameTreesHardCore <- function(fTrees, xmax, ymax,
2  + myData, denom) {
3  + numberFtrees <- (xmax * ymax) * fTrees / 10000
4  + myData <- myData[order(myData$dbh, decreasing = TRUE), ]
```

```
 5  + ncand <- trunc(length(myData$treeno) / denom)
 6  + helpindex <- rep(0, ncand)
 7  + d <- matrix(0, ncol = ncand, nrow = ncand)
 8  + for (i in 1 : ncand) {
 9  +   for (j in i : ncand) {
10  +   d[i, j] <- simpleEuclideanDistance(myData$x[i],
11  +   myData$y[i], myData$x[j], myData$y[j])
12  +   d[j, i] <- d[i, j]
13  +   if (i == j)
14  +     d[i, j] <- 10^6
15  +   }
16  + }
17  + nremove <- 0
18  + while(nremove < (ncand - numberFtrees)) {
19  +   minpair <- 10^3
20  +   for (i in 1 : (ncand - 1)) {
21  +     for (j in (i + 1) : ncand) {
22  +       if ((d[i, j] < minpair) & (helpindex[i] == 0) &
23  +       (helpindex[j] == 0)) {
24  +         minpair <- distin[i, j]
25  +         mini <- i
26  +         minj <- j
27  +       }
28  +     }
29  +   }
30  +   if (myData$dbh[mini] > myData$dbh[minj])
31  +     helpindex[minj] <- 1
32  +   if (myData$dbh[mini] < myData$dbh[minj])
33  +     helpindex[mini] <- 1
34  +   if (myData$dbh[mini] == myData$dbh[minj]) {
35  +     mink <- sample(c(mini, minj), 1)
36  +     helpindex[mink] <- 1
37  +   }
38  +   nremove <- nremove + 1
39  + }
40  + for (i in 1 : ncand)
41  +   if (helpindex[i] == 0)
42  +     myData$status[i] <- "F"
43  + return(myData)
44  + }
```

In the main R script, the function `selectFrameTreesHardCore` needs to be initialised and called like in the example below:

```
> fTrees <- 250
> xfrac <- 3
> trees$status <- "M"
> trees <- selectFrameTrees(fTrees, xmax, ymax, trees, xfrac)
```

Figure 7.5 shows an application of the above code to a beech (*Fagus sylvatica* L.) woodland in Switzerland (Pommerening and Särkkä 2013). On the left-hand side a regular dispersion of frame trees was simulated and a clustered dispersion with groups of 1–3 large frame trees per cluster on the right.

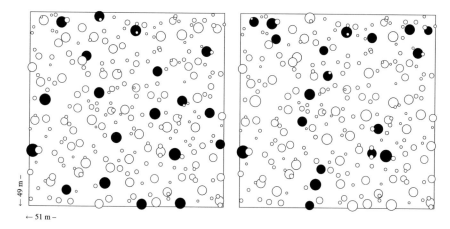

Fig. 7.5 Simulation of two different frame tree dispersion patterns in European beech (*Fagus sylvatica* L.) at Embrach (Switzerland). 19 trees out of 262 were selected as frame trees corresponding to 76 frame trees/ha. The most important criteria were size followed by distance, see Sect. 3.6.1. Modified from Pommerening and Särkkä (2013)

Nearest Neighbour Indices

As an objective reference for local thinning methods Johann (1982), for example, proposed the A-thinning index (Eq. 7.1). It was intended for selecting competitor trees in thinnings and has been implemented in some forest growth simulators. Pommerening and Sánchez Meador (2018) noted that the similarity of this index to competition indices used in forest ecology and management is striking and thus confirms that the ecological concept of competition has indeed had a strong influence on forest management.

The index defines a critical distance cd_j between tree i and its nearest neighbours depending on the thinning intensity parameter A:

$$cd_j = \frac{h_i}{A} \cdot \frac{d_j}{d_i} \qquad (7.1)$$

Any neighbouring tree j being located closer to tree i than the critical distance cd_j needs to be removed. Apart from the thinning intensity parameter A the index uses the height-diameter ratio (see Eq. 2.6) of tree i and the diameter d_j of the neighbouring tree j. The A-thinning index is sensitive to the h/d ratio of tree i: Trees with a larger h/d ratio are relatively more heavily released than those with a smaller h/d ratio. The values of A can range from 4 to 8 with decreasing thinning intensity,[1] although theoretically A is continuous and can take decimal numbers as well. Johann (1982) recommended values of 4, 5 and 6 for even-aged pure Norway spruce (*Picea abies* (L.) KARST.) forests which he considered to be synonymous with heavy, moderate and

---

[1] $A = 4$—very heavy, $A = 5$—heavy, $A = 6$—moderate, $A = 7$—weak, $A = 8$—very weak.

light release. A-values of 4 and 6 are frequently used values in thinning experiments (Hasenauer et al. 1996; Pretzsch 2009, p. 172f.).

Like competition indices (e.g. Biging and Dobbertin 1992; Moravie et al. 1999) the A-thinning index attempts to identify competitors of trees and to put thinning intensity on a quantitative basis. Hasenauer et al. (1996) and Pommerening and Sánchez Meador (2018) have demonstrated how this index can be used in the analysis of human-induced disturbances to quantify tree competition before and after thinning. The thinning intensity parameter A can also be interpreted as a proportionality factor between the height of tree i and the critical distance. Pretzsch (2009, p. 174ff.) pointed out that this proportional relationship does not hold for young forest stands with small diameters and older stands with larger diameters. In the first case thinnings turn out to be too weak and the latter they become too heavy. His recommendation was to modify the formula cd_j in the following way

$$cd_j = \begin{cases} 2 \cdot \frac{d_j}{d_i} & \text{for } \frac{h_i}{A} \le 2 \text{ m}, \\[2ex] 6 \cdot \frac{d_j}{d_i} & \text{for } \frac{h_i}{A} \ge 6 \text{ m}, \\[2ex] \frac{h_i}{A} \cdot \frac{d_j}{d_i} & \text{otherwise}. \end{cases} \tag{7.2}$$

However, in young forest stands, it may anyway be best not to remove competitors selectively but rather to fell all other trees within a certain radius around each frame tree, see Sect. 3.6.1. The A-thinning index was originally developed for monospecies even-aged forests. For mixed species woodlands with different light requirements different A-values can be applied to each species or species group.

Alternatively the A-thinning index can be applied by means of the re-arranged Eq. (7.3).

$$A_j = \frac{h_i}{dist_j} \cdot \frac{d_j}{d_i} \tag{7.3}$$

For all neighbours of tree i the individual A_j value is calculated according to Eq. (7.3) where $dist_j$ is the observed distance between tree i and neighbour j. The larger A_j the stronger the competition pressure of tree j on tree i. All neighbours of tree i can then be sorted from high to low values according to their A_j values. A decision can be made to remove only one, two or three competitors from the top of this list. In the example of Fig. 7.6, it is also possible just to check the A_j values. As $A = 5$ is the thinning intensity selected, every tree with $A_j > 5$ needs to be removed.

The A-thinning index is often used in individual tree growth simulators to simulate local thinnings (Hanewinkel and Pretzsch 2000; Hasenauer 2006). The index also has a high educational value when developing practical experience with local thinnings.

Below a simple R code is provided that calculates critical distance, cd_j, (Eq. 7.1) and A_j value (Eq. 7.3) for neighbouring tree no. 3 in Fig. 7.6.

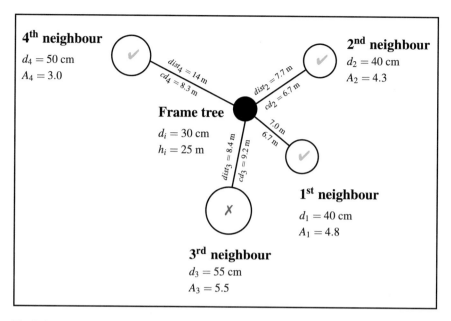

Fig. 7.6 A worked example of the A-thinning index involving a frame tree, its four nearest neighbours and $A = 5$ (heavy thinning). The critical distances, cd_j, and the A_j values were calculated based on Eqs. (7.1) and (7.3), respectively. Ticked trees are not considered as competitors and will remain in the forest stand whereas a cross means that the corresponding tree will be removed. Modified from Pommerening and Sánchez Meador (2018)

```
1  > hi <- 25
2  > di <- 30
3  > dj <- 55
4  > dist <- 8.4
5  > A <- 5.0
6  >
7  > (cd <- hi / A * dj / di)
8  [1] 9.166667
9  > (Aj <- hi / dist * dj / di)
10 [1] 5.456349
```

The input values are specified in lines 1–5. For easier recognition the variable names are loosely based on the symbols used in the text of this section. Critical distance is calculated in line 7 and the A_j value in line 9. The results are given in lines 8 and 10.

Vorobyov Mean

Stoyan et al. (2018b) suggested another reference marking based on set-theoretic methods: Trees can be considered as part of a reference marking, if they were included in the selection of at least u test persons. This can be interpreted as a *wisdom of crowd* approach in psychology (Surowiecki 2004), where the wisdom of the crowd is the collective opinion of a group of individuals rather than that of a single person. The method can also be understood as a vote or rating by several individuals, as it includes the most frequently selected trees. As such the results are likely to be closer to a ground truth than single judgements.

As preparation for applying these set-theoretic methods the trees j are ranked according to s_j, i.e. the number of test persons that selected tree j. Thus s_j offers information on the passive rating frequencies of trees. Trees with larger s_j are ranked lower than those with smaller s_j, whilst the ranking of trees with equal s_j does not matter. As a result the s_j form a decreasing sequence.

The R code listed below demonstrates the aforementioned data preparation which is crucial to the analysis methods described in this chapter. The comments in the code explain the purpose of the code and the variable names follow the notation used in the text.

```
> # Select marking scores from data
> myData <- tdata[, 9 : 32]
> ni <- colSums(myData)

> # Sort test persons according to ni
> myData <- myData[order(ni, decreasing = T)]

> # Sort trees according to marking frequencies
> sj <- rowSums(myData)
> myData <- myData[order(sj, decreasing = T), ]
```

Assume there is a set E of n trees, $\{1, 2, \ldots, n\}$ (Stoyan et al. 2018b). The authors now considered subsets of E, i.e. $X_1, X_2, \ldots, X_r$ that occur randomly. In the context of this chapter, X_i is the set of trees marked by test person i. Subsets were considered because each test person only selects n_i trees where $n_i < n$. Characteristic n_i gives information on the marking activity of test person i.

An important summary characteristic of a random set X is its *coverage function* $p_X(j)$ which empirically can be defined as

$$\hat{p}_X(j) = \frac{s_j}{r} \text{ for } j = 1, 2, \ldots, n. \tag{7.4}$$

The ranking of trees implies that $\hat{p}_X(j)$ decreases in j (see Fig. 7.7 for two examples). The coverage function is used to determine the *Vorobyov mean* $\overline{X}$ (Vorobyov 1984; Molchanov 2017) and the idea of this characteristic is that of a subset of E with m elements.

$\overline{n}$ is the mean number of trees selected in the experiment and lies between 1 and n in an interval with integer end points where $\hat{p}_X(j)$ is constant. The right end point of that interval is m. Thus $\overline{X}$ is the set of all trees with at least u 1-marks where $u = r\hat{p}_X(m)$, see Fig. 7.7 (left). For more details on the associated set-theoretic theory see Stoyan et al. (2018b).

Following on from the previous code listing in this section, the next code example shows how to calculate Eq. (7.4). s_j is re-calculated in line 4 to reflect the new rank

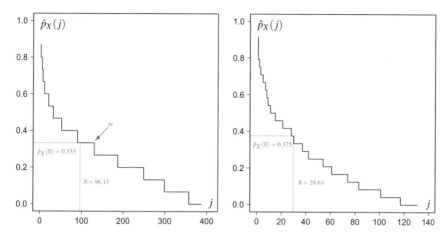

Fig. 7.7 Empirical coverage function (Eq. 7.4) for the marteloscopes at Coed y Brenin (plot 7, Wales, UK) and Dundrum Forest (Co. Tipperary, Ireland). For a given tree rank number j the function gives the proportion of test persons who marked tree j. The maximum number of marks are 13 and 22, respectively, and the minimum is 0. $\hat{p}_X(1) = 13/15$ and $\hat{p}_X(358) = 0$ for Coed y Brenin (plot 7) and $\hat{p}_X(1) = 22/24$ and $\hat{p}_X(118) = 0$ for Dundrum Forest

order of the trees (see Fig. 7.7). dim(myData)[2] in line 6 gives the number of test persons, r, which is the second dimension of the data matrix.

```
1  > # Sort trees according to marking frequencies
2  > sj <- rowSums(myData)
3  > myData <- myData[order(sj, decreasing = T), ]
4  > sj <- rowSums(myData)
5  > # Calculate coverage function
6  > p_j <- sj / dim(myData)[2]
```

Finally, to appear like in Fig. 7.7, the principle of right continuity has to be applied to p_j.

Two examples are considered here, a marteloscope experiment at Coed y Brenin in North Wales in 2006 and another one at Dundrum Forest in Ireland in 2007. At Coed y Brenin there were $r = 15$ test persons and $n = 387$ trees, whilst at Dundrum Forest we had $r = 24$ test persons and $n = 131$ trees. The mean number of trees marked per test person was $\bar{n} = 96.13$ at Coed y Brenin (plot 7) and $\bar{n} = 29.63$ at Dundrum Forest. These numbers fall into the interval [91, 130] (marked by five test persons) and [29, 30] (marked by nine test persons), respectively, where $\hat{p}_X(j)$ takes the constant values 0.333 and 0.375, see Fig. 7.7. Following the definition by Stoyan et al. (2018b) the Vorobyov means $\overline{X}$ are sets $1, 2, \ldots, 130$ and $1, \ldots, 30$, respectively. In other words, $\overline{X}$ is the set of all trees marked by at least $u = 5$ (Coed y Brenin) and $u = 9$ (Dundrum Forest) test persons. This can be interpreted as the set of trees the 15 and 24 test persons definitely want to select. The tree numbers referred to here are not the numbers originally attached to them in the field but their rank numbers.

To study the difference in tree marking between expert and Vorobyov mean in greater detail, we can quantify the difference as distance

$$\delta(X, \overline{X}) = \sum_{j=1}^{n} |\mathbf{1}_X(j) - \mathbf{1}_{\overline{X}}(j)|, \qquad (7.5)$$

where $\mathbf{1}_X(j)$ is an indicator function and X is again the random set of trees selected by one test person. $\mathbf{1}_X(j) = 1$, if a tree from X was selected by a test person, otherwise $\mathbf{1}_X(j) = 0$. It is, of course, also possible to calculate the distances between each other test person's tree selection and the Vorobyov mean as shown in Stoyan et al. (2018b). The distance between expert marking and Vorobyov mean is 123 at Coed y Brenin and only 42 at Dundrum Forest. When divided by the number of trees, n, the relative distances are same, i.e. 0.32. Incidentally, the expert was the same person in both marteloscopes.

If in any given case circumstances allow us to assume that the expert has really provided an optimised, best practice marking, his marking pattern in relation to that of the Vorobyov mean gives us an idea whether the instructions and/or the training course delivered prior to the marteloscope experiment were successful. For our two experiments used as examples we can state that both experiments were equally successful.

Conformity Numbers

Based on the idea of using trees that are frequently selected by test persons as a wisdom-of-crowd reference as discussed in the previous paragraphs, we can quantify the tendency of a test person i to conform with the general tree selection tendency. Stoyan et al. (2018b) introduced the *conformity number* c_i

$$c_i = \frac{1}{n_i} \sum_{j=1}^{n} \mathbf{1}_{X_i}(j) \cdot s_j \text{ for } i = 1, 2, \ldots, r. \qquad (7.6)$$

Here X_i is the set of trees selected by test person i whilst r as before is the number of test persons. The conformity number c_i simply is the mean of numbers s_j of trees selected by test person i. The quantity is more suitable for comparisons when transformed to the *relative conformity number* r_i:

$$r_i = \frac{c_i}{C_i} \text{ with } C_i = \frac{1}{n_i} \sum_{j=1}^{n_i} s_j \text{ for } i = 1, 2, \ldots, r \qquad (7.7)$$

Quantity C_i is the conformity number of an opportunist who marks n_i trees as the observed test person i, but s/he selects the n_i trees with the largest numbers s_j from the list of all trees. r_i gives positive numbers smaller than one and a large value of r_i indicates a high degree of conformity of test person i with the whole group of all other test persons.

The listing below provides the calculation of Eqs. (7.6) and (7.7). Lines 1–11 repeat previous listings for completeness. Equation (7.6) is calculated in line 14 and Eq. (7.7) in lines 17–18.

```
1  > # Select marking scores from data
2  > myData <- tdata[, 9 : 32]
3  > ni <- colSums(myData)
4  >
5  > # Sort test persons according to ni
6  > myData <- myData[order(ni, decreasing = T)]
7  >
8  > # Sort trees according to marking frequencies
9  > sj <- rowSums(myData)
10 > myData <- myData[order(sj, decreasing = T), ]
11 > sj <- rowSums(myData)
12 >
13 > # Calculation of c_i
14 > c <- t(t(as.matrix(myData))%*%sj) / ni
15 > C <- NA
16 > for (i in 1 : dim(myData)[2])
17 +   C[i] <- sum(sj[1 : ni], na.rm = T) / ni
18 > ri <- c / C
```

Let us denote the relative conformity number of the expert by r_e. Assuming again that a given expert performed a tree selection independent of the test persons of an experiment and assuming further that s/he achieved a near perfect marking, a large value of r_e means that the test persons selected trees in a similar way as the expert while a low number suggests that the expert's results are quite different from the tendency of the test persons. In the context of a training course that concluded with a marteloscope experiment, a low r_e could mean that the training did not fully achieve the anticipated purpose.

Relative conformity r_e of the expert at Coed y Brenin was 0.74 and 0.68 at Dundrum Forest. Apparently these results suggest that the test persons at Coed y Brenin marked trees slightly more closely to the selection of the expert than at Dundrum Forest, but both values are not too different.

7.2.4 Active and Passive Rating Behaviour

Most basically tree selection is influenced by two processes, an *active* and a *passive* process: 1. the test person activity performed from the point of view of the test persons. A simple indicator of this activity is the number of marks given by a single test person. There may be test persons that mark many and others that mark only few trees.

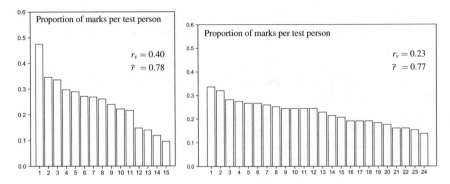

Fig. 7.8 Rating bar charts from the marteloscope experiments at Coed y Brenin (plot 7, North Wales, left) and Dundrum Forest (Co. Tipperary, Ireland, right). The test persons are ranked and arranged on the abscissa according to their n_i and the symbols are explained in the text

The second process 2. is the passive attraction evoked by the trees. A simple indicator of this passive process is the number of test persons selecting a given tree. In any forest stand, there are trees where the decision is evident, whilst for others it is much less obvious even to experts.

A first natural step to understand these two processes is to use bar charts. They represent the marginal distributions of the selection data matrix and give valuable information on the selection behaviour.

For process 1, depicting the test-person activity we can create a chart showing the proportions n_i/n of trees selected, where n_i as previously defined is the number of trees selected by test person i. Naturally, this results in r bars and Pommerening et al. (2018) referred to this bar chart as the *rating bar chart*, see Fig. 7.8.

From the rating bar chart descriptive statistics can be derived. We considered the coefficient of variation, r_v, of the proportions of the rating bar chart and the arithmetic mean of the aforementioned relative conformity number (Eq. 7.7).

In the rating bar charts, we see clear differences in the rating intensity of the test persons calculated as $n_i/387$ and $n_i/131$, respectively (Fig. 7.8). The method is reminiscent of species rank/abundance or Whittaker plots (Magurran 2004, 21ff.). Test person no. 1 from the Coed y Brenin experiment showed somewhat extreme behaviour by selecting 184 trees whilst test person no. 15 marked only 37 trees. Also the first two test persons at Dundrum Forest selected markedly more trees (44 and 42) than their colleagues, but the general descent towards test person 24 is more gradual than in the Coed y Brenin marteloscope experiment. This is reflected by the coefficient of variation of the proportions of the rating bar chart, r_v. This number is much higher for the Coed y Brenin marteloscope than for the one at Dundrum Forest, whilst the mean relative conformity numbers $\bar{r}$ are almost the same.

The passive marking frequency of the trees (process 2) can be analysed by a bar chart showing the proportions z/n of trees selected, where z is the number of marks "1" assigned by different test persons with $z = 0, 1, \ldots, r$. With r test persons there are potentially $r + 1$ bars, as some trees can also be selected by no test person. To this

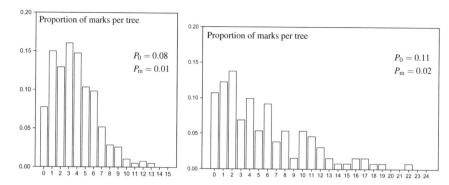

Fig. 7.9 Marking bar charts from the marteloscope experiments at Coed y Brenin (plot 7, North Wales, left) and Dundrum Forest (Co. Tipperary, Ireland, right). The marks per tree are listed on the abscissa and the symbols are explained in the text

bar chart Pommerening et al. (2018) referred to as the *marking bar chart*, see Fig. 7.9. The marking bar chart essentially is the empirical distribution of the proportions of trees with mark "1".

One of the parameters derived from the marking bar chart is the proportion of trees marked "0" by all test persons, P_0. This proportion constitutes a kind of negative agreement on unselectable trees. It typically includes trees that even to the eyes of a layman suggest the risk of worsening stand conditions, ecosystem goods and services as well as biodiversity, if they are eventually removed from the forest. A complementary characteristic from the marking bar charts is the proportion of trees marked in the 20% highest classes of the marking bar chart, P_m.

In the Coed y Brenin marteloscope, there were 30 and at Dundrum Forest 22 unmarked trees that were accounted for in the bar labelled "0" (Fig. 7.9). This corresponds to values of P_0 of 0.08 and 0.11, respectively. None of the trees received the possible maximum scores of 15 and 14 at Coed y Brenin and there was a similar situation at Dundrum Forest. Accordingly the values of P_m were both low.

Pommerening et al. (2018) found that the marking bar charts from marteloscopes, where the test persons were required to mark for low thinnings, often tended to be U-shaped, i.e. P_m was markedly larger than in marteloscopes used to train people in crown thinnings (see Fig. 7.10, right). The marking bar charts relating to marking for crown thinning rather tended to have an exponential shape. This is also the situation in the two example marteloscope results shown in Fig. 7.9. Larger values of P_m typically indicate more agreement between the test persons, also note the high mean relative conformity number $\bar{r}$ at Cannock Chase (Fig. 7.10, left). Naturally low thinning methods do not necessarily need to lead to greater agreement in tree selection than crown thinning methods. However, in the UK and Ireland this is typically the case, because many forest practitioners are much more familiar with low thinnings and crown thinning as a new approach causes confusion and hence less agreement. The zero classes in Figs. 7.9 and 7.10 are curious. They seem to suggest that all test persons were in perfect agreement here with regard to the trees in this class. However,

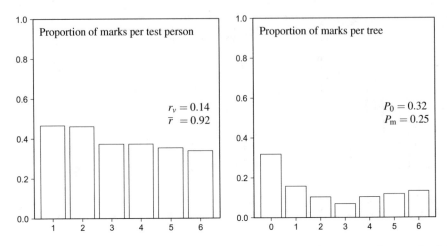

Fig. 7.10 Rating (left) and marking (right) bar charts from the marteloscope experiments related to low thinning at Cannock Chase (UK in 2012) involving $r = 6$ test persons and $n = 204$ trees. The test persons are ranked and arranged on the abscissa according to their n_i (left) and the marks per tree are listed on the abscissa (right). The symbols are explained in the text. Modified from Pommerening et al. (2018)

as previously discussed this is only a kind of pseudo or passive agreement (Stoyan et al. 2018b). The situation of trees that are marked by no test person is not unusual, see Pommerening et al. (2018), the discussion in Zucchini and Gadow (1995) and Sect. 7.2.2.

Active and passive processes interact in a complicated way. Therefore it is difficult to disentangle them and to characterise their joint effects by simple statistical characteristics.

Stoyan et al. (2018b) pointed out that the number of trees marked by test person i (n_i) and the conformity number (c_i, Eq. 7.6) are correlated, see Fig. 7.11. The correlation is negative, i.e. active test persons are less conform than passive ones. Incidentally, similar results can be achieved using the *latent class analysis* (LCA), see Collins and Lanza (2010) and Uebersax and Grove (1993). From this analysis statistical indicators, the so-called *specificity* and *sensitivity* can be calculated, which perform in a very similar way as n_i and c_i in Fig. 7.11, however, the latter are much easier to compute.

7.2.5 Agreement

When selecting trees, regardless of purpose or management objective, a major decision is taken that affects the dynamics of a forest stand for many years if not decades to come. This is where the importance of selecting trees lies, particularly in management types like continuous cover forestry that much depends on individual-tree

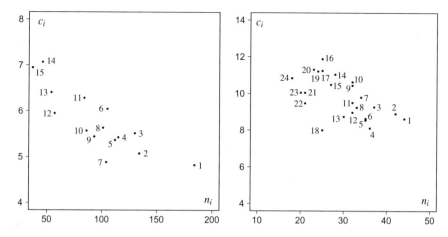

Fig. 7.11 Scatterplot of the number of trees marked by test person i and the average number of trees marked by test person i (conformity number), i.e. c_i over n_i for Coed y Brenin (plot 7, left) and Dundrum Forest (right). The numbers denote the test persons' rank number like in Fig. 7.8

selection and local thinnings (see Chap. 3). A single management operation following a marking of trees can indeed severely affect the dynamics of a forest stand, since it induces a disturbance in the natural development of a forest comparable to pathogen infestations and sporadic fire. With ongoing climate change, increasing importance of forest conservation and an emphasis on balancing ecosystem goods and services, the question of human tree selection behaviour has gained renewed attention. As previously mentioned, until recently, both in research and industry it was assumed that thinnings and other management activities were sufficiently defined so that tree marking would lead to almost unanimous results and hardly any variation would occur if the staff in question had the same education and instructions (Pommerening et al. 2018). In reality many factors influence the marking of raters in forests, even the seemingly unrelated childhood and upbringing in rural as opposed to urban environments. For example, test persons used to dense plantations of introduced conifers from the days of their childhood naturally mark conifers versus broadleaves differently than those who grew up in the midst of natural broadleaved forests.

The variability in tree selection also plays an important role in forest models simulating the development of forests over time (Burkhart and Tomé 2012; Pretzsch 2009; Weiskittel et al. 2011). Such model simulations are carried out to identify, for example, consequences of climate change, of invasive species colonising a site and for production forecasts to name but a few purposes. Also in these models, it has commonly been assumed that forest managers and machine operators mark trees according to theoretical rules published in textbooks or as best practice recommendations (Stoyan et al. 2018b). In previous studies, however, authors have found little evidence for agreement in the marking behaviour among forestry professionals (Zucchini and Gadow 1995; Füldner et al. 1996; Daume et al. 1997; Spinelli et al. 2016; Pommerening et al. 2018).

This begs the question, why experienced forest managers and operators should not be allowed to deviate from one another in terms of selecting individual trees as long as the overall objectives and targets are met. Popular opinion for a long time suggested that the general trend rather than the individual tree is important and allowing people's decisions to differ would spread the risk of fatal decisions. Though intuitively this makes sense, there is no firm evidence supporting this opinion and there is a fundamental research interest in studying the selection behaviour of different persons and how this behaviour is influenced by individual trees and their neighbourhood and by other factors.

The question of agreement between professionals judging an object of interest is not unique to forest science, but very common in medicine (Cao et al. 2016; Stoyan et al. 2018a). Here quantifying agreement is part of assessing reliability and reproducibility as well as quality assurance (Cao et al. 2016). It is interesting to know whether there is any agreement at all among test persons and if so, to which degree the test persons have arrived at similar conclusions. For two test persons ($r = 2$) agreement in this context simply means a high number of equal decisions whilst for more than three raters agreement is difficult to describe. Studying agreement between individuals selecting trees has so far largely been neglected.

Fleiss' Kappa

There is a standard characteristic for measuring the degree of agreement in a collective of r test persons (with $r > 2$) and this characteristic is referred to as Fleiss' kappa, κ, (Fleiss 1971; Fleiss et al. 2003). It is frequently used in applied statistics (Stoyan et al. 2018a).

The concept of kappa is based on pairwise comparisons and has its roots in the one-way analysis of variance. Fleiss' kappa can be expressed in different equivalent forms, which highlight various aspects of the nature of this statistical characteristic. The first form is given in Eq. (7.8).

$$\kappa = \frac{p_0 - p_e}{1 - p_e}, \tag{7.8}$$

where p_0 is the observed proportion of ratings in agreement and p_e is the expected proportion of ratings in agreement. The formula for p_0 is given by

$$p_0 = \frac{2}{r(r-1)} \sum_{i=1,j>i}^{r} e_{ij}. \tag{7.9}$$

Here e_{ij} is n_{ij}/n, where n_{ij} is the number of trees which were assigned the same mark ("0" or "1") by both test persons i and j. Equation (7.9) shows one aspect of the nature of kappa: p_0 is a mean closely related to agreement in pairwise comparisons. For the second term, p_e, Fleiss (1971) set

$$p_e = p^2 + (1 - p)^2, \tag{7.10}$$

where $p = N_1/nr$ and N_1 is the total number of marks "1" given in the experiment. The second form Fleiss' kappa can take is

$$\kappa = 1 - \frac{\frac{1}{n}\sum_{j=1}^{n} s_j(r - s_j)}{r(r - 1)\, p(1 - p)}, \tag{7.11}$$

where s_j is the number of marks "1" of tree j. The term $s_j(r - s_j)$ is a good choice for characterising agreement, as it takes extreme values for the cases $s_j = r/2$ and $s_j = 0$ or $s_j = r$. We see that κ only depends on the s_j's, i.e. on the passive rating frequencies of the trees. This demonstrates the strongly passive nature of kappa (Pommerening et al. 2018).

Kappa can be calculated with the R package `irr`. After loading the package (line 2) a data matrix containing the marking scores needs to be created (line 3). Fleiss' kappa can now be calculated by setting the option `exact = FALSE` in function `kappam.fleiss()`. The purpose of repeating variable `kappa` in line 6 is to print the results on screen.

```
1  > # install.packages("irr", dep = T)
2  > library(irr)
3  > myData <- tdata[,9 : 32]
4  > kappa <- kappam.fleiss(myData, exact = FALSE,
5  + detail = FALSE)
6  > kappa
```

As far as the interpretation of kappa is concerned, Landis and Koch (1977) were the first to suggest guidelines for interpreting κ, which were revised by Stoyan et al. (2018a), see Table 7.2.

In terms of our two example marteloscopes Coed y Brenin 7 and Dundrum Forest the kappa values were 0.102 and 0.194, respectively. Both results correspond to slight agreement according to Table 7.2. Pommerening et al. (2018) found that slight agreement was the most common agreement score in 36 marteloscope experiments related to crown thinning across Britain. When low thinning methods were required in the instructions, agreement according to κ was fair to moderate. The authors also compared their results with published kappa values in medicine and found forestry kappas to be considerably lower than than those reported in medicine.

Pommerening et al. (2018) also tried another variant of κ, i.e. the Conger-Hubert-Schouten kappa, that includes more information on the active rating behaviour than

Table 7.2 Interpretation of k values proposed by Stoyan et al. (2018a)

k	Interpretation
<0.10	Poor agreement
0.10–0.33	Slight agreement
0.33–0.50	Fair agreement
0.50–0.67	Moderate agreement
0.67–0.90	Substantial agreement
≥0.90	Almost perfect agreement

the original kappa discussed in this section. However, the authors found hardly any difference between the values of the two kappas. Most likely this was related to the fact that rating bar charts were sufficiently close to a uniform distribution, i.e. all test persons marked with similar intensities. In that case both kappas lead to very similar results (Stoyan et al. 2018a).

Incidentally, the Conger-Hubert-Schouten kappa can be computed by setting the option exact = TRUE in function kappam.fleiss():

```
> kappa <- kappam.fleiss(myData, exact = TRUE,
+ detail = FALSE)
```

Pommerening et al. (2018) computed Fleiss' kappa for each of the 36 marteloscope included in their study. The results (Fig. 7.12) clearly showed that the crown thinning experiments featured at the lower end of the κ distribution and the low thinning experiments at the upper. There was poor to fair agreement in crown thinning experiments and fair to moderate agreement in low thinning experiements. In general, there were no cases of substantial and (almost) perfect agreement, the majority of experiments were between slight and fair agreement. In 4 out of 36 experiments, even poor agreement occurred.

Independent of management type the variability of selecting individual trees is always considerable, even if good instructions and training are provided. The results in Fig. 7.12 highlighted that low thinning apparently is the traditional method in the country and that forestry staff in the UK need more training in crown thinnings, since the latter method is considered an important element of continuous cover forestry, see Chap. 3.

Fig. 7.12 The empirical distribution of Fleiss' kappa values scored in 36 marteloscope experiments in Great Britain according to Table 7.2. Black—low thinning, red—crown thinning. Modified from Pommerening et al. (2018)

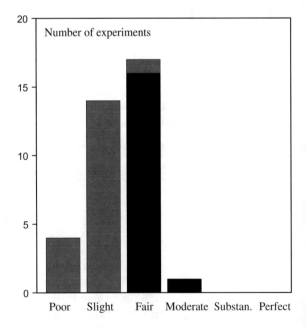

7.2.6 Impact Intensity and Type of Impact

Murray and Gadow (1991) suggested the proportion of the basal area of selected trees, P_G as an expression of *impact intensity*. Naturally basal area can also be replaced by other measures such as the number of trees, volume or biomass. Consider the simple example in the following R code:

```
> G_0 <- 55
> G_sel <- 10
> (P_G <- G_sel / G_0)
[1] 0.1818182
```

In this example, 18% of the initial basal area (G_0) was scheduled for removal (G_sel) by marking individual trees of a forest stand. Kassier (1993) suggested the ratio of P_G and P_N, the proportion of the number of selected trees, as a measure of impact type:

$$B = \frac{\text{Proportion of the number of trees selected}}{\text{Proportion of basal area of selected trees}} = \frac{P_N}{P_G} \qquad (7.12)$$

This measure quantifies the tree selection strategy or *impact type* by comparing numbers of trees selected with their cumulative size. If $B < 1$, a smaller proportion of trees has been selected compared to their proportion of cumulative basal area. In a thinning context (see Sect. 3.6), this typically indicates a crown thinning and the trees selected show a tendency of being in the upper part of the empirical diameter distribution. A larger proportion of trees is selected compared to their proportion of basal area, if $B > 1$. In a thinning context, this is consistent with a thinning from below and trees were preferably selected in the lower part of the empirical diameter distribution (Pommerening et al. 2018). A result $B \approx 1$ is often a consequence of natural disturbances, schematic and random thinnings. Table 7.3 gives an example data set from the UK.

The mixed Sitka spruce (*Picea sitchensis* (BONG.) CARR.)—birch (*Betula spp.*) woodland was thinned to release birch from oppressive Sitka spruce competition. To achieve this, the thinning mainly targeted spruce trees and other conifers. The thinning was also carried out as frame-tree based crown thinning. Consequently the removal rate of trees other than birch ranged from 20–30%, see Fig. 7.13 (left). Measure B clearly indicated crown thinnings for all non-birch trees. A few birch trees

Table 7.3 Thinning in Coed y Brenin, plot 1 (North Wales, UK) in 2003. G and N are basal area and number of trees, respectively. The indices "init" and "post" refer to before and after thinning. SS—Sitka spruce, BI—birch

	G_{init} (m^2 ha^{-1})	G_{post} (m^2 ha^{-1})	N_{init} (ha^{-1})	N_{post} (ha^{-1})	P_G	P_N	B
SS	33.4	23.5	1066	849	0.30	0.20	0.69
BI	5.6	5.2	1038	962	0.07	0.07	1.03
Others	3.4	2.5	500	444	0.26	0.11	0.42
Total	42.4	31.2	2604	2255	0.26	0.13	0.51

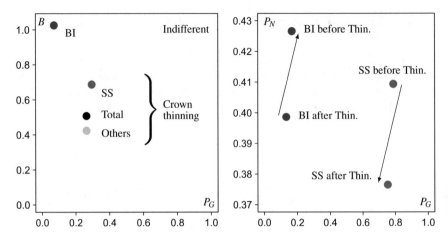

Fig. 7.13 Visualisation of P_G and B of Table 7.3

were taken out by accident and as a result the removal rate of this species was rather low and B suggested an indifferent impact as expected. The code below illustrates the calculation of P_G and B.

```
1   > G.init <- c(33.4, 5.6, 3.4, 42.4)
2   > G.post <- c(23.5, 5.2, 2.5, 31.2)
3   > N.init <- c(1066, 1038, 500, 2604)
4   > N.post <- c(849, 962, 444, 2255)
5   >
6   > plot1 <- data.frame(cbind(G.init, G.post, N.init, N.post))
7   >
8   > (plot1$P_G <- (plot1$G.init - plot1$G.post) / plot1$G.init)
9   [1] 0.2964071856 0.0714285714 0.2647058824 0.2641509434
10  > (plot1$P_N <- (plot1$N.init - plot1$N.post) / plot1$N.init)
11  [1] 0.2035647280 0.0732177264 0.1120000000 0.1340245776
12  >
13  > (plot1$B <- plot1$P_N / plot1$P_G)
14  [1] 0.686773931 1.025048170 0.423111111 0.507378758
```

Number of trees and basal area are inputted as vectors in lines 1–4 and converted to a data frame in line 6. P_G and P_N are calculated in lines 8–9 and 10–11, respectively, and B in lines 13–14. Figure 7.13 shows possibilities of how to illustrate the results of Table 7.3. The graph on the left-hand side simultaneously tells us about thinning intensity (abscissa) and thinning type (ordinate). In the graph on the right-hand side, P_N is depicted over P_G and gives an impression of the relative changes for the main species. In species-rich Chinese ecosystems, Hui and Pommerening (2014) found an interesting saturation relationship between P_N and P_G of the ten most abundant (in terms of P_N) tree species and described it using the Michaelis-Menten saturation curve (Michaelis and Menten 1913; Bolker 2008):

$$P_N = \frac{a \cdot P_G}{b + P_G}, \tag{7.13}$$

where a and b are model parameters of nonlinear regression which should be determined from the data. Model parameter a can be interpreted as the asymptote of the saturation curve, i.e. maximum P_N, whilst b represents the point where the curve achieves the half maximum. The authors found that there were always 1–2 lead species with P_G well in excess of 0.2 determining the asymptote. From rarest to commonest species the abundances eventually increased more in P_G than in P_N, i.e. the most frequent species had individuals of larger size than the rarer species (Fig. 7.14). The authors of this book found this saturation relationship also for other tree species-rich forest ecosystems in different parts of the world and it is another example of an allometric relationship, see Sect. 6.2.4.

Going back to our example marteloscope results from Coed y Brenin (plot 7) and Dundrum Forest, we could see more variability in the former than in the latter, see Fig. 7.8. This can also be confirmed by the coefficient of variation, which is 0.28 and 0.09 for B and 0.27 and 0.25 for P_G. At Coed y Brenin, only 27% of the test persons have marked for a low thinning contrary to the instructions whilst it was 58% at Dundrum Forest. These percentages refer to the data points above the dashed horizontal line running through 1 (Fig. 7.15). The mean measure of impact type, $\bar{B}$, was 0.89 in the Coed y Brenin and 1.02 at the Dundrum Forest marteloscope. This supports the previously mentioned impression that there was a stronger trend towards crown thinning in the marking at Coed y Brenin than at Dundrum Forest, where $\bar{B}$ indicated indifferent marking as the average of all test persons. Incidentally the expert (no. 9 and no. 4, respectively) scored $B = 0.69$ at Coed y Brenin and $B = 0.97$ at Dundrum Forest. In a sense these results suggest that he followed the trend of the mean and therefore the wisdom of the crowd or more likely the crowd followed him (Fig. 7.15).

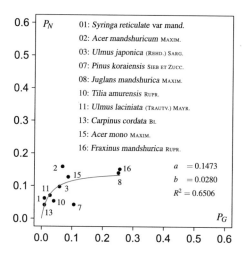

Fig. 7.14 The (allometric) relationship of P_N and P_G in the species-rich forest ecosystem of the Dongdapo Natural Reserve, northern China. The results from plot F are shown here. The numbers represent the original species codes and the parameters a and b are those of the Michaelis-Menten saturation function (Eq. 7.13) used as trend line (red). Modified from Hui and Pommerening (2014)

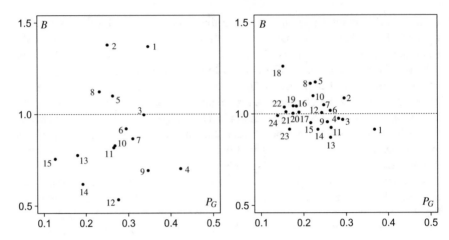

Fig. 7.15 Scatterplot of size marking intensity P_G and impact type characteristic B (Eq. 7.12) for the marteloscopes at Coed y Brenin (plot 7, left) and Dundrum Forest (right). The numbers denote the test persons' rank number like in Fig. 7.8

There was also considerable variability in P_G, i.e. the impact intensity. The range of P_G did not differ too much between the two experiments, it was mostly between 13% and just over 40%. Values > 35% certainly qualify as heavy interventions here. Incidentally, the expert suggested 35% for Coed y Brenin and 28% for Dundrum Forest (Fig. 7.15).

Staupendahl and Puumalainen (1998) and Álvarez-González et al. (2002) successfully related B to the parameters of the Weibull distribution of stem diameters after thinning, which supports the importance of this measure.

A similar measure of impact type is Magin's k factor. Wenk et al. (1990, p. 138f.) define a variant of this measure as the ratio of the mean volume of trees marked for thinning and the mean volume of all trees before marking.

$$k = \frac{\bar{v}_{sel}}{\bar{v}_{init}} \tag{7.14}$$

Considering a human disturbance, according to Wenk et al. (1990) $k < 1$ indicates a thinning from below, $k = 1$ an indifferent thinning and $k > 1$ a crown thinning. In analogy it is also possible to use arithmetic or quadratic mean diameters, see also Fig. 7.22, and to define many other, similar ratios based on, for example, biomass or leaf area index. Alternatively it is also an option to plot the Shannon and Simpson diversity indices (Magurran 2004) calculated for simple proportions against the same index calculated for basal area proportions.

A traditional way of assessing the effect of impacts was that of using stacked empirical diameter distributions. According to this method the parts of the histogram bars relating to, for example, trees marked for removal are depicted in a colour different from those of the remaining forest stand. Figure 7.16 illustrates the principle.

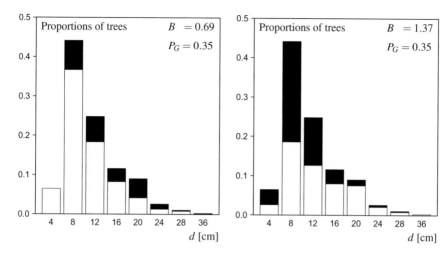

Fig. 7.16 Empirical stacked diameter distributions achieved by the marking of two test persons (left: no. 9, right: no. 1) participating in a marteloscope experiment at Coed y Brenin (plot 7) in North Wales (UK) in 2006. Black: Proportion of trees marked for removal. White: Proportions of remaining trees. Black and white parts of the bars together constitute the proportions of trees before marking

Comparing both stacked diameter distributions and the associated B and P_G values it is obvious that both participants adopted a very different thinning type whilst removing exactly the same proportions of basal area, although this is harder to see in the empirical diameter distributions than by studying B. The left graph reflects a test person intending to remove trees preferably from the right-hand side of the diameter distribution. This typically leads to a crown thinning. On the other hand Fig. 7.16 (right) clearly shows a marking behaviour that results in a thinning from below: Here considerably more trees have been marked in smaller diameter classes than by the participant whose results have produced the left graph.

Naturally stacked diameter distributions can also be applied to natural disturbance events. In this case we would expect an indifferent "thinning type", i.e. the majority of dead trees would be near the mean basal area tree, d_g.

If both frame and competitor trees are marked, it is possible to depict the proportions of both types of trees along with that of the residual stand (see Fig. 7.4 in Sect. 7.2.2). Here one would expect that the frame trees are usually recruited from larger diameter classes and also that the majority of competitors are approximately of the same size as the frame trees.

In a similar way, box plots can be used for analysing the size distributions of trees selected and of residual trees, see Figs. 6.2 and 6.3.

Another line of analysis can include nearest neighbour summary characteristics (NNSS, Sect. 4.4.7.1). For this we computed the individual-tree indices for all trees before thinning and then subset according to the marks given by the test persons. Test person no. 9, for example, selected trees from the upper end of the dominance

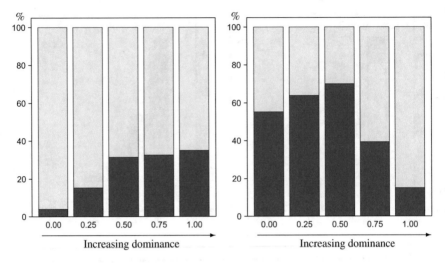

Fig. 7.17 Percentage of residual trees (light) and trees selected for thinning (dark) in the classes of the dominance mark distribution at Coed y Brenin (plot 7) in North Wales (UK) in 2006. Left: Results of two test person no. 9. Right: Results of test person no. 1. The mark dominance distribution is based on four nearest neighbours

mark distribution, i.e. 33 and 38% of all trees in the second highest classes 0.75 and 1.00 were marked by this person with only very few percentages in classes 0.00 and 0.25 (Fig. 7.17).

However, the selection pattern of test person no. 1 showed large percentages of marked trees (55 and 64%) in the lower dominance classes and only few percentages in classes 0.75 and 1.00. Once more we see that test person no. 9 selected considerably fewer trees than test person no. 1.

A similar analysis can be done for spatial species mingling (see Sect. 4.4.7.1). In this case the species trait groups broadleaves and conifers were used rather than the original nine species.

We can see that both test persons adopted a similar strategy, i.e. they favoured trees in higher mingling classes and predominantly marked trees in the lower mingling classes (Fig. 7.18). This is particularly evident for test person no. 1. He selected broadleaved trees in clusters of other broadleaves and followed the same pattern for conifers. The percentages of selected trees in the first three mingling classes are almost uniform for test person no. 9, however, he marked 30% of all trees in class 0.50. These trees have two trees of a different trait group among the four nearest neighbours. Test person no. 9 marked very few trees in the two highest mingling classes.

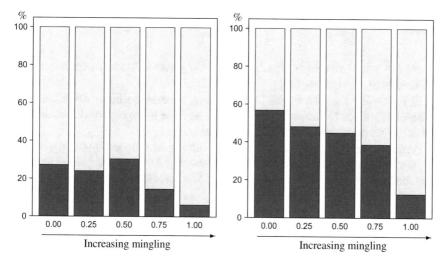

Fig. 7.18 Percentage of residual trees (light) and trees selected for thinning (dark) in the classes of the mingling mark distribution at Coed y Brenin (plot 7) in North Wales (UK) in 2006. Left: Results of two test person no. 9. Right: Results of test person no. 1. The mark mingling distribution is based on four nearest neighbours

7.2.7 Tree Selection Probabilities

A key interest in analysing disturbances and tree selection behaviour is in uncovering factors that have influenced the selection of particular individual trees. This gives insights into the decision making of humans working in forests and in the way how the tree selection is likely to modify the forest under consideration (Füldner et al. 1996; Daume et al. 1997).

In analysing these factors we can draw on experience and knowledge from mortality modelling and insurance statistics. Based on the definitions made at the beginning of Sect. 7.2.1 we can use *logistic regression*, where the probability of success can be related to a set of predictors. In the simplest case we just select stem diameter as a proxy of size for a start. However, at advanced stage we can include multiple explanatory variables in the regression to explain the behaviour of a particular test person as best as possible. Stem diameter, for example, is an appropriate factor influencing thinnings, as it is closely related to thinning types and intensity, see Sect. 3.6. Crown thinnings for example require the removal of large sized trees whilst predominantly small sized trees are marked in thinnings from below. Also, stem diameter d is easily accessible and therefore inexpensive marteloscope experiments can be set up based on numbered and callipered trees only without spatial reference if necessary.

The binary selection data for each tree suggests the use of simple logistic regression (see also Sect. 4.4.7.1):

$$P_i^{(s)} = \frac{e^{\beta_0 + \beta_1 \cdot d}}{1 + e^{\beta_0 + \beta_1 \cdot d}}, \tag{7.15}$$

where $P_i^{(s)}$ is the tree selection probability of test person i. Model parameter β_0 is an expression of impact intensity.

In R, logistic regressions can be fitted using *generalised linear models* and the corresponding `glm()` function. The response variable is the observed outcome, i.e. the actual marking carried out by a test person.

As an example we again used the marteloscope data from plot 7 at Coed y Brenin. We started by analysing the marking behaviour of the expert (test person no. 9) in the Coed y Brenin marteloscope experiment. The basic R code is given below.

```
> marking.9 <- glm(TestPerson9 ~ dbh, family = binomial,
+ data = myData)
```

`myData$TestPerson9` is a vector containing the marking scores of test person 9 as a sequence of "0"s and "1"s as previously discussed. The option `family = binomial` indicates that our tree marking data are binomial and that a logit link function will be used. This statement is necessary because the `glm()` function includes a wide range of regression types. The model parameters β_0 and β_1 are estimated based on the maximum likelihood (ML) method.

We can now examine the plot diagnostics with the function `summary(marking.9)` and check the significance of the regression coefficients.

```
Call:
glm(formula = TestPerson9 ~ dbh, family = binomial,
data = tdata)

Deviance Residuals:
Min        1Q    Median        3Q       Max
-1.5605   -0.7236   -0.5895   -0.5188    1.9892

Coefficients:
Estimate Std. Error z value Pr(>|z|)
(Intercept) -2.58468    0.31883    -8.107 5.20e-16 ***
dbh          0.11984    0.02357     5.084 3.69e-07 ***
---
Signif. codes:  0 '***' 0.001 '**' 0.01 '*' 0.05 '.' 0.1 ' ' 1

(Dispersion parameter for binomial family taken to be 1)

Null deviance: 426.81  on 386  degrees of freedom
Residual deviance: 399.35  on 385  degrees of freedom
AIC: 403.35

Number of Fisher Scoring iterations: 3
```

The generalised likelihood ratio test was used to determine the significance of the model parameters. In the case of test person no. 9, stem diameter (dbh) was highly significant, i.e. it has definitely been a factor influencing the test person's marking

Fig. 7.19 Tree selection probabilities of five test persons participating in a marteloscope experiment at Coed y Brenin (plot 7, North Wales, UK) and their dependence on stem diameter d, see Table 7.4. Three fundamentally different behaviour types were highlighted in colours

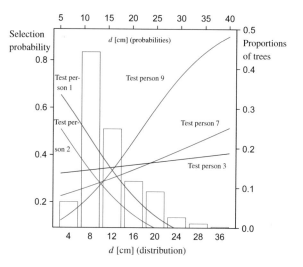

decisions. The slope parameter $\beta_1 = 0.11984$ of test person no. 9 in fact tells us that the selection probability increases by $e^{0.11984} = 0.0754$, i.e. by 8% for an increase of stem diameter of 1 cm.

For clarity and better contrasts we selected five test persons who participated in a marteloscope experiment and showed contrasting behaviour. Based on Eq. (7.15), Fig. 7.19 gives their selection probabilities. The four scales relate to the fact that we overlaid a bar plot with the empirical stem-diameter distribution.

Figure 7.19 clearly shows that test persons 1, 2, 7 and 9 have been influenced by stem diameter whilst test person 3 has not responded much to stem diameter. For this test person stem diameter has not been an important criterion. With test persons 7 and 9 the selection probability increases with increasing stem diameter. This indicates a tendency towards a crown thinning. Test persons 1 and 2 show a tendency reflecting thinning from below, as the tree selection probability increases with decreasing stem diameters. These results perhaps show particularly clearly how person-specific, selective thinning and harvesting strategies as well as their variability can be modelled to be incorporated in individual-based tree models.

Table 7.4 gives the parameters of the logistic regression model of the five test persons shown in Fig. 7.19. Comparing model parameter β_0 with B it is obvious that all β_0 are negatively signed for $B < 1$. By contrast, all β_0 are positively signed for $B > 1$. Positive values of β_1 are related to values of $B < 1$ and negative values of β_1 to values of $B > 1$. Obviously there is a high correlation between model parameters β_0 and β_1 on one hand and B on the other.

P_G does not vary much between the five test persons. Test persons 1 and 2 have approximately the same slope parameter β_1 but different intercepts β_0. In this case the intercept expresses different thinning intensities: Test person 1 has marked more trees than test person 2, i.e. the two curves approximately run in parallel, the one associated with test person 1 is above that of test person 2.

Table 7.4 Model parameters, P_G and B of the five test persons of Fig. 7.19. The test person numbers are rank numbers according to the principle explained in Fig. 7.8

Test person	β_0	β_1	P_G	B
1	1.2785	−0.1243	0.3471	1.3698
2	0.6560	−0.1199	0.2511	1.3792
3	−0.8033	0.0107	0.3371	0.9964
7	−1.4275	0.0371	0.3104	0.8658
9	−2.5847	0.1198	0.3469	0.6928

We can now examine the scatterplots of the two model parameters β_0 and β_1 over B, see Fig. 7.20. For this purpose the full set of 15 test persons was analysed rather than the selection of five that were used for Fig. 7.19 and Table 7.4.

Figure 7.20 clearly shows the high correlation between the B ratio and the parameters of the logistic regression model. This means that the model parameters can substitute the B ratio whilst revealing additional information at the same time. The differently signed slopes of the linear relationship also illustrate that a negative intercept and a positive slope parameter are related with crown thinnings whilst positive intercepts and negative slopes correspond to thinnings from below.

In analogy to and replacing stem diameter other factors can now be investigated such as for example the dominance index (Aguirre et al. 2003, see Sect. 4.4.7.1), a spatial variant of traditional crown classes. The aforementioned generalised likelihood ratio test can then help to identify the most significant factors influencing tree marking decisions. For example, using the data of the marteloscope at Dundrum Forest (Co. Tipperary, Ireland), we explored the dependence of marking decisions on the spatial dominance measure U_i' (Eq. 4.23; Albert 1999).

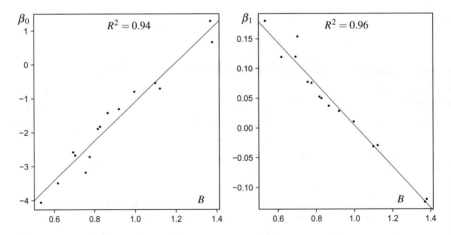

Fig. 7.20 Relationship between measure B and the parameters of the logistic regression model. The data points represent 15 participants in a marteloscope experiment at Coed y Brenin (plot 7, North Wales, UK)

Fig. 7.21 Tree selection probabilities of 24 test persons participating in a marteloscope experiment at Dundrum Forest (Co. Tipperary, Ireland) in 2007 and their dependence on height dominance U_i' (Eq. 4.23). Three fundamentally different behaviour types were highlighted in colours

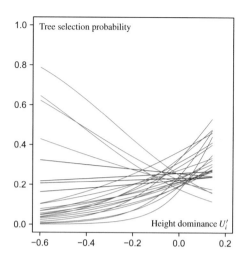

For this analysis, first U_i' was calculated for each tree using total tree height as size characteristic and periodic boundary conditions (Eq. 4.36). Then logistic regression was carried out separately for each test person using U_i' as explanatory variable. The results clearly show that U_i' is a good explanatory variable which was significant for 13 test persons ($p < 0.05$) according to the generalised likelihood ratio test. Studying the pattern of the 24 curves suggests that there are three main behavioural types: The 16 curves highlighted in blue with positive $\beta_1 > 1$ have in common that the corresponding test persons selected dominant trees with increasing probability. By contrast four curves highlighted in red with $\beta_1 < -1$ indicate a common behaviour where the corresponding test persons selected dominated trees with increasing probability. Another four test persons were quite indifferent to the spatial dominance measure U_i', i.e. dominance or suppression did not matter to them when making their decisions. As a consequence the corresponding curves highlighted in black are rather flat and have small absolute values of β_1 (Fig. 7.21).

7.2.8 Growth Rates and Growth Projection

Growth Sustainability

One of the earliest and most fundamental requirements of sustainable forestry was to strike a balance between periodic stand absolute growth rate (AGR, see Chap. 6) and tree removal. If standing volume or basal area have accumulated for a long time without natural disturbances or human interventions, this can—from a human point of view—negatively affect woodland structure. As a consequence an undesired uniform structure can potentially develop that is mainly supported by shade tolerant tree species and important rare and desired light demanding tree

Fig. 7.22 Quadratic mean
diameter over basal area of
the trees marked for thinning
of five participants in the
marteloscope experiment at
Coed y Brenin (plot 7, North
Wales, UK). The absolute
stand growth rate of 8.7 m^2
ha^{-1} was observed for the
period 2006–2011

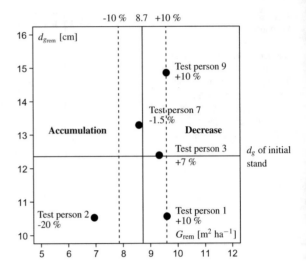

species, shrubs and ground vegetation may be lost in a certain area. Invasive plant
species may spread more easily in such conditions. Also, tree mortality increases at
the same time, which—from a forest management point of view—can be considered
as uncontrolled and wasteful tree decline. On the other hand, an over-cutting can also
prevent a diverse woodland structure.

Considering this it may therefore be interesting to study previous stand growth
rates with the personal tree selection results in a marteloscope experiment: Does the
marking of a particular test person imply over- or undercutting? In the light of past
growth performance the outcomes of this comparison can then be judged on. In this
comparison, observed stand AGR acts as a reference.

To be in a position to carry out such an analysis, it is, for example, useful to set up
a marteloscope experiment in an existing long-term research plot or in a plot where
the trees have been re-measured at least once. Increment boring and stem analyses
are an alternative, otherwise there is the option and recommendation to re-measure
new marteloscope plots every 5–10 years.

First, stand AGR needs to be calculated. Then the quadratic mean diameter of
the trees removed is depicted over the basal area of the removed trees. Alternatively
volume or biomass can be used. Note the similarity to Magin's k factor in Eq. (7.14).
Figure 7.22 gives an example using the same five test persons that have already
featured in Fig. 7.19 and Table 7.4.

All participants above the horizontal line marking the initial quadratic mean diameter performed a tree marking corresponding to a crown thinning. The two test persons
1 and 2 below this line made decisions leading to a thinning from below. The vertical
continuous line marks the stand AGR of the last five years and is accompanied by
two dashed vertical lines that give a region of allowance of ±10%. Assuming that no
additional thinning will be carried out within the next five years other than the one
defined by the test persons, basal-area values smaller than 8.7 m^2 lead to an accu-

mulation of basal area. Values larger than 8.7 m^2 result in a decrease of stand basal area. The marking of test person 7, a university student without forestry education, was closest to the observed stand growth rate whilst test person 2, a professional forester, marked trees so that basal area will further accumulate. All others carried out a marking that would decrease stand basal area, which makes sense in this very dense forest stand. Interestingly test persons 9 and 1 both marked trees to amount to 10% more than the basal area absolute growth rate of the last five years, however, one of them carried out a crown thinning and the other a thinning from below. This illustrates that information on thinning intensity or residual stand basal area is not sufficient to define the residual size structure of a forest stand.

Growth Projection

Repeatedly surveying the sites of marteloscope experiments also offers the opportunity of modelling growth locally and using the local model for growth projections. Also regional tree and growth models can, of course, be used to project stand development based on individual tree markings. However, a much simpler local growth model can be employed with the added benefit that it is more accurate for a given site. All that is required is a projection of tree stem diameters (and/or derived measures such as basal area, volume and biomass), since thinnings have been defined by the test persons and mortality is unlikely or negligible in the first 5–10 years after a thinning. We can also often assume that for young and middle-aged forest stands no regeneration/ingrowth processes take place. This approach has the advantage that local growth information is used, which has been collected from the same plot, where the marteloscope experiment is located. Even if long-term growth records are available, it may be better to include only recent measurements in the modelling. This ensures a good temporal extrapolation of growth processes with up-to-date information. If the system of twin plots as described in Sect. 7.2.2 is used, it is, of course, a good idea to pool the recent growth rates of both plots in the modelling process. In the simplest case, the linear relationship between tree size at the beginning of the growth period and the corresponding AGR or RGR can be used for modelling. To make the model more sophisticated a competition or structural index can be included, see also Sect. 4.4.7.1.

For illustration we chose the simplest and most effective case of a linear relationship between tree size at the beginning of the growth period and the corresponding AGR, i_k:

$$i_k = a + b \cdot y + \varepsilon \qquad (7.16)$$

In our application, i_k was stem diameter AGR, y was stem diameter and ε was an error term. This primary model we used in a linear regression. In a second step we computed RGR through the relationship

Fig. 7.23 Mean annual RGR $\overline{p}_k$ based on stem diameter of conifers (red) and broadleaves (blue) dependent on stem diameter. The data are from the marteloscope experiment at Coed y Brenin (plot 7, North Wales, UK)

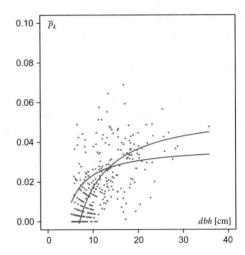

$$\overline{p}_k = \log\left(\frac{a}{y} + b + \frac{\varepsilon}{y} + 1\right) \qquad (7.17)$$

that is explained in the footnote relating to Eq. (2) in Table 6.4 (Chap. 6). The species-group specific curves in Fig. 7.23 show an increasing $\overline{p}_k$ with increasing size. In single growth-rate surveys, such a trend is possible as discussed in Sect. 6.3. Originally nine different species occurred in this woodland and we decided to organise them in two species trait groups, broadleaves and conifers. The curves show the differences between the species groups: In the broadleaves, the increase of RGR is much more moderate than in the conifers and the blue broadleaved curve levels off faster. The *RMSE* is slightly lower for conifers compared to broadleaves but the difference is small (Table 7.5).

The error term ε was quantified as the standard deviation of residuals of the linear regression. In the simulations, random numbers were generated from a normal distribution with a mean of 0 and a standard deviation matching ε.

The R coding for linear regression separately for conifers (lines 1–4) and broadleaves (lines 6–9) is shown below. The summary function applied in lines 3 and 8 extracts the regression results whilst `sigma()` gives the standard deviation of residuals.

```
1  > fit3.1 <- lm(AGR[speciesGroup == "C"] ~ dbh[speciesGroup ==
2  + "C"], data = growthRegres)
3  > summary(fit3.1)
4  > sdres3.1 <- sigma(fit3.1)
5  >
6  > fit3.2 <- lm(AGR[speciesGroup == "B"] ~ dbh[speciesGroup ==
7  + "B"], data = growthRegres)
8  > summary(fit3.2)
9  > sdres3.2 <- sigma(fit3.2)
```

Table 7.5 Model parameters, *Bias* and *RMSE* relating to stem-diameter RGR as estimated from Eqs. (7.16) and (7.17) for the marteloscope experiment at Coed y Brenin (plot 7, North Wales, UK)

Species	a	b	Bias	RMSE
Conifers	−0.40142	0.05728	−0.00102	0.01168
Broadleaves	−0.14937	0.03855	−0.00149	0.01252

This simple model can now be employed to project growth for five or ten years. For this purpose we used the 2006 survey data and removed those trees that were marked for thinning according to a selected test person. Obviously there are many more possibilities and methods of projecting stand dynamics in marteloscope plots and for assessing the outcomes. If spatial growth data from more surveying periods were available, it would also be possible to apply individual-based models (Sect. 5.2). For marteloscopes in old-growth forest stands, for example, birth processes need to be included. Naturally there are also plenty of measures that can be applied to assessing the outcomes of model projections. This section just illustrates the potential of projecting thinning results in the analysis of marteloscope data.

In the R listing below, function `estRGRstoch()` calculates RGR separately for the species trait groups conifers and broadleaves according to Eqs. (7.16) and (7.17). In line 15, the residual trees of a certain test person are selected for growth projection. Finally a `for` loop projects the stem diameters of the residual trees iteratively for ten years using the concept of the growth multiplier (Eq. 6.16) in line 21.

```
1  > estRGRstoch <- function(size, species, paramC, paramB, sd_C,
2  + sd_B) {
3  + RGR <- NA
4  + for(i in 1 : length(size)) {
5  +   if(species[i] == "C")
6  +     RGR[i] <- log(paramC[1] / size[i] + paramC[2] +
7  +     rnorm(1, 0, sd_C) / size[i] + 1)
8  +   else
9  +     RGR[i] <- log(paramB[1] / size[i] + paramB[2] +
10 +     rnorm(1, 0, sd_B) / size[i] + 1)
11 + }
12 + return(RGR)
13 + }
14 >
15 > testPerson <- subset(testPerson, testPerson[, 7] == 0)
16 >
17 > for(i in 1 : 10) {
18 +   RGR <- estRGRstoch(testPerson$dbh, testPerson$speciesGroup,
19 +   summary(fit3.1)$coefficients, summary(fit3.2)$coefficients,
20 +   sdres3.1, sdres3.2)
21 +   testPerson$dbh <- testPerson$dbh * exp(RGR)
22 + }
```

As an example we projected the growth of the stand at Coed y Brenin (plot 7) using the residual trees as marked by test persons no. 9 and no. 1 (rank numbers, see

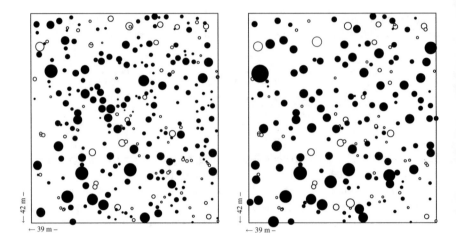

Fig. 7.24 Marteloscope plot 7 at Coed y Brenin (North Wales, UK) according to the tree marking of test person no. 9 (left) and test person no. 1 (right) and projected for ten years. Broadleaves are shown as open and conifers as closed circles

Fig. 7.8). From earlier results in this section, we remember, whilst test person no. 9 performed a crown thinning by marking few big trees, test person no. 1 contrary to the instructions ended up with a thinning from below selecting many small trees. In terms of thinning intensity both suggested removing the same 35% of the stand basal area. Since the relative growth model of Eqs. (7.16) and (7.17) is stochastic, we here present the results of a sample simulation only. Quite opposite thinning strategies are also evident from the plot maps after ten years of growth projection in Fig. 7.24, where among other things we can see that the residual number of trees was larger with test person no. 9.

Next it is interesting to study the mark or empirical size distribution. The empirical diameter distributions after ten years also show the impact of removing predominantly larger as opposed to smaller trees. Test person no. 9 achieved a more pronounced negative exponential diameter distributions with many more remaining small trees than test person no. 1. By contrast the marking of test person no. 1 led to a diameter distribution with more trees towards the middle and upper end of the diameter range.

The marking of test person no. 1 has favoured conifers slightly more than broadleaves. Both the shapes of the two empirical diameter distributions and the associated coefficients of variation clearly show that the marking of test person no. 9 has led to greater size diversity as a consequence of tree removal and ten years of growth since the simulated intervention.

The results of person-specific growth projections cannot only be used for assessing the long-term impact of tree selection but also helps to keep forest data up to date.

Finally it is also possible to use the projected stand data for spatial analysis. Since woodland managers are often interested in size development, we selected the mark

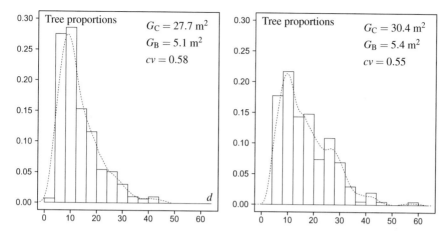

Fig. 7.25 Empirical diameter distributions at Coed y Brenin, plot 7 (North Wales, UK) after thinnings marked by test person no. 9 (left) and test person no. 1 (right) and projected for ten years. G_C and G_B are conifer and broadleaved stand basal area whilst cv is the diameter coefficient of variation. The histograms are overlaid by an Epanechnikov kernel density function with a bandwidth of $h = 2.5$ cm (see Eq. 4.28). d is stem diameter in cm

variogram (see Sect. 4.4.7.2) that offers insights on the spatial correlation of marks, in this case stem diameter. In this application, it is interesting not to normalise the mark variogram so that the differences in mark variance are visible.

The results clearly show that the mark variance is different. It is 59.3 cm² using the data from projecting the tree selection of test person no. 9 and 88.2 cm² when applied to the data of test person no. 1. These results differ from those of the coefficient of variation (Fig. 7.25), because variance is an absolute and the coefficient of variation is a relative dispersal measure. The difference in variance can be explained by the fact that the low-thinning marking of test person no. 1 left more residual large-sized trees behind than that of test person no. 9 (see Fig. 7.25). The general trend of the mark variograms is the same for the tree data after 10 years of simulation, i.e. the variogram curve indicates positive mark association up to $r = 20$ m, where trees of the same size (either both small or both large) are spatially associated with each other. However, in the case of test person no. 9, this trend was slightly stronger and partly even significant at small distances up to $r = 5$ m (Fig. 7.26).

Naturally it is also possible to carry out such an analysis with other spatial characteristics. For an example using the mark connection function in order to study spatial species relationships before and after a thinning, see Fig. 4.39 in Sect. 4.4.7.2.

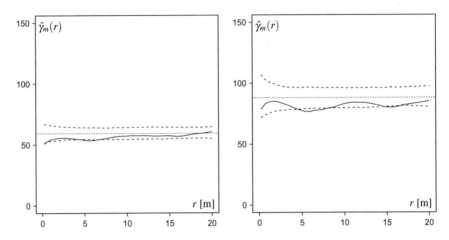

Fig. 7.26 Mark variograms $\hat{\gamma}_m(r)$ estimated from the tree coordinates at Coed y Brenin, plot 7 (North Wales, UK) and the corresponding tree stem diameters projected for ten years and based on the tree selection by test person no. 9 (left) and test person no. 1 (right). A bandwidth of $h = 1.3$ m and the Epanechnikov kernel (Eq. 4.28) were used in both cases. The 95% pointwise envelopes are from 999 random labelling simulations

References

Aguirre O, Hui GY, Gadow K, Jiménez J (2003) An analysis of spatial forest structure using neighbourhood-based variables. For Ecol Manag 183:137–145

Albert M (1999) Analyse der eingriffsbedingten Strukturveränderung und Durchforstungsmodellierung in Mischbeständen [Analysis of thinning-induced changes in stand structure and modelling of thinnings in mixed-species stands]. PhD thesis, Göttingen University. Hainholz Verlag Göttingen, 195 p

Álvarez-González JG, Schröder J, Rodríguez-Soalleiro R, Ruíz Gonzáles AD (2002) Modelling the effect of thinnings on the diameter distribution of even-aged maritime pine stands. For Ecol Manag 165:57–65

Assmann E (1970) the principles of forest yield study: studies in the organic production, structure, increment and yield of forest stands. Pergamon Press, Oxford, 506 p

Biging GS, Dobbertin M (1992) A comparison of distance-dependent competition measures for height and basal area growth of individual conifer trees. For Sci 38:695–720

Bolker BM (2008) Ecological models and data in R. Princeton University Press, Princeton, 396 p

Brams S, Fishburn P (1978) Approval voting. Am Polit Sci Rev 72:831–847

Brzeziecki B, Pommerening A, Miścicki S, Drozdowski S, Żybura H (2016) A common lack of demographic equilibrium among tree species in Białowieża National Park (NE Poland): evidence from long-term plots. J Veg Sci 27:460–469

Burkhart HE, Tomé M (2012) Modeling forest trees and stands. Springer, New York, 457 p

Cao H, Sen PK, Peery AF, Dellon ES (2016) Assessing agreement with multiple raters on correlated kappa statistics. Biom J 58:935–943

Collins L, Lanza ST (2010) Latent class and latent transition analysis. Wiley, Hoboken, 330 p

Daume S, Füldner K, Gadow Kv (1997) Zur Modellierung personenspezifischer Durchforstungen in ungleichaltigen Mischbeständen [Modelling person-specific thinnings in uneven-aged mixed stands]. Allgemeine Forst- und Jagdzeitung 169:21–26

Fleiss JL, Levin B, Paik MC (2003) Statistical methods for rates and proportions, 3rd edn. Wiley, New York, 760 p

Fleiss JL (1971) Measuring nominal scale agreement among many raters. Psychol Bull 76:378–382

Füldner K, Sattler S, Zucchini W, Gadow Kv (1996) Modellierung personenabhängiger Auswahlwahrscheinlichkeiten bei der Durchforstung [Modelling person-specific tree selection probabilities in a thinning]. Allgemeine Forst- und Jagdzeitung 167:159–162

Gadow Kv (1996) Modelling growth in managed forests—realism and limits of lumping. Sci Total Environ 183:167–177

Gadow Kv (2005) Forsteinrichtung-Analyse und Entwurf der Waldentwicklung [Forest planning—analysis and outline of forest development]. Universitätsverlag Göttingen, Göttingen, 342 p

Gibson DJ (2002) Methods in comparative plant population ecology. Oxford University Press, Oxford, 352 p

Hanewinkel M, Pretzsch H (2000) Modelling the conversion from even-aged to uneven-aged stands of Norway spruce (Picea abies (L.) Karst.) with a distance-dependent growth simulator. For Ecol Manag 134:55–70

Hasenauer H (ed) (2006) Sustainable forest management: growth models for Europe. Springer, Heidelberg, 398 p

Hasenauer H, Leitgeb E, Sterba H (1996) Der A-Wert nach Johann als Konkurrenzindex für die Abschätzung von Durchforstungseffekten [Johann's A-value used as competition index for determining thinning effects]. Allgemeine Forst- und Jagdzeitung 167:169–174

Hecker S, Haklay M, Bowser A, Makuch Z, Vogel J, Bonn A (2018) Citizen science: innovation in open science, society and policy. UCL PRESS, London, 542 p

Helms JA (ed) (1998) The dictionary of forestry. Society of American Foresters, Bethesda, 210 p

Hornby AS (2010) Oxford advanced learner's dictionary of current English, 8th edn. Oxford University Press, Oxford, 1952 p

Hui G, Pommerening A (2014) Analysing species and size diversity patterns in multi-species uneven-aged forests of northern China. For Ecol Manag 316:125–138

Illian J, Penttinen A, Stoyan H, Stoyan D (2008) Statistical analysis and modelling of spatial point patterns. Wiley, Chichester, 534 p

Johann K (1982) Der A-Wert–ein objektiver Parameter zur Bestimmung der Freistellungsstärke von Zentralbäumen [The A-thinning index–an objective parameter for the determination of release intensity of frame trees]. Tagungsbericht der Jahrestagung 1982 der Sektion Ertragskunde im Deutschen Verband Forstlicher Forschungsanstalten in Weibersbrunn, pp 146–158

Kassier HW (1993) Dynamics of diameter and height distributions in commercial timber plantations. PhD thesis University of Stellenbosch. Stellenbosch, 190 p

Kimmins JP (2004) Forest ecology-a foundation for sustainable management, 3rd edn. Pearson Education Prentice Hall, NJ, 700 p

Kramer H (1988) Waldwachstumslehre [Forest growth and yield science]. Verlag Paul Parey, Berlin, 374 p

Landis JR, Koch GG (1977) The measurement of observer agreement for categorical data. Biometrics 33:159–174

Magurran AE (2004) Measuring biological diversity. Blackwell Publishing, Oxford, 256 p

Mandallaz D (2008) Sampling techniques for forest inventories. Applied environmental statistics. Chapman and Hall/CRC, Boca Raton, 256 p

Matonis MS, Binkley D, Franklin J, Johnson KN (2016) Benefits of an "undesirable" approach to natural resource management. J For 114:658–665

Michaelis M, Menten ML (1913) Die Kinetik der Invertinwirkung [The kinetics of invertase action]. Biochemische Zeitschrift 49:333–369

Molchanov I (2017) Theory of random sets, 2nd edn. Springer, London, 696 p

Moravie M-A, Durand M, Houllier F (1999) Ecological meaning and predictive ability of social status, vigour and competition indices in a tropical rain forest (India). For Ecol Manag 117:221–240

Murray DM, Gadow Kv (1991) Relationships between the diameter distributions before and after thinning. For Sci 37:552–559

Newton AC (2009) Forest ecology and conservation: a handbook of techniques. Oxford University Press, Oxford, 454 p

Oliver CD, Larson BC (1996) Forest stand dynamics, Update edn. Wiley, New York, 520 p

Otto H-J (1994) Waldökologie [Forest ecology]. Ulmer, Stuttgart, 391 p

Perry DA, Oren R, Hart SC (2008) Forest ecosystems, 2nd edn. The Johns Hopkins University Press, Baltimore, 632 p

Pommerening A, Murphy ST (2004) A review of the history, definitions and methods of continuous cover forestry with special attention to afforestation and restocking. Forestry 77:27–44

Pommerening A, Sánchez Meador AJ (2018) Tamm review: tree interactions between myth and reality. For Ecol Manag 428:164–176

Pommerening A, Särkkä A (2013) What mark variograms tell about spatial plant interactions. Ecol Model 251:64–72

Pommerening A, Pallarés Ramos C, Kędziora W, Haufe J (2018) Rating experiments in forestry: How much agreement is there in tree marking? PLOS ONE 13:e0194747

Pommerening A, Vítková L, Zhao X, Pallarés Ramos C (2015) Towards understanding human tree selection behaviour. For Facts 9:6 p

Poore A (2011) The marteloscope—a training aid for continuous cover forest management. Woodl Herit 2011:28–29

Pretzsch H (2009) Forest dynamics, growth and yield. from measurement to model. Springer, Heidelberg, 664 p

Puettmann K, Coates KD, Messier C (2009) A critique of silviculture. Island Press, Washington, 204 p

Röhrig E, Bartsch N, Lüpke B, v., (2006) Waldbau auf ökologischer Grundlage [Silviculture on an ecological basis]. Verlag Eugen Ulmer Stuttgart, Stuttgart, 479 p

Schütz JP, Pommerening A (2013) Can Douglas fir (Pseudotsuga menziesii (Mirb.) Franco) sustainably grow in complex forest structures? For Ecol Manag 303:175–183

Soucy M, Adégbidi HG, Spinelli R, Béland M (2016) Increasing the effectiveness of knowledge transfer activities and training of the forestry workforce with marteloscopes. For Chrona 92:418–427

Spinelli R, Magagnotti N, Pari L, Soucy M (2016) Comparing tree selection as performed by different professional figures. For Sci 62:213–219

Staupendahl K, Puumalainen J (1998) Modellierung des Einflusses von Durchforstungen auf die Durchmesserverteilung von gleichaltrigen Fichtenreinbeständen [Modelling the influence of thinnings on diameter distributions of pure even-aged Norway spruce forest stands]. Centralblatt für das gesamte Forstwesen 116:249–269

Sterba H (2010) Forstliche Ertragslehre [Forest growth and yield science]. Lecture notes. BOKU University Vienna, Vienna, 120 p

Stoyan D, Pommerening A, Hummel M, Kopp-Schneider A (2018a) Multiple-rater kappas for binary data: models and interpretation. Biom J 60:381–394

Stoyan D, Pommerening A, Wünsche A (2018b) Rater classification by means of set-theoretic methods applied to forestry data. J Environ Stat 8:1–17

Surowiecki J (2004) The wisdom of crowds. Random House, New York, 295 p

Susse R, Allegrini C, Bruciamacchie M, Burrus R (2011) Management of irregular forests: developing the full potential of the forest. Azur Multimedia, Saint Maime, 144 p

Uebersax JS, Grove WM (1993) A latent trait finite mixture model for the analysis of rating agreement. Biometrics 49:823–835

Vítková L, Ní Dhubháin Á, Pommerening A (2016) Agreement in tree marking: what is the uncertainty of human tree selection in selective forest management? For Sci 62:288–296

Vorobyov O (1984) Mean-value modelling. Nauka, Moscow, 373 p

Weiskittel AR, Hann DW, Kerschaw JA, Vanclay JK (2011) Forest growth and yield modeling. Wiley Blackwell, Chichester, 415 p

Wenk G, Antanaitis V, Šmelko Š (1990) Waldertragslehre [Forest growth and yield science]. Deutscher Landwirtschaftsverlag. Berlin, 448 p

Zucchini W, Gadow Kv (1995) Two indices of agreement among foresters selecting trees for thinning. For Landsc Res 1:199–206

Appendix A
Qualitative Forest Description

The basic method of forest management planning at stand level includes four distinctive steps.

1. **Analysis of current state**

   - Description of site (elevation, exposition, climate, soil), vegetation and fauna (if possible and relevant).
   - Current state of the forest, stand description, inventory and quantitative analysis.

2. **Anticipation of forest dynamics**

   - "Anamnesis": What has influenced forest dynamics in the past? Any clues from historical records or current tree morphology? Stand origin, thinning history, silvicultural objectives, past forest development.
   - How will the ecosystem change? In which direction and what is the likely pace of change?

3. **Assessment of forest development pathways**

   - Reference scenario: What would happen without human interventions?
   - What vegetation types and forest structures are possible in the future? What should be the target diameter range, the rotation period?

4. **Selecting the silviculturally appropriate techniques to meet the objectives**

   - What are important sustainability criteria for this site?
   - How much input is necessary (compared to zero intervention as a reference) and justifiable? Intervention types, intervention cycles, intervention intensity.
   - Optimising the solution.

A key element of silvicultural planning and in fact of many aspects of research, is the description of the current state of a given forest unit. This is always the beginning and the basis for subsequent planning and research. Qualitative forest description is also an important aspect of silvicultural education and training, because it is a useful

© Springer Nature Switzerland AG 2019
A. Pommerening and P. Grabarnik, *Individual-based Methods in Forest Ecology and Management*, https://doi.org/10.1007/978-3-030-24528-3

exercise for developing and enhancing observational skills. The importance of such skills cannot be emphasised enough because they foster the ability to anticipate future forest development. These skills are required for deciding what silvicultural or conservation action to take if any.

After careful observation in the field and a detailed analysis of environmental factors the analyst starts with a qualitative description of the current state. This provides the analyst and the reader of the silvicultural plan/the research work with an easy access to the woodland in question. There are many possible schemes and templates for stand descriptions. In this book, as an example, the modified structure of a stand description is presented that was originally developed at the Institute of Silviculture, Göttingen University (Germany) by U. Weihs and colleagues (see also Weihs 1999). The elements of stand description draw on traditional ways of classifying forests (see for example Köstler 1956; Bauer 1962) that cannot be attributed to a single author.

The analyst first establishes the general stand type (mixed species or pure stand) and describes the principle species of the forest or stand (see Table A.1). This is followed by general characteristics, the main tree species and age. Then a reference to the stage of stand development is made using traditional forestry terms that typically vary from country to country and are only defaults.

The numbers given in Tables A.1 and A.2 may also differ from region to region and need to be adapted to what is commonly used in the geographic area where the stand description is made. In certain situations also depending on the analyst's preferences, it may be more suitable to use the ecologically motivated, qualitative development stages defined by Oliver and Larson (1996, p. 148f):

Stand initiation or formation stage: After a disturbance, new individuals and species continue to appear for several years.

Stem exclusion stage: After several years, new individuals do not appear and some of the existing ones die. The surviving ones grow larger and express differences in height and diameter, first one species and then another may appear to dominate the stand.

Understorey reinitiating stage: Later, forest floor herbs, shrubs and advance regeneration again appear and survive in the understorey, although they grow very little.

Old growth stage: Much later, overstorey trees die in an irregular fashion, and some of the understorey trees begin growing to the overstorey.

Providing more quantitative criteria, Emborg et al. (2000) have suggested the following forest development stages for Suserup Skov, a near-natural, temperate mixed beech forest in Denmark:

Innovation phase: Starts with the occurrence of well established regeneration in gaps, more than 5 vigorous plants larger than 20 cm per m^2. *Average duration*: 14 years.

Table A.1 Characteristics for describing the main species of a forest stand. Modified from Institute of Silviculture (2004) and Guest (2004, p. 55f.)

Principal tree species		
Characteristic	Item	Description
Title		General characteristics of the stand (main species before admixture, e.g. mixed oak-beech forest)
Main tree species	Exact botanical description	Tree species, on which management emphasis lies
Age[a]	Average age, planting year (if known)	For example $\frac{16}{11-20}$ years or $p\frac{72}{68-75}$
Stage of stand development	Seedlings/saplings	From establishment until canopy closure ($\sim$2 m total height)
	Young stand	From canopy closure (2 m total height) to 7 cm dbh
	(a) Thicket stage	Canopy closure to beginning of natural self pruning
	(b) Young growth	Natural self-pruning (branchless stem >3 m) to 7 cm dbh
	Pole wood	Average dbh of dominant trees 15–20 cm
	Small wood	Average dbh of dominant trees 20–35 cm
	Medium wood	Average dbh of dominant trees 35–50 cm
	Large wood	Average dbh of dominant trees >50 cm
Establishment	Planted	
	Direct seeding	
	Natural regeneration	Initial spacing, provenance, planting stock, afforestation
	Coppice	
	Beating up/refilling	
Growth rate	Vigorous	
	Slow growth rate	For the principal tree species
	Stunted	
Dominant trees	*Stem length*	
	– Long	Crown base above 2/3 of tree total height
	– Medium	Crown base above 1/2 of tree total height
	– Short	Crown base above 1/3 of tree total height
	Stem shape	
	– Valuable timber	For mature oak, beech and other valuable hardwoods as well as valuable conifers, e.g. Douglas fir, larch and pine
	– Straight, swept, crooked, etc.	Deviations from the average stem shape
	– Forked	High fork >9 m; intermediate fork 6–9 m; low fork <6 m
	– Ecological features	Cavities, epiphytes (ferns, lichens, mosses), ivy, mistletoe, fruiting bodies of fungi, nesting boxes, nest holes etc.

(continued)

Table A.1 (continued)

Characteristic	Item	Description
	Stem shape	
	– Branchiness	Pruned? (important with trees which tend not to self-prune, e.g. most conifers), light/heavy branching, swellings on the stem; branch defects: pegs, knots, knot scars, e.g. "Chinese beards" on beech, epicormic shoots
Dominant trees	– Damages	Felling and skidding damage, frost and drought cracks, browsing damage, root and butt rot, canker, bark-stripping, browsing and fraying damage
	Crown	
	– Shape	Large, narrow, onesided, squashed, harvesting damage
	– Damage	Mildew, frost, insects, effects of emissions, broken top/crown snap
	– Health	Needle loss, chlorosis etc.
	– Ecology	Nests, dreys, epiphytes etc.

[a] The "fraction" gives the average stand age or average planting year in the "numerator" and the range of these variables in the "denominator". In Britain, the planting year (abbreviated with the letter p) is preferred to stand age

Aggradation phase: Starts when regeneration has control of the herbal vegetation which is usually the case when regeneration plants are larger than 3 m. *Average duration*: 56 years.

Early biostatic phase: Starts when trees have reached the upper canopy layer, i.e. a total height of 25 m. *Average duration*: 96 years.

Late biostatic phase: Starts when trees are aging, start collecting wounds and scars and tend to become more vulnerable to biotic and abiotic damage. Usually when trees reach a dbh[1] of 80 cm. *Average duration*: 108 years.

Degradation phase: Starts when degrading trees cause more permanent gaps in the main canopy, large enough to encourage regeneration, i.e. gaps $> 100\,m^2$, which cannot be filled by lateral crown growth of adjacent trees. *Average duration*: 10 years.

In Switzerland, Schütz (2003) has suggested a strictly quantitative system for defining stand development phases (see Table A.3).

[1] Stem diameter at breast height, usually at 1.3 m above soil level.

Table A.2 Characteristics for describing admixed species in a forest stand. Modified from Institute of Silviculture (2004) and Guest (2004, p. 55f.)

Admixed tree species		
Characteristic	Item	Description
Mingling	*Horizontal mingling*	
	– Individual trees	Individual tree mixtures
	– Small groups	Group diameter ≤15 m (∼1/2 tree length)
	– Groups	Group diameter 15–30 m (∼1 tree length)
	– Large groups	Group diameter 30–60 m (∼2 tree lengths)
	– Areas	Group diameter >60 m
	– Rows	Tree species mixed in rows
	– Strips	Several rows of one tree species up to 30 m wide
	Vertical mingling	The admixed tree species can have different storeys in relation to the main species e.g., beech under-storey (upper, lower, mid)
The characteristics age, development stage, origin, dominant trees should be described in a similar way to the main tree species		
Growth rate (the likely future must be considered here)	Catching up	The visually assessed growth rate of the admixed tree species is always compared with the main tree species
	Faster growth	
	Similar	
	Suppressed	
	Left behind	
Other tree species	Scattered	Tree species with a mixture proportion <10% only need to be named; minority tree species with a high conservation value should be emphasised
Canopy closure	– Dense	Crowns intersect
	– Closed	Crowns touch each other
	– Loose	Crowns are separated by half of the crown diameter
	– Light	Crowns are separated by the diameter of a whole crown
	– Scattered	Crowns separated by a few crown diameters
	Additional descriptions	
	– Regeneration gaps	Beating up or replanting may be required
	– Openings	Open areas in older stands
	– Holes	Disruption of canopy which are unlikely to close
	– Scattered	Older stands with SD^a of 0.1–0.3
	– Bogs or windblows	Unstocked or SD^a < 0.1 stocked with trees

(continued)

Table A.2 (continued)

		Admixed tree species
Characteristic	Item	Description
	Secured regeneration	Secured regeneration under main canopy
	Beating up/refilling	Artificial introduction of tree species in a middle-aged stand, which is supposed to become part of the main stand, e.g. Douglas fir in an unsuccessful pine polewood
	Understorey	Storey to protect stems in the upper storey or the soil
Special features	Remaining seed trees/retention of standards	Remnants of canopy trees from the previous forest generation which are still present on site, either isolated or at a SD[a] of 0.1–0.3
	Underplanting	Artificial regeneration of species under the canopy of a mature stand
	Nurse (crop)	Use of pioneer species to nurse desired future stand
		Structure, afforestation, habitats, aesthetically pleasing "character trees", other tree species, ground vegetation, degree of tending, recreation pressure, forest margins, reserve/seed trees etc.

[a] SD—stocking degree: $SD = \frac{\text{Observed basal area/ha}}{\text{Norm basal area/ha}}$; norm basal area/ha can be defined as a corresponding yield table/model basal area or as the maximum basal area of an unthinned control (natural stocking degree)

To assess the history of stand development the origin of the main canopy species is established. Then judging by the visual tree characteristics the growth performance and potential is described. This information has a bearing on the options for future stand development and tending.

Following on from this, the morphology of the dominant trees is described separately for stem and crown. This assessment includes general, economically important and ecological aspects.

Table A.3 System of stand development phases after Schütz (2003)

Stage	Top diameter[a] (cm)	Top height[b] (m)
Young growth		0.3–1.3
Thicket	0–10	1.3–8.0
Small pole wood	10–20	>8.0
Large pole wood	20–30	<18
Small timber stand	30–40	>18
Medium timber stand	40–50	
High timber stand	>50	

[a] Quadratic mean diameter of the 100 largest diameter trees per hectare
[b] Stand height corresponding to top diameter

The stand description is then continued using Table A.2 for any admixed species. This refers to the most important (in terms of trees per hectare or basal area/ha) 1-2 species after the principle species. First the type of horizontal mingling in relation to the principle and other tree species is determined. At the same time the analyst indicates to which canopy storey the species belong. Naturally the assessment of horizontal and vertical mingling should also be applied to the main species in uneven-aged complex forest stands.

In Switzerland, three distinctive mingling terms are used in stand description, i.e. *mingling type*, *mingling degree* and *mingling form* (Schütz 2003, p. 44f.). The mingling type simply refers to the tree species occurring in the stand under study whilst the mingling degree gives the absolute abundances of the species (in terms of stand area, basal area, volume or number of trees). Finally, the mingling form describes horizontal mingling in the narrow sense of the word as defined in Table A.2.

For a quantitative assessment of storeys Assmann (1970, p. 91) suggested that all trees with a total height greater than 80% of the height of the tallest tree in the stand or of the top height belong to the overstorey (sometimes also referred to as upper storey). Trees between 50 and 80% of maximum tree height are considered as part of the middle or mid storey and all trees with a total height smaller than 50% of the height of the tallest tree are understorey or lower-storey trees. Again these numbers can be adjusted to meet local conditions better. On p. 94, Assmann (1970) used the classes >90, 70–90 and <70% instead.

Next the characteristics age, development stage, origin and dominant trees of Table A.1 should be applied to the main admixed species. This is followed by an assessment of the absolute growth rate of the admixed tree species in relation to the main species. Other tree species which make up less than 10% of stand density only need to be named. However, tree species with a high conservation value should be emphasised independent of their relative numbers. This can, for example, be single middle-aged or old oak trees in spruce plantations, sub-dominant yew trees (*Taxus baccata* L.) in beech (*Fagus sylvatica* L.) stands and scattered individuals of Montpellier maple (*Acer monspessulanum* L.) in Portuguese oak (*Quercus faginea* LAM.) forests.

Finally canopy closure and special features are described as suggested in Table A.2. Canopy closure and the description of tree crowns help to understand stand density and thinning urgency. Naturally not all aspects of Tables A.1 and A.2 apply in all woodlands. Both tables are only meant as guidelines and it is possible to use some, all or additional elements of description depending on the objectives of the stand analysis. Throughout the two tables it is also possible that combinations of more than one item applies in a single stand, for example, small wood and medium wood. The stand description should be brief and precise, thus enabling a reader, who has not yet visited the site, to develop a good idea of the stand under study.

Example A.1 is only loosely orientated towards the guidelines in Tables A.1 and A.2. The text also includes information about current ecosystem goods and services. Separate descriptions were prepared for each storey and the ground vegetation which in this case was very effective, as the management plan for the stand under consideration was prepared with the objective to identify suitable methods for transformation to continuous cover forestry management where a special assessment of canopy layers is very useful.

Example A.1 Isle of Anglesey (Wales, UK), Newborough Forest, Compartment 13, subcompartment A (Guest 2008, p. 13):

Current use
Conservation/Protection : Recreation : Production: 4:4:2

Stand description
Overstorey: Aesthetically pleasing 59-year-old slow growing mature Corsican pine large wood stand. Valuable stand with good stem form (some high forking), however, with relatively large dead branches.
Midstorey: Occasional scattered individual Sitka spruce and lodgepole pine.
Understorey: High species diversity. Scattered individuals and groups of birch, elder, sycamore, oak, hawthorn, willow, cherry and wild service tree.
Ground vegetation: Moderate—dense. Bramble and fern.

Example A.2 is from the Estonian boreal forest at Järvselja, the experimental forest of the Estonian University of Life Sciences, Tartu, see also Fig. A.1.

Example A.2 Compartment 228, Järvselja (Estonia):

Stand description
Mixed birch—common alder—aspen wood, approximately 50–60 years old, small to medium wood from natural regeneration after clearfelling. Main species vigorous with long, straight stems and short, narrow crowns. Admixed species individually mixed and occasionally in small groups, the same age, development stage, origin and growth rate as birch. Aspen is occasionally faster growing than birch. Dense lime understorey that has been cut back during the last thinning. Norway spruce scattered in under- and midstorey with signs of moose damage. Main canopy loose to closed.

In addition it would seem appropriate to comment on aspects of infrastructure, i.e. forest roads and rides, extraction racks, roundwood stacking locations, topography, exposition and ownership, if this information is relevant to the purpose of the stand description.

Fig. A.1 Mixed
birch—common
alder—aspen wood at
compartment 228, Järvselja
experimental forest in
Estonia (see Example A.2)

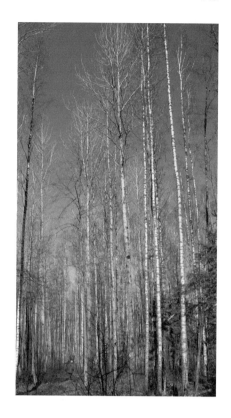

References

Assmann E (1970) The principles of forest yield study. Studies in the organic production, structure, increment and yield of forest stands. Pergamon Press, Oxford, 506 p

Bauer FW (1962) Waldbau als Wissenschaft. Waldbauliche Wisssenschaftslehre und Grundlegung [Silviculture as science. Scientific theory and basics of silviculture.], vol 1. BLV Verlagsgesellschaft, München, 183 p

Emborg J, Christensen M, Heilmann-Clausen J (2000) The structural dynamics of Suserup Skov, a near-natural temperate deciduous forest in Denmark. For Ecol Manag 126:173–189

Guest CJ (2004) Quantifying the response of naturally regenerating sessile oak (Quercus petraea LIEBL.) to silvicultural systems in the Pfälzer Forest (Germany). BSc thesis, Bangor University, Bangor, 69 p

Guest CJ (2008) Newborough forest management plan. Bangor, 72 p

Institute of Silviculture (2004) Forest stand description. Göttingen University, Göttingen, 2 p

Köstler J (1956) Silviculture. Oliver and Boyd, Edinburgh, 416 p

Oliver CD, Larson BC (1996) Forest stand dynamics, Update edn. Wiley, New York, 520 p

Schütz JP (2003) Waldbau I. Die Prinzipien der Waldnutzung und der Waldbehandlung. Skript zur Vorlesung Waldbau I. [Silviculture I. The principles of forest exploitation and forest management. Notes accompanying the lectures in silviculture I.] Unpublished manuscript. ETH Zürich, 212 p

Weihs   U   (1999)   Waldpflege.   Ein   geeignetes   Instrument   zur   nachhaltigen Sicherung der vielfältigen Waldfunktionen. [Forest management. A suitable method for sustaining multiple forest functions.] Förderverein des Fachbereichs Forstwirtschaft und Umweltmanagement, Göttingen, 308 p

Appendix B
Survey Protocol for the Establishment of Permanent Forest Research Plots

Based on the authors' own experience and that of other researchers (e.g. Pretzsch 2009, p. 112ff.), a general and basic survey protocol is presented here, which is suitable for multiple purposes including

- Woodland structure research and spatial tree interactions,
- Analysis of the effects of natural disturbances and human interventions (including environmental change) on forest structure and biodiversity,
- Sampling simulation,
- Tree modelling,
- Marteloscopes,
- Best-practice demonstration plots,
- Monitoring,
- Classic factor and block experiments,
- Teaching, training, life-long learning,
- PR, open-day, team-building events and research dissemination.

The main focus of this survey protocol is on mature, individual trees, not on entire forest stands or tree populations in the first instance. For very small plants, e.g. seedlings and saplings or ground vegetation, other survey protocols apply. Depending on the objectives of specific projects this protocol naturally needs to be adapted and/or extended.

Information is collected on growth and biomass allocation of individual trees dependent on tree properties, the immediate vicinity of each tree, environmental factors and impact/disturbance effects. The change in stem diameter, total height, crown morphology and mortality (or survival probability) of individual trees has to be measured along a sufficiently wide gradient of intertree interaction and neighbourhood situations for all tree species involved. To achieve this, the research plots should also include extreme tree neighbourhood scenarios where some trees are exposed to exceptionally high or low competition pressure or interaction intensity.

© Springer Nature Switzerland AG 2019
A. Pommerening and P. Grabarnik, *Individual-based Methods*
in Forest Ecology and Management, https://doi.org/10.1007/978-3-030-24528-3

Research experience, particularly in spatial analyses, suggests that it is desirable to include a minimum of 150–200 trees in every plot during its whole lifetime. For marteloscope research it is crucial that the plot area is sufficiently large so that test persons marking trees do not influence each other.

Although the individual tree and individual test person, rather than the forest stand, is the basic unit of information, square or rectangular plots with an extent of 0.6–1.5 ha are desirable, because it is easier and cheaper to measure and monitor trees in a defined area. Also in spatially explicit approaches, interaction and edge effects can then more easily be taken care of.

B.1   Site Selection

First, research objectives need to be identified followed by the selection of a suitable study area. Before further steps are taken to select specific sites, the local authorities in charge of the likely study area should be informed and asked for comment, permission and any support they may be able to offer. It is crucially important for the success of a research project to secure the support of the local forester/officer and/or landowner.

An initial field reconnaissance should be carried out together with representatives of the local landowner to select suitable sites. Taking into account the research objectives of the project (including environmental conditions, target tree species, age/height range etc.) 2–3 alternative sites should be identified. To ensure a good potential for research and publications every plot should have at least one replication. In marteloscope research, not trees or plots but the test persons marking the trees for thinning constitute the replicates. However, it is recommended to set up at least two marteloscope plots at the same site (twin plots), as one of the two plots in turns may be affected by recent thinnings and can only be used for demonstration purposes during the next 5–8 years.

The following items should be considered:

- As part of the initial field reconnaissance the plot boundaries should be roughly marked with flagging tape. In temperate and boreal forests, an approximate size of 100 m × 100 m has turned out to be a good standard.
- Each prospective forest site should be described using the templates of Tables A.1 and A.2 in Appendix A. Sample measurements of tree diameter and total height help to establish the forest development stage and the tree densities involved. Digital photographs may be useful to refresh your memory back in the office.
- The proportion of differing (non-target) tree species should be small. Differing tree species are those which are not a typical element of the research objectives and/or of the studied woodland community, e.g. Sitka spruce (*Picea sitchensis* (BONG.) CARR.) is unusual/not natural in a European stand of oak (*Quercus spp.*) and ash (*Fraxinus spp.*), whilst rowan (*Sorbus aucuparia* L.) or birch (*Betula spp.*) would be acceptable.

- For marteloscope research, only select sites that have not been thinned during the past 8–15 years.
- All tree species relevant to the research project should be found in the main canopy layer, preferably in even proportions. As mentioned, heterogeneous stand structures including locally variable tree density are advantageous. Environmental conditions (particularly soil and topography) should, however, be as uniform as possible.

After a pre-selection of 2–3 alternative sites a final decision based on stand descriptions, initial survey data and another site visit, if necessary, should be made. At this point a written permit should be obtained from the local landowner.

B.2   Plot Establishment

Research plots typically consist of a core area and a surrounding outer buffer (of 5–10 m width). All tree locations should be inside the core area or the buffer and surveys should always take place outside the vegetation period, preferably in the same season as used for plot establishment.

Research plots should not share a boundary with open fields or other fundamentally different vegetation or land-use types. They also need to be kept well away from roads and rides. Extraction racks should only be included, if they are an essential part of the experiment, e.g. in marteloscope-based research.

All trees should be permanently marked with a unique reference number and a stem-diameter (dbh, see Sect. B.3.3) line before any measurements are taken.

It is essential to obtain information about past forest development including human and natural disturbances from the relevant forestry or conservation database. Also the environmental conditions should be described and monitored as accurately as possible.

It is recommended that all survey work activities are recorded. This record should ideally include number of staff and hours worked and the equipment used. With this information it should be possible to plan future work and to judge on data quality some time in the future.

B.2.1   Marking Plot Boundaries

The corners of the plot core area (and, if necessary, plot edges) should be marked with wooden posts. To ensure some permanence it is recommended to use marking devices that attract as little attention as possible and that are difficult to remove. If possible the boundary posts should be marked with station numbers (e.g. stn1, stn2, …). Internal theodolite survey points may be established within the plot boundary as necessary and should be marked in the same way. It is important that all boundary posts and internal survey points (e.g. sti1, sti2, …) are maintained as permanently as possible to allow efficient re-measurements. Boundary posts may be complemented by small trenches or walls pointing either way to the next posts.

The trees in the buffer can be marked with a contrasting colour to that used in the main plot. These markings have the purpose of alerting operators working in the forest to the presence of a research plot and thus safeguard the trees. Yellow and orange have been found to be satisfactory for this purpose. Marking can for example encircle buffer trees at a height of 1.5 m. Buffer trees are marked with numbers well out of sequence with the trees in the plot core area, e.g. >900, if the number of trees in the plot is markedly smaller than 900, otherwise the marking of buffer trees starts with numbers >9000. Apart from that trees in the buffer should be recorded in the same way as any other tree in the plot (see Pretzsch 2009, p. 114).

B.2.2   Plot Identification Number

On one of the buffer trees, on a sign or on the plot corner posts the unique plot identification number should be painted, so as to be visible from inside the plot.

B.3   Individual-Tree Measurements

B.3.1   Tree Numbers

All trees with a dbh value greater than 4–5 cm should be numbered. As part of plot establishment it is best to mark the location of dbh measurement first followed by painting the tree number above the dbh line before moving on to the next tree. Tree number and dbh line should be close to each other and at the same side of the tree. Stem diameter permitting tree numbers should be painted large enough so that they can be identified from afar. This is particular important in marteloscope and demonstration plots. In such experiments, resources permitting it may be even useful to have tree numbers on two sides of a tree to facilitate tree recognition from different angles.

Where possible exterior grade white paint should be used. Prior to any painting the bark should be cleaned. The methods will depend on species and may range from using a rag on smooth and thin barked species to partially removing bark with a billhook or a slasher on thick-barked species such as pine. This preparation has a strong effect on the durability of the marks but should not be done so as to damage the tree. Painting should not be considered when the bark is wet or in frosty weather.

Numbers should preferably be painted horizontally and only vertically where the stem size does not allow otherwise. In the latter case, tree number 123 should for example be painted as $\frac{1}{2}$.

Fig. B.1 Example of a tree number and a dbh line from a permanent research plot at Artist's Wood in North Wales (UK)

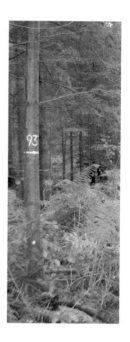

Where trees are too small to be painted, numbered aluminum discs can be attached to a branch of the tree using strong, clear sticky tape.

It has been found advantageous to divide the plot into strips of approximately 3–5 m (older forest stands 10 m) running parallel to two of the plot boundaries and to number the trees in the strips in sequence (Pretzsch 2009). This facilitates later tree recognition and data collection. Numbers and marks should be discrete, e.g. not visible from foot paths and roads so as not to draw undue attention.

On a practical note, it is also recommended to paint number "1" on trees always in the English way as a simple vertical line for better contrast with number "7". The number "3" is easier to recognise when painted as in Fig. B.1.

dbh marks and numbers should be checked and repainted prior to every re-measurement.

During the lifetime of a long-term research plot, eventually some trees die and others are removed from site. At the same time new offspring trees reach maturity so that they can be included in the survey. To avoid confusion and miscalculations unique new numbers outside the original range of numbers should be assigned to these trees, i.e. if the maximum original number was 400, a new ingrowth tree should be given the number 401 rather than that of a dead tree.

Depending on research objectives, lying and standing dead trees can be numbered in a similar way.

B.3.2   Tree Species

Tree species should be recorded using simple unique species codes to expedite the survey work.

B.3.3   Stem Diameter at Breast Height

Stem diameter at breast height (dbh) should be applied at 1.3 m above ground level (on a slope this should be on the uphill side). Care should be taken with older trees, e.g. pine trees, because a thick humus cover at the base formed by for example detached bark pieces could cause the measuring point to be higher than it should be. Figures in forest mensuration books, e.g. Avery and Burkhart (2002), van Laar and Akça (2007), Philip (1994) and West (2009) may help to identify the dbh locations of trees in critical situations.

Stem diameter at breast height should be measured to nearest 0.1 cm (e.g. dbh = 16.7 cm) preferably using diameter tapes rather than callipers. If for some reason callipers need to be used, a short additional line perpendicular to the dbh line should indicate the direction of the first calliper measurement (a second one should be taken at an angle of 90° to the first).

B.3.4   Total Tree Height and Height to Base of Crown

At least 20–40 or as many as possible total height (h) and height to base of crown-records per tree species should be taken across the whole stem diameter range and measured to the nearest 0.1 m (e.g. $h = 12.4$ m). As part of the first survey (plot installation) it is useful to include all trees in the height survey if affordable. If the forest is clearly divided into different layers, e.g. understorey of beech (*Fagus sylvatica* L.) in a stand of mature oak (*Quercus spp.*)/beech, tree heights should be collected separately for each canopy layer.

The same sample trees should be used in every re-measurement and complemented by appropriate substitutes for dead trees.

B.3.5   Tree Locations

Tree locations are useful to survey for multiple reasons, even if they are not directly used as part of a current research project. Applying a computer-based theodolite x, y and z Cartesian coordinates should be produced from polar coordinates. Devices with a reflector like a theodolite are preferred to ensure the correct measurement of tree coordinates. For measuring angles, the reflector is held at a central point on the stem surface directly facing the theodolite. The distance measurement is taken by moving the reflector to a lateral position on the stem surface towards the stem centre. For certain research objectives it can be useful to additionally survey the locations of recent tree stumps and of boundary/survey points. Lying deadwood requires two sets of coordinates, one at the base and the other at the tip.

Tree locations are usually defined as stem centre locations, however, in studies of tree interactions, it can sometimes be useful to define alternative or additional tree locations (e.g. tree tip locations projected down to the forest floor).

B.3.6 Crown Measures

To establish crown morphology, it is recommended to measure crown radii in at least four, preferably in eight cardinal directions (N, NE, E, etc.). Crown mirrors and spherical densiometer can be used for this purpose. It has been found that a simple "look-up method" involving a measuring tape is quite satisfactory, however, the results of this method should be checked or calibrated against those using proper measuring devices. Crown radii measurements should always be based on the sample trees that are selected for measuring total tree height and height to base of crown (see Sect. B.3.4). The main tree species of the plot should be well represented in the sample.

Where a tree is leaning, the centre of gravity of the crown will not lie directly over the tree's stem centre location. In such a case, it is necessary to determine the projection of the centre of gravity or of the crown tip onto the ground and mark this with a ranging rod. The crown radii are then taken from this point. The location of the ranging rod, in relation to the tree location (distance and angle), should be measured and noted.

Visibility and wind regime permitting terrestrial LiDAR devices and digital cameras in connection with photogrammetric software can be employed for complex and more precise surveying of various aspects of crown morphology including past growth rates of crown measures and even shoot growth rates.

B.4 Additional Measurements and Observations

B.4.1 Growth Rates, Volume and Age

Growth rates are most precisely established from subsequent measurements of the same trees. Depending on measuring devices and growth velocity of the trees under study it often requires 3–10 years before any re-measurement can produce reliable results.

If time is an issue, growth rates can be established from off-plot sample trees adjacent to the plot buffer by using destructive methods. Additional permission from local landowners may be required for this.

Increment cores should then be taken from 20–40 trees per species or from as many as possible. They should cover the whole dbh range. Two increment cores (if possible) should be taken from every sample tree, one from NE, one from SW preferably at a height of 1.3 m above ground level (boring height should be recorded). The use of 8-mm borers is preferable.

Stem analysis is a more precise method to establish past growth patterns. The tree processed for stem analysis as well as all neighbouring trees affecting its growing space in recent years should be numbered (using a previously unused range of tree numbers) and measured in a circular sample plot centered at the stem-analysis tree. For neighbouring trees, tree locations, species, dbh and total height should be recorded. A sketch should be drawn of this circular sample plot to show its location in relation to the large research plot.

On standing trees, north should be indicated on the stem before felling. The stem should then be marked for disk sampling. Disks should be taken using absolute 2-m intervals, starting at 1.3 m height (i.e. 1.3, 3.3, 5.3, 7.3 m etc.). Additional disks should represent 0.3 m and 10% of total tree height, the latter to provide data for the true form factor. North should be marked at each disk before cutting them. Disks are to be labelled with plot number, tree number, and disk location. The use of an electric planer has proved to facilitate further analysis. Small disks may be planed on a lathe. Analysis or scanning of the disks should be done not later than 48 hours after sampling.

Windblown, thinned and other dead trees from inside the research plot should also be used for stem analysis. If volume-dbh-height relationships and/or tree age are unknown, increment cores and stem analyses can also be used to determine these measures.

B.4.2   Diameter at Stump Height/Root Collar Diameter

To reconstruct dbh and total height of trees recently thinned before the first survey, stem diameters at stump height can be measured on at least 30 live trees per species and across the entire diameter range. Stump height should be considered in the preliminary site inspection and will be above the point of root buttressing (usually at 30 cm above ground level). This location roughly corresponds to the location of root collar.

B.4.3   Particularities

Additional observations that may add to an understanding of the site should be recorded, e.g. tree morphology, tree health, biotic and abiotic damage, animal presence etc.

B.4.4   Additional Marteloscope Requirements

In marteloscope plots, a complete survey and/or estimation of tree-based volume, habitat value, timber quality and stem damage may be useful to allow more detailed analyses of the marking behaviour of test persons.

B.4.5   Open-Grown Trees

If the plot data are used for tree modelling including the potential-modifier approach (see Sect. 5.2.5), it can be recommended to sample a range of open-grown trees outside the forest near the research plots growing in comparable soil conditions. These trees should never have had tree neighbours throughout their lifetime and can also be re-measured in the same way as the plot trees inside the forest following the same survey protocol. The measurements from open-grown trees, particularly stem diameters and crown measures, will allow defining growth potentials (Hasenauer 1997).

B.4.6   Upper Stem Diameters

Stem diameters measured at locations higher than 1.3 m above ground level, e.g. at 7 m, can help to establish stem morphology and timber quality.

B.4.7   Trees of Special Scientific Interest

As part of the study it may be necessary to identify trees of special scientific interest, e.g. frame trees, see Sect. 3.6.1. These trees should also be marked in the field using ribbons of varying colours and this information should also be entered in the database. However, in marteloscope plots, for obvious reasons such trees should only be recorded on file and their special nature should not be apparent to test persons in the field.

B.4.8   Maintenance

If silvicultural or conservation interventions are necessary, researchers should do the tree marking or should at least be involved. Any plans for interventions should previously be discussed with the responsible local landowner.

It is recommended to check research plots immediately after any (likely) impact, i.e. after storm events have subsided, e.g. in early spring, after every human intervention (even if trees selected for removal were previously marked) to monitor trees that have recently been damaged or died and to record the causes.

B.4.9   Soil Survey

On each experimental plot a soil pit should be dug in the approximate centre of the plot. The pit should be large enough to allow adequate description and sampling, and be constructed in such a way to allow easy entrance and exit and escape for small creatures. The headwall of the pit should be at least two thirds the crown radius away from any tree. The soil should be described using standard soil survey procedures. If permission is obtained, the pit should be left open for teaching and demonstration purposes. In this case, it should be fenced to avoid accidents. Soil heterogeneity should be checked over the whole plot and any major variations described and sampled as appropriate.

References

Avery TE, Burkhart HE (2002) Forest measurements, 5th edn. McGraw-Hill, Inc., New York, 456 p

Hasenauer H (1997) Dimensional relationships of open-grown trees in Austria. For Ecol Manag 96:197–206

Philip MS (1994) Measuring trees and forests, 2nd edn. CABI Publishing, Wallingford, 310 p

Pretzsch H (2009) Forest dynamics, growth and yield. From measurement to model. Springer, Heidelberg, 664 p

van Laar A, Akça A (2007) Forest mensuration. Manag For Ecosyst (Springer, Dordrecht) 13:383 p

West PW (2009) Tree and forest measurement, 2nd edn. Springer, Dordrecht, 192 p

Appendix C
Brief Introduction to the R Language

For many quantitative methods introduced in this book listings in R are provided. R is a program and computer language for scientific computing including data analysis and modelling. Originally R was developed by Robert Gentleman and Ross Ihaka between 1992 and 1995 and was based on the S language, a commercial software created by John Chambers in 1976. Now the R program is maintained by an international core team. Working with R has become a standard in plant sciences. As a free and powerful open-source programming environment its significance in natural sciences, particularly in plant sciences, is constantly rising. The software is platform independent, i.e. it runs on the most important operating systems including MS Windows, Mac OS, Linux and Ubuntu. R is also compatible with the higher programming languages Fortran and C/C++, i.e. it is possible to write functions in these languages stored in external files. The compiled code can then be used in R.

Whilst most programs nowadays use interactive graphical user interfaces, R is mainly command-driven. The user has to type in sequences of commands and to request R to execute them. This is something one needs to get accustomed to, however, it has the advantage that the user is more flexible for creative and complex tasks such as the development of sophisticated analysis routines and simulation models. With menu-based programs we much depend on the particular organisation of that program (Braun and Murdoch 2007) and have limited choices.

The following pages have been designed to ease the process of getting used to the command-line approach of the R software. They are a hands-on introduction for readers who are unfamiliar with R to offer just enough material to get started and to motivate beginners to explore and experiment with the program.

Download R from http://cran.r-project.org and select the "CRAN mirror" for your country of residence. Click on the download link for your operating system and on the subfolder "base". It is sufficient for the purpose of this book to download and install a binary (precompiled) version. Then click on the download link and launch the installation program. (Double) clicking on the R icon will launch the program.

With no prior knowledge of R it is recommended to follow the examples below for 1–3 days to get started. Some of the R code introduced in the following sections you can find on https://github.com/apommerening/R-course. The introductory chapters

© Springer Nature Switzerland AG 2019
A. Pommerening and P. Grabarnik, *Individual-based Methods*
in Forest Ecology and Management, https://doi.org/10.1007/978-3-030-24528-3

of Braun and Murdoch (2007), Bolker (2008), Dalgaard (2008), Jones et al. (2009) and Robinson and Hamann (2010) can help to expand the basic knowledge given in this appendix.

C.1 Basics

The sign that looks like a greater-than operator (>) is in fact a prompt symbol indicating that R is ready for user inputs. When this appears in the console window you can type commands. For example, you can simply use R as a calculator in the following way

```
> 1 + 2
[1] 3
```

The number in square brackets in the output line gives the index number of the first element. Operators can also be nested, e.g.

```
> (8 - 5) * 3
[1] 9
```

first 5 is subtracted from 8 and then the result is multiplied by 3.

Although all possible R commands can be typed and run at the prompt, it is recommended to write so-called scripts in the document window of the graphical user interface (GUI) or in the workspace window of RStudio. Scripts include a collection of commands for data operations similar to small computer programs. They can be saved on your computer drive (commonly with the extension *.R) and will eventually serve as a valuable collection of numerical recipes that you may like to come back to at a later stage. Scripts can be exchanged between colleagues thus enhancing professional collaboration. Also, saved R scripts are a good reproducible documentation and repository of your data manipulation and analysis work. They can, for example, be attached to B.Sc., M.Sc. or Ph.D. theses and scientific papers as supplementary material.

In the R console, commands are executed by hitting the Enter button. By contrast, commands typed in the R script editor need to be highlighted followed by pressing Ctrl-R in MS Windows and Cmd-Enter in Mac OS for execution. Alternatively you can click on the corresponding icon in the GUI. It is possible to run every code line separately and also to highlight several lines and to execute them at the same time. You can even highlight and run excerpts from one line of code only.

Continuing lines are automatically indicated by the + sign, when the first line is incomplete.

```
> 5 *
+ 2^3
[1] 40
```

Often the appearance of + in the console means that parentheses or quotes need to be balanced (Robinson and Hamann 2010, p. 7). A summary of basic operators and functions can be found in Table C.1.

Table C.1 Basic arithmetic operators and functions

Operator/function	Description
+, -	Addition and subtraction
*, /	Multiplication, division
^	Power
abs()	Absolute
exp()	Exponential function
log()	Natural logarithm
logb(x, base = 2)	Logarithm to the base 2
sqrt()	Square root
round()	Rounds decimal numbers
floor()	Rounds decimal numbers down
ceiling()	Rounds decimal numbers up
sin(), cos(), tan()	Trigonometric functions
integrate()	Calculates the integral of a function
<, >	Smaller, greater than
==, !=	Equal, unequal
<=, >=	Smaller equal, greater equal
&, |	And, or
is.na()	Missing?
round(x, digits = 3)	Rounding to three decimal digits

Any alphanumeric character including "_" and "." (but no white spaces) that start with a letter can freely be selected as variable names (Bolker 2008, p. 23), however, some letters and words have been reserved by R and should be avoided, e.g. "F" (= False), "T" (= True) and "data". Values are assigned to variables using the <- sign, the assignment operator, because the equal sign (=) is reserved for other purposes.

As demonstrated in the second and third line of the code below, x has the value of 3 and can be used in subsequent calculations.

```
> x <- 3
> x
[1] 3
```

Typing and running the variable name again will allow you to see its value. Alternatively you can execute the command print(x). Inside loops (see Sect. C.5) only the command print(x) produces the desired output in the R console.

Comments are useful to remember what you had in mind when writing your code. They should be marked with # (hash key) to inform the compiler that what follows in the corresponding line is non-executable code that should be ignored. The hash key can also be used to disenable lines of code.

```
> sin(pi / 2) # This is a comment.
[1] 1
```

It is important to be aware of the fact that R is case-sensitive, i.e. variable names
involving lower-case and upper-case versions of the same letter essentially constitute
different variables and confusing them can cause errors:

```
> dbh <- 16.5
> Dbh
Error: object 'Dbh' not found
```

Almost all objects in R are internally represented by vectors, even if they contain only
one number. The round brackets in the listing below force R to print the vector dbh
after assigning the value of 5.6 to it, where dbh is a simple variable name borrowed
from the abbreviation of tree stem diameters (dbh). The round brackets save typing
another command line for displaying the value of dbh.

```
> (dbh <- 5.6)
[1] 5.6
```

In R, functions always require round brackets containing no, one or more arguments
and return results without any additional prompt. Using the function c() (= concatenate) you can easily create vectors with multiple values, e.g. a list of tree stem
diameters. A strength of R is that it can handle entire data vectors as single objects
(Dalgaard 2008, p. 4).

```
> (dbh <- c(5.6, 10.3, 14.5, 27.8, 48.5))
[1] 5.6 10.3 14.5 27.8 48.5
```

Vectorisation and vector arithmetics are an important feature of R to make data
processing more efficient. The function length(dbh) returns the length of a vector.
The command mode(dbh) gives you the data type.

```
> length(dbh)
[1] 5
```

By the way, R can also read data that you type into the console and assign them to a
vector using the command dbh <- scan():

```
> dbh <- scan()
1:
```

Numbers followed by colons prompt you to input data in the console. After typing a
value you press Enter. The data gathering procedure is finished after pressing Enter
without previously typing a value.

To access a particular stem diameter of the vector dbh, e.g. the second one, type

```
> dbh[2]
[1] 10.3
```

Using the function c again allows selecting several values at the same time, e.g. the
second, fourth and fifth value:

```
> dbh[c(2, 4, 5)]
[1] 10.3 27.8 48.5
```

In R, square brackets are always applied to select a subset of data by introducing a
condition. Negative indices can be used to suppress certain elements. You can, for
example, select all but the second stem diameter:

```
> dbh[-2]
[1] 5.6 14.5 27.8 48.5
```

It is also possible to print all stem diameters larger than 15 cm with the following code.

```
> dbh[dbh > 15]
[1] 27.8 48.5
```

The same result you obtain by using the command subset(dbh, dbh > 15). Vectors can be manipulated by using basic arithmetic operators, e.g. we can let the stem diameters grow using a growth multiplier of 1.3 (see Eq. (6.16)):

```
> dbh * 1.3
[1] 7.28 13.39 18.85 36.14 63.05
```

As a result all elements of the vector length(dbh) have been multiplied by 1.3. Naturally vectors can be modified by any other operator or mathematical function. We can now apply the first summary characteristics to vector dbh. For this purpose we use functions that are written in a similar way as in MS Excel and other programs. Minimum and maximum dbh we can for example identify in the following way:

```
> min(dbh)
[1] 5.6
> max(dbh)
[1] 48.5
> range(dbh)
[1] 5.6 48.5
```

The range command produces minimum and maximum at the same time. min, max and range are functions that are part of the common functionality of R. A summary including similar characteristics can be produced with the command summary(dbh).

```
> summary(dbh)
Min. 1st Qu. Median Mean 3rd Qu. Max.
5.60 10.30 14.50 21.34 27.80 48.50
```

Table C.2 Basic arithmetic operators and functions

Operator/function	Description
var(x)	Variance of x
quantile(x, p)	p quantile of x
cor(x, y)	Correlation between x and y
prod(x)	Product of x
sum(x)	Sum of x
diff(x)	Vector with differences x[i] - x[i - 1]
factorial(x)	Factorial of number x, i.e. x!

More sophisticated descriptive statistics include the arithmetic mean, the median, the standard deviation and the coefficient of variation as given in the code below.

```
> mean(dbh)
[1] 21.34
> median(dbh)
[1] 14.5
> sd(dbh)
[1] 17.29026
> sd(dbh) / mean(dbh)
[1] 0.8102276
```

However, when using concrete numbers as opposed to variables you need to resort to the concatenate function, e.g. mean(c(4, 6, 8, 9)) to obtain 6.75. Other frequently used statistical functions are provided in Table C.2.

Another frequent application in statistics is the ranking of observations according to their size. Consider a vector with various stem-diameter values:

```
> dbh <- c(27.8, 5.6, 48.5, 10.3, 14.5)
> rank(dbh)
[1] 4 1 5 2 3
```

Function rank() provides the required ranking. Often we can have observations with the same values, so-called "ties". Using the default of the rank() function we obtain

```
> dbh <- c(27.8, 5.6, 5.6, 10.3, 14.5)
> rank(dbh)
[1] 5.0 1.5 1.5 3.0 4.0
```

average ranks for stem diameters 2 and 3 (both 5.5 cm) whilst method "min" gives us

```
> dbh <- c(27.8, 5.6, 5.6, 10.3, 14.5)
> rank(dbh, ties.method = "min")
[1] 5 1 1 3 4
```

equal ranks for both observations.

In analogy to numeric vectors, character vectors are also possible. However, the text strings need to be wrapped in quote symbols. Consider the following code:

```
> myNames <- "Peter"
> myNames <- c(myNames, "John", "Lucy")
> myNames
[1] "Peter" "John" "Lucy"
```

In the first line, Peter's name is stored to vector myNames. Then perhaps the idea has come up to add John's and Lucy's name to the vector myNames, however, without overwriting the current contents which is Peter's name. That is why the vector myNames itself is included on the right hand side of the assignment.

Finally it can be useful to create simple vectors by using the seq and rep functions. The command

```
> seq(from = 1, to = 17, by = 2)
[1] 1 3 5 7 9 11 13 15 17
```

creates a sequence of odd numbers between 1 and 17. The optional parameter `by` specifies the step width. As a shortcut you can, of course, simply write `seq(1, 17, 2)`.

We can now assign the sequence of odd numbers to a variable, `ad`, and use the function `rev` to reverse the order of elements (lines 1–2). The same effect can be achieved by reversing the index using the command `ad[length(ad) : 1]` (line 4):

```
1  > ad <- seq(1, 17, by = 2)
2  > rev(ad)
3  [1] 17 15 13 11 9 7 5 3 1
4  > ad[length(ad) : 1]
5  [1] 17 15 13 11 9 7 5 3 1
```

The command `rep(7, 7)` on the other hand repeats the value '7' 7 times:

```
> rep(7, 7)
[1] 7 7 7 7 7 7 7
```

Simple sequences can also be produced by the following command:

```
> c(1, 7 : 9)
[1] 1 7 8 9
```

The sample function `sample` can be used to return a random permutation of a vector. Consider a vector x of integers from 1 to 10.

```
> x <- 1 : 10
>
> sample(x)
[1] 4 3 6 5 10 2 9 7 1 8
```

Incidentally, the command `sample(10)` has exactly the same effect. Using the `size` argument we can now draw a subsample of vector x.

```
> sample(x, size = 4)
[1] 10 9 1 7
```

Finally, the `replace` argument allows us to perform sampling with replacement, i.e. each number of vector x can be drawn more than once. In that case the sample size can also exceed the length of the vector. Incidentally, we can check the arguments of any R function with the command `args()`, e.g. `args(sample)`.

```
> sample(x, size = 20, replace = T)
[1] 2 2 4 2 8 3 4 4 4 8 10 10 5 1 3 3 2 6 4 1
```

Sometimes it is necessary to delete large variables and objects to free up computer memory or to ensure that old variable definitions do not interfere with new ones that by accident may involve the same variable name. This can be achieved with the remove command, i.e. `rm(x)`.

Logical expressions and binary data can also be accommodated in R. For example, after assigning values to variables a and b, we can check logical relationships:

```
1  > a <- 3
2  > b <- 4
3  > a == b
```

```
4  [1] FALSE
5  > a != b
6  [1] TRUE
```

Logical equal is expressed by "==" and unequal by "!=". Such logical expressions play an important role in if statements, see Sect. C.5. It is also interesting to note the close relationship between logical data types and binary data that can only take values of zero and one:

```
1  > logicalVector <- c(TRUE, TRUE, FALSE, FALSE)
2  > logicalVector
3  [1] TRUE TRUE FALSE FALSE
4  > sum(logicalVector)
5  [1] 2
```

In line 1, a logical vector including values of TRUE and FALSE was created. Superficial reading seems to suggest that these values appear to be characters, but no quotation marks were used. Summing up the logical values of vector logicalVector gives a result of 2, because by implicit type coercion values of TRUE are converted to one and values of FALSE to zero. This is a very useful property when working with binary data.

New R packages can be downloaded and installed using the function install.packages(). Here it is useful to switch on the option dep = TRUE, since then also other dependent packages are downloaded and everything is fully functional once the download is complete:

```
1  > # install.packages("moments", dep = TRUE)
2  > library(moments)
3  > dbh <- c(27.8, 5.6, 5.6, 10.3, 14.5)
4  > skewness(dbh)
5  [1] 0.9573732
```

Once the new package is installed, there is no need to repeat the download in your next R session and the corresponding line can be disenabled using the hashtag. The function library() loads the package into the computer's memory. In this example, we used the function skewness() from the package moments.

Help and explanations relating to any function or operator, e.g. log can be called on by typing help(log) or ?log. For code examples only, you can type example(log). There is also a growing community of R users throughout the world and carefully passing your R related question on to an internet search machine may give you quick and useful answers. The same applies to error messages that you feel unable to interpret.

Ctrl–C or Esc stops any processing, which currently is underway. Incidentally, earlier commands can be retrieved in the console by pressing the arrow keys (up and down) of the keyboard. The reasons for any error message can be analysed with the function traceback() and to quit your R session type

```
> q()
```

After running q() R enquires whether it should save the workspace image, i.e. the data and the sequence of commands of the current session. In the authors' experience this is usually not necessary as every session can easily and quickly be reconstructed from the script used so that it suffices to save the script file. Only after lengthy simulations it can be recommended to save intermediary and final results.

C.2 Data Frames

Consider two tree variables of interest, stem diameter (dbh), d, and total tree height, h. The corresponding data columns can be represented by and stored in two separate columns or vectors, dbh and h.

```
1   > dbh <- c(33.5, 40.5, 39.0, 54.0, 38.8, 32.4, 29.7, 31.0,
2   + 55.5, 26.1)
3   > h <- c(28.9, 30.0, 26.6, 30.7, 27.0, 26.2, 27.8, 25.5, 31.7,
4   + 24.8)
5   > myData <- data.frame(dbh, h)
6   > str(myData)
7   'data.frame': 10 obs. of 2 variables:
8   $ dbh: num 33.5 40.5 39 54 38.8 32.4 29.7 31 55.5 26.1
9   $ h  : num 28.9 30 26.6 30.7 27 26.2 27.8 25.5 31.7 24.8
```

In lines 1–4, 10 stem diameter and corresponding height values are assigned to the vectors dbh and h. Note that for successful calculations both vectors should have the same length. Also the order of dbh and h values matters so that corresponding values (from the same individuals) should occur at the same locations in the two vectors. As they form a common data set, the vectors can be combined as two columns in a data frame entitled myData (line 5). The command str(myData) is useful to check up on or to remind ourselves of the structure of the data frame. For accessing individual columns you now have to use the name of the data frame plus the column name separated by a $ sign, e.g. myData$h. Alternatively you can, for example, use the command with(myData, mean(dbh)) instead of mean(myData$dbh).

A data frame is a two-dimensional structure for storing vectors. Each column corresponds to a variable and each row to an observation. A common task in working with data sets is to sort the data in an ascending or descending way. This can be accomplished using the following code, in which we sort descendingly according to stem diameter.

```
> (myData.s <- myData[order(myData$dbh, decreasing = TRUE), ])

    dbh    h
9  55.5 31.7
4  54.0 30.7
2  40.5 30.0
3  39.0 26.6
5  38.8 27.0
1  33.5 28.9
6  32.4 26.2
```

```
  8   31.0 25.5
  7   29.7 27.8
 10 26.1 24.8
```

The comma in the command ensures that all columns are correctly included in the sorting process. Again the round brackets prompt R to print the data in `myData.s` on screen.

For checking up on your computations you can list a subset of the total data frame by using indices, e.g. the code

```
> myData.s[1 : 5, ]
```

```
  dbh    h
9 55.5 31.7
4 54.0 30.7
2 40.5 30.0
3 39.0 26.6
5 38.8 27.0
```

gives you the first five rows of the data set `myData`. This is again a subsetting operation and the comma at the end of the expression in the squared brackets indicates that you wish to display all columns of the data set. Alternatively use the commands `myData.s[2]` or `myData.s["h"]` to select the tree height column only. There is also the possibility to print the first and the last six lines of a data frame using the commands `head(myData.s)` and `tail(myData.s)` (in our case here).

`sapply()` is one of many functions in R that have been designed to work with vectors by using *implicit loops* (Dalgaard 2008, p. 26), which—if programmed manually in R—would otherwise consume a lot of computation time. `sapply()` allows us to apply a function of our choice (including user-defined ones) simultaneously to all columns of a data frame. In the listing below we calculate the arithmetic mean of both data columns.

```
> sapply(myData, mean)
dbh h
38.05 27.92
```

Alternatively the commands `apply(myData, 1, mean)` and `apply(myData, 2, mean)` calculate the row and column means, respectively.

A new column or vector within a data frame can simply be created by specifying a new vector name and assigning values to it. We can, for example, calculate the h/d ratio (see Eq. (2.6)) in the following way:

```
> myData$hd <- 100 * myData$h / myData$dbh
> myData[1 : 3, ]
```

```
  dbh    h       hd
1 33.5 28.9 86.26866
2 40.5 30.0 74.07407
3 39.0 26.6 68.20513
```

A selection of data can be made by using a conditional expression, e.g.

```
> myData[myData$dbh > 35, ]

  dbh    h       hd
2 40.5 30.0 74.07407
3 39.0 26.6 68.20513
4 54.0 30.7 56.85185
5 38.8 27.0 69.58763
9 55.5 31.7 57.11712
```

As a result all data have been selected where dbh > 35 cm. It is also possible to use more than one condition linked with a logical "and" (&):

```
> myData[myData$dbh > 30 & myData$hd > 80, ]

  dbh    h       hd
1 33.5 28.9 86.26866
6 32.4 26.2 80.86420
8 31.0 25.5 82.25806
```

A logical "or" is expressed with the symbol |.

C.3   Input and Output

Often the data we wish to process are too many to input in R manually or are already available in digital format elsewhere. For the purpose of this book, it can be recommended to edit and to maintain data externally in MS Excel or in similar spreadsheet or database programs. The data to be analysed in R should include a header line and can then be conveniently converted to ASCII format. Every header should consist of a single word with continuous letters. Numeric and string values should not be mixed in a single column. If all data cells have valid entries, it is easiest to convert the data to text tabs delimited (*.txt) in MS Excel. If some data cells are empty the conversion option text comma delimited (*.csv) should be preferred.

In a short comment line at the beginning of your R script, you may want to describe the purpose of your code, when you wrote it and the date of last modification. It is also useful to start every new R script with the command rm(list = ls()), which removes all pre-existing objects and data. In line 4f. of the following code snippet, the ASCII data saved in file TreeData.txt are read by R and assigned to the data frame myData.

```
1 > # This script is for basic tree analysis. Ap - 01.04.2019.
2 Last modified on 10.04.2019.
3 > rm(list = ls())
4 > myData <- read.table("/MyDataAnalysis/TreeData.txt",
5 + header = T)
```

```
6    > # myData <- read.csv("/MyDataAnalysis/TreeData.csv",
7    > # header=T)
8    > dim(myData)
9    [1] 56 6
10   > names(myData)
11   [1] "treeno" "species" "x" "y" "dbh" "h"
```

In lines 6f., the alternative code for comma delimited data is given. header = T indicates that the first row of the data file contains headers. The use of forward slashes is common practice in R irrespective of the operating system. The directory names are case sensitive and ideally should not contain blank spaces. When working in MS Windows, a drive name, e.g. c: (without backslash) needs to be added immediately following the first quotation mark. It is also possible to substitute each forward slash by a double backslash ($\backslash\backslash$).

In our case at hand, myData is a data frame and the data can be printed by highlighting myData and pressing Ctrl–R or Cmd–Enter:

```
> myData
   treeno species    x    y   dbh    h
1     197      3 49.2 21.3 26.0 18.8
2     198      3 40.2 19.7 19.3 16.5
3     199      3 31.2 20.2 27.1 20.8
4     208      3 34.1 24.3 21.0 16.3
5     209      3 39.1 22.7 23.0 17.6
6     210      3 44.7 22.5 21.4 17.1
7     211      3 49.2 23.8 23.2 19.1
8     232      3 50.0 25.4 13.6 13.3
9     235      3 34.3 26.9  8.4  9.3
10    236      3 33.2 26.9 25.4 20.0
11    241      3 40.4 28.6 28.5 20.3
12    242      3 49.3 29.9 28.3 17.8
13    243      3 49.5 28.1 22.0 20.5
14    264      3 47.1 30.9 15.1 15.8
15    267      3 39.0 32.9 24.9 18.1
16    273      3 32.8 38.4 26.8 17.5
17    274      3 38.6 38.3 28.3 19.8
18    298      3 46.6 39.8 28.6 17.9
19    138     12  0.4  0.7 42.5 26.0
20    139     12 18.0  0.7 34.4 25.0
21    140     12 23.5  0.8 45.7 29.3
22    141     12 38.3  0.3 47.1 27.3
23    152     12 33.7  3.2 51.9 28.9
24    153     12 27.7  3.2 36.8 25.6
25    154     12 15.1  3.5 32.8 23.9
26    155     12  4.5  3.7 43.0 26.8
27    156     12  1.0  7.7 43.9 27.6
```

```
28    157    12 28.9  7.5 36.0 24.5
29    158    12 43.6  7.2 28.1 22.8
30    166    12 38.1  8.8 28.8 24.1
31    167    12 23.5  9.0 38.3 27.1
32    168    12 12.3  8.9 59.2 28.8
33    169    12  6.4  8.9 32.7 23.3
34    170    12 42.8 10.1 35.3 22.9
35    172    12 31.6 11.7 39.4 25.5
36    173    12 45.6 12.9 45.4 26.7
37    180    12 40.4 14.4 40.5 22.4
38    181    12 17.2 14.5 31.4 24.5
39    182    12  4.2 14.8 35.1 29.8
40    183    12  9.7 16.3 44.8 28.2
41    184    12 25.9 16.0 37.5 26.8
42    200    12 28.5 21.9 37.8 24.1
43    201    12 21.8 20.5 29.8 25.6
44    202    12 17.8 21.8 32.3 25.2
45    203    12 13.5 22.0 35.6 29.3
46    204    12  5.0 22.1 29.7 26.9
47    205    12  9.5 24.8 48.8 28.9
48    206    12 22.1 24.4 32.7 24.1
49    207    12 26.5 24.3 37.2 23.7
50    237    12 16.8 27.6 36.2 27.3
51    238    12  5.8 31.0 35.4 27.4
52    239    12 20.8 28.6 26.9 22.4
53    269    12 28.9 31.6 39.2 27.8
54    270    12 18.4 33.5 49.0 27.7
55    271    12  8.7 38.4 41.3 28.4
56    272    12 29.4 38.4 33.7 20.5
```

You can copy and paste these data and save them in a suitable file format as described above. Alternatively you can access them on https://github.com/a-pommerening/R-course/Data in `Data1.txt`.

Using the `spatstat` package (see Chap. 4) a map of the data can be produced, where the two species are shown in different colours and the approximate size of the trees is indicated by the radii of the circles denoting the trees' stem-centre coordinates (Fig. C.1).

Ideally "." is always set as standard decimal separator in MS Excel, however, if commas were used, the argument `dec = ","` separated by a comma in lines 4 or 6 will perform an automatic conversion.

The commands `dim` and `names` produce information on the dimensions of the new data frame and give the headers which simultaneously serve as vector names.

Missing data, which can originate from unmeasured characteristics, are represented in R by a logical constant with the value NA (**N**ot **A**vailable) and any operations on NA also yield NA as a result (Dalgaard 2008, p. 14). In that case a special

Fig. C.1 Map of a
subwindow of the Sitka
spruce (*Pinus sitchensis*
(BONG.) CARR.) plantation
forest stand at Cefn Du
(Clocaenog Forest, plot 2,
North Wales, UK) with an
admixture of lodgepole pine
(*Pinus contorta* DOUGL. ex
LOUD.) in 2002. The
subwindow includes 56 trees

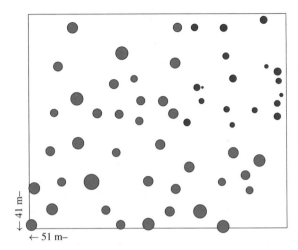

41 m → ← 51 m–

command can limit calculations to valid observations, i.e. missing values are then
removed.

```
> mean(myData$dbh, na.rm = T)
```

T is short for TRUE. In R, it is possible to use both T or TRUE and F or FALSE, respectively. Alternatively records with no entry, i.e. with the value NA, can be removed
beforehand using the following command.

```
> myData <- myData[!is.na(myData$dbh), ]
```

After modifying the data frame the data can be saved to ASCII files using one of the
following commands. Naturally it is recommended to use a file name different from
that of the input file to avoid overwriting, since original data files should never be
modified.

```
> write.table(myData, file = "/MyDataAnalysis/TreeData/
+ TreeDataMod.txt")
> write.csv(myData, file = "/MyDataAnalysis/TreeData/
+ TreeDataMod.csv")
```

As discussed in Sect. C.1, subsets can be created in two different ways, by using
1. conditional statements in square brackets and 2. the subset function. In the following example, lodgepole pine trees (*Pinus contorta* DOUGL. ex LOUD.) are selected
for species-specific analysis. In this context, the length function serves as a simple
check up that both operations yield the same results. The comma towards the end of
the first line is again responsible for selecting all data columns.

```
> myDataLP1 <- myData[myData$species == 3, ]
> length(myDataLP1$treeno)
[1] 18
> myDataLP2 <- subset(myData, species == 3)
> length(myDataLP2$treeno)
[1] 18
```

Similar to `sapply`, `tapply` allows the use of an implicit-loop command for exploring the number of trees per species. Again implicit loops are shortcuts to what otherwise would need to be programmed as long-winded loops.

```
> tapply(myData$treeno, myData$species, length)
3 12
18 38
```

In this example, there are 18 lodgepole pine (*Pinus contorta* DOUGL. ex LOUD., coded as 3) and 38 Sitka spruce (*Picea sitchensis* (BONG.) CARR., coded as 12) trees in the data frame.

As we have already seen in the case of subsetting, the same results can be obtained in R from more than one set of commands. In this case, the command `table(myData$species)`, for example, gives the same information.

Finally it is worth mentioning that not all code that you require for some data operation needs to be in one R script only. It is also possible to source code from an external script either written by yourself or by another person. In the example below, two assignments and a multiplication are carried out in the external R script `ExternalExample.R` (lines 3–5). In line 6, the final result is printed in the console.

```
1  > source("/MyDataAnalysis/TreeData/ExternalExample.R",
2  + echo = TRUE)
3  > a <- 5
4  > b <- 6
5  > result <- 5 * 6
6  > cat("The result is", result, ".", "\n")
7  The result is 30.
```

C.4 Graphs and Regressions

Graphs are essential elements of any data analysis. They visualise important relationships and help to spot mistakes. Graphs are a particular strength of R and convince with high quality that is only limited by the user's knowledge of how to program and to fine-tune them.

Following on with the data frame introduced in the last section, the diameter histogram is presented first. A histogram is a chart for displaying grouped continuous data, in which the width of each bar is proportional to the class interval and the area of each bar is proportional to the frequency it represents (Porkress 2004, p. 118). All graphic commands are wrapped in the statements `pdf()` and `dev.off()`. This is a way to direct the graphical output to a pdf file for use in other computer programs such as LaTeX, MS PowerPoint or Apple Keynote. Other file formats are, of course, also possible, e.g. `png("*.png")`. If a screen output is intended, lines 1 and 9 can be removed or disenabled with the # sign. Graphical outputs directly printed to files usually have a higher quality than saved screen outputs and should therefore be preferred for publications.

```
 1  pdf(file = "/MyDataAnalysis/TreeData/histExample.pdf")
 2  > hist1 <- hist(myData$dbh, breaks = seq(8, 60, by = 4),
 3  + include.lowest = T, right = F, plot = FALSE)
 4  > hist1$counts <- hist1$counts / length(myData$dbh)
 5  > par(mar = c(2, 4, 1, 2))
 6  > plot(hist1, las = 1, cex.axis = 1.7, ylim = c(0, 0.20),
 7  + main = "", xlab = "", ylab = "")
 8  > box(lwd = 2)
 9  > dev.off()
10  null device
11  1
```

In principle the command hist(myData$dbh) is sufficient to produce a basic histogram. In the above code, the histogram is, however, assigned to the variable hist1 for further manipulation. The parameter breaks = seq(8, 60, by = 4) defines the diameter classes. The first two values give the minimum and maximum classes and can be established from the diameter range (range(myData$dbh)). The argument by = 4 defines 4-cm diameter classes and the parameters include.lowest = T and right = F determine specific boundaries of diameter classes.

In line 4, the absolute frequencies in each diameter class are transformed to proportions for better comparison with other forest stands. This is accomplished by dividing the absolute frequencies in each class by the total number of trees.

The plot margins are defined in line 5. From left to right the numbers represent the bottom, left, top, right margins of the plot and are interpreted in units of character widths (Jones et al. 2009).

Finally the plot command in line 6f. commits R to produce the actual histogram using the modified histogram variable hist1. The argument las = 1 organises the values on the ordinate in a horizontal way which is good for presentations and lectures. The argument cex.axis defines the size of the axes labels. ylim determines the extent of the abscissa, a similar command xlim also exists but is not necessary here. The histogram title and the axes labels can be determined with the arguments main, xlab and ylab. Many more parameters exist to fine-tune histograms and the online help in R provides options and examples.

As a last step, a box with line width 2 has been added to the graph. Figure C.2 shows the result.

Bar charts are simple graphs that display single sets of numbers. In contrast to histograms the bars correspond to each number in the vector (Porkress 2004). In Sect. 4.4.7.1, we discussed how to compute spatial species mingling and the empirical mark distribution of this characteristic. For depicting this distribution graphically we typically use bar charts:

```
 1  > names <- seq(0, k, 1) / k
 2  > names <- format(names, dig = 2)
 3  > pdf(file = "/MyDataAnalysis/TreeData/barExample.pdf")
 4  > par(mar = c(2, 3, 0.5, 0.5))
 5  > barplot(mh, beside = TRUE, ylim = c(0, 1), ylab = "",
 6  + names.arg = names, cex.names = 1.7, col = "white",
 7  + main = "", las = 1, cex.axis = 1.7)
 8  > box(lwd = 2)
```

```
9   > dev.off()
10  null device
11  1
```

The number of nearest neighbours is k and names stores the labels on the abscissa. Vector mh contains the proportions of the empirical mark mingling distribution. We computed this distribution for the example data from Clocaenog Forest (plot 2) and the result is shown in Fig. C.3.

Another important graph in data analysis is the scatterplot. We will apply this type of graph to visualise the relationship between stem diameters and total height in tree populations based on the same data frame as before.

```
1   > pdf(file = "/MyDataAnalysis/TreeData/scatterExample.pdf")
2   > par(mar = c(2, 3, 0.5, 0.5))
3   > plot(myData$dbh, myData$h, xlim = c(0, 65), ylim = c(0, 35),
4   + pch = 16, xlab = "", ylab = "", axes = FALSE)
5   > axis(1, lwd = 2, cex.axis = 1.8)
6   > axis(2, las = 1, lwd = 2, cex.axis = 1.8)
7   > box(lwd = 2)
8   > dev.off()
9   null device
10  1
```

Many parameters and arguments in the above code are already known from the histogram example. A scatterplot is produced using the plot function. First the abscissa values (stem diameter) are specified followed by the ordinate values (total tree height). The command axes = FALSE suppresses the drawing of the axes at this stage. This is performed separately by the following two axes commands. pch = 16 defines the plotting characters as small filled circles. Other definitions are, of course, possible, pch = 17 for example yields filled triangles.

Fig. C.2 Example of a diameter histogram based on a subwindow including 56 trees from a mixed Sitka spruce-lodgepole pine forest stand at Cefn Du (Clocaenog Forest (plot 2), North Wales)

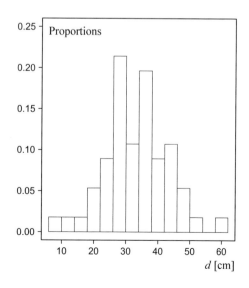

Fig. C.3 Example of an empirical species mingling bar chart based on a subwindow including 56 trees from a mixed Sitka spruce-lodgepole pine forest stand at Cefn Du (Clocaenog Forest (plot 2), North Wales)

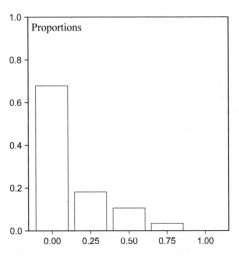

It is now possible to define a trend curve and to display this curve in the scatterplot. This is a common application in data analysis and modelling. For this purpose we have to use nonlinear regression applied to a height-diameter model. This can be achieved with the following code.

```
> nls.Petterson <- nls(h ~ 1.3 + (dbh/(a + b * dbh))^3,
+ data = myData, start = list(a = 0.5, b = 3.8), trace = T)

  28201.54 :   0.5 3.8
  20851.01 :   33.8030885 -0.3563551
  20756.15 :   33.6571018 -0.3536527
  20567.28 :   33.3663958 -0.3482686
  20192.88 :   32.790018 -0.337583
  19456.83 :   31.657130 -0.316537
  18031.2  :   29.4687529 -0.2757102
  15335.76 :   25.3866524 -0.1988602
  10422.76 :   18.3055084 -0.0627713
  2790.814 :   8.035270 0.145125
  838.3544 :   0.9757181 0.3110218
  254.7894 :   1.8406893 0.2965715
  238.5269 :   2.1459689 0.2887622
  238.468  :   2.1665622 0.2882068
  238.468  :   2.1671261 0.2881906
  238.468  :   2.1671405 0.2881902
> summary(nls.Petterson)

Formula: h ~ 1.3 + (dbh/(a + b * dbh))^3

Parameters:
Estimate Std. Error t value Pr(>|t|)
a 2.167141    0.184550    11.74    <2e-16 ***
b 0.288190    0.005458    52.80    <2e-16 ***
---
```

```
Signif. codes:  0 '***' 0.001 '**' 0.01 '*' 0.05 '.' 0.1 ' ' 1

Residual standard error: 2.101 on 54 degrees of freedom

Number of iterations to convergence: 15
Achieved convergence tolerance: 2.408e-07
```

In the first two lines, the model equation is specified followed by the data definition and the list of starting model parameters. `trace = T` confirms our intention to follow the individual iterations of the regression, which we can see in the following lines. Finally, the results are presented. Dalgaard (2008, p. 275ff.) provides a whole chapter with useful information on nonlinear regression in R.

The model parameters shown in the paragraph with the header "`Parameters:`" can now be used to superimpose the trend curve on the scatterplot. For this purpose we employ the `curve` function. This function allows the direct drawing of function graphs from equations.

```
> curve(1.3 + (x/(summary(nls.Petterson)$coefficients[1] +
+ summary(nls.Petterson)$coefficients[2] * x))^3,
+ from = min(myData$dbh), to = max(myData$dbh),
+ lwd = 4, lty = 1, col = "grey", add = TRUE)
```

The command `summary(nls.Petterson)$coefficients[1]` gives the first and `summary(nls.P etterson)$coefficients[2]` the second regression coefficient. The rest of the code is quite self-explanatory. Parameter `add = TRUE` ensures that the scatterplot is not overwritten and `lty = 1` defines the line type, which in our case should be a simple continuous line. This code needs to be included before the command `dev.off()` after the regression. The final results can be seen in Fig. C.4.

In some cases, often when more than two model parameters are involved, the `nls` routine stops processing or only produces results after several new attempts of trying

Fig. C.4 Example of a scatterplot with a superimposed nonlinear trend curve based on a subwindow including 56 trees from a mixed Sitka spruce-lodgepole pine forest stand at Cefn Du (Clocaenog Forest (plot 2), North Wales)

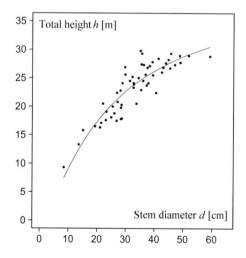

new starting parameters, which can be awkward. In that case it can be recommended
to make use of the `optim` function as outlined in Jones et al. (2009).

As part of this alternative to `nls`, first a loss function needs to be defined, which
is in lines 7–11 in the below code. In line 8, the Petterson function of lines 14–17 is
called. The deviation between observed and estimated total tree heights is calculated
in line 9 and returned to `optim` in line 10. In line 19, a vector with the starting values
is defined.

```
1  > par(mar = c(2, 3, 0.5, 0.5))
2  > plot(myData$dbh, myData$h, xlim = c(0, 65), ylim = c(0, 35),
3  + pch = 16, xlab = "", ylab = "", axes = FALSE)
4  > axis(1, lwd = 2, cex.axis = 1.8)
5  > axis(2, las = 1, lwd = 2, cex.axis = 1.8)
6  >
7  > loss.L2 <- function(abdn, xdata) {
8  + yh <- xh(abdn[1 : 2], xdata)
9  + xdev <- xdata$h - yh
10 + return(sum(xdev^2, na.rm = TRUE))
11 + }
12 >
13 > # Petterson
14 > xh <- function(abdn, xdata) {
15 + yh <- 1.3 + (xdata$dbh/(abdn[1] + abdn[2] * xdata$dbh))^3
16 + return(yh)
17 + }
18 >
19 > abdn0 <- c(0.5, 3.8)
20 > abdn.L2 <- optim(abdn0, loss.L2, xdata = myData,
21 + control = list(maxit = 30000, temp = 2000,
22 + trace = TRUE, REPORT = 500))
23 >
24 > abdn.L2$par
25 [1] 2.1679653 0.2881626
26 >
27 > curve(1.3 + (x/(abdn.L2$par[1] + abdn.L2$par[2] * x))^3,
28 + from = min(myData$dbh), to = max(myData$dbh), lwd = 1,
29 + lty = 1, col = "black", add = TRUE)
30 >
31 > axis(1, lwd = 2, cex.axis = 1.8)
32 > axis(2, las = 1, lwd = 2, cex.axis = 1.8)
33 > box(lwd = 2)
```

Finally `optim` is run in lines 20–22 and the model parameters are produced by the
command in line 24. The `curve` command in lines 27–29 adds the model curve to the
plot. Another alternative for difficult data situations is *robust regression* as provided
by the R package MASS.

A box plot (or "box-and-whisker plot") is an alternative to a histogram providing
a visualisation of the main features of a data set (Braun and Murdoch 2007, p.
36f.). The bold horizontal line marks the median and the upper and lower edges of
the box give the upper and lower quartiles. About 50% of the data lies within the
box, which defines the *interquartile range* (IQR). The dashed lines and end lines,

the whiskers, lead to the smallest/largest value that is no smaller/no larger than 1.5 IQR below/above the lower/upper quartile. When data are drawn from the normal distribution or other distributions with a similar shape, about 99% of the observations fall between the whiskers. Outliers (observations that are very different from the rest of the data) are plotted as separate points (Braun and Murdoch 2007, p. 37). Box plots are convenient for comparing distributions of data in two or more categories.

In the code example below, we compare the distributions of the dbh measurements between the two species, lodgepole pine (*Pinus contorta* DOUGL. ex LOUD.) and Sitka spruce (*Picea sitchensis* (BONG.) CARR.).

```
1  > my.labels <- c("LP", "SS")
2  > par(lab = c(length(my.labels), 5, 7), mar = c(2.5, 4, 0.5,
3  + 0.5))
4  > boxplot(dbh ~ species, data = myData, boxwex = 0.5, lwd = 2,
5  + axes = FALSE)
6  > axis(1, at = 1 : 2, labels = my.labels, lwd = 2,
7  + cex.axis = 1.8)
8  > axis(2, las = 1, lwd = 2, cex.axis = 1.8)
9  > box(lwd = 2)
```

Note that the abscissa labels are defined in line 1 and used in lines 2 and 6. boxwex is a scaling factor, which can be used to make the boxes narrower when there are a few groups to compare. An additional argument horizontal = TRUE allows the drawing of horizontal box plots which is sometimes useful. Figure C.5 shows the box plots produced from the above R code. They reveal that both species have quite different median diameters and diameter ranges. Sitka spruce ($N = 38$) has larger diameter trees and a wider range of tree sizes than lodgepole pine ($N = 18$).

In R, it is also possible to visualise a mathematical function directly without the need to compile a table of function values beforehand. This is very useful for visualising functions that we would like to consider as trend curves or models. As an

Fig. C.5 Example of a box plot comparing two tree species of the same example forest stand (subwindow including 56 trees from a mixed Sitka spruce-lodgepole pine forest stand at Cefn Du (Clocaenog Forest (plot 2), North Wales) in terms of diameter distribution and the meaning of the box plot features. LP: lodgepole pine (*Pinus contorta* DOUGL. ex LOUD.), SS: Sitka spruce (*Picea sitchensis* (BONG.) CARR.). *d* is stem diameter (dbh) in cm

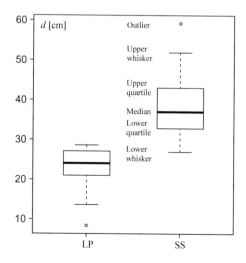

example, we use here the Chapman–Richards growth function (see Chap. 6, Pienaar and Turnbull 1973). In the following code, first the three function parameters are specified and then the graph is produced using the curve command.

```
# Specify parameters of Chapman-Richards growth function
> A <- 35.204
> k <- 0.0235
> p <- 1.237
> # Draw the curve of the growth function
> par(mar = c(4.5, 4.5, 2, 0.5))
> curve(A * (1 - exp(-k * x))^p, from = 5, to = 120,
+ xlab = "Age [years]", ylab = "Top height [m]",
+ main = "SP (YC 14, ITh, 1-8m)", axes = FALSE, lwd = 2)
> axis(1, lwd = 2, cex.axis = 1.8)
> axis(2, las = 1, lwd = 2, cex.axis = 1.8)
> box(lwd = 2)
```

This example of top height development over age is taken from the British yield table system (Hamilton and Christie 1973), i.e. Scots pine (*Pinus sylvestris* L.), yield class 14, intermediate thinning Thinning and 1×0.5 m initial spacing. The result is given in Fig. C.6, this time using the original R axes labels.

As a summary the most important graph functions are listed in Table C.3. Graph parameters can be found in the R online help. Incidentally, several graphs can be simultaneously displayed on screen or in a file using the graphical parameters par(mfrow = c(1, 2)). In this case, two graphs are shown in one row and two columns, which is helpful for visual comparisons.

For completeness let us also consider the case of a simple linear regression. For this purpose we will work with the following two vectors of stem diameters in cm and the corresponding absolute diameter growth rates (also in cm):

```
> dbh <- c(42.4, 54.0, 32.2, 39.8, 26.1, 30.4, 39.9, 45.5,
+ 37.9, 31.7)
> id <- c(5.5, 7.2, 4.0, 5.1, 3.1, 3.8, 5.1, 6.0, 4.8, 4.0)
```

Fig. C.6 Visualising the Chapman–Richards growth function

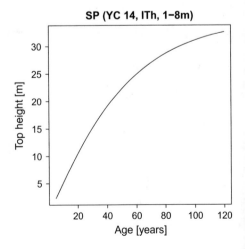

Table C.3 Important graph functions

Function	Description
plot()	Scatterplot (and more)
hist()	Histogram
barplot()	Barplot graph
boxplot()	Boxplot graph
lorenz()	Lorenz curve
pie()	Pie chart

These are sample data from a Sitka spruce (*Picea sitchensis* (Bong.) Carr.) forest stand at Clocaenog forest in North Wales. The cycle of repeated stem-diameter measurements that form the basis of the growth-rate values is 5 years.

A simple linear regression between the initial stem diameters, dbh, i.e. the diameters at the beginning of the growth period, and diameter AGR, id (see Sect. 6.2.2), as independent variable can be performed with the following code:

```
1  > lm.inc <- lm(id ~ dbh)
2  > summary(lm.inc)

   Call:
   lm(formula = id ~ dbh)

   Residuals:
   Min        1Q        Median     3Q        Max
   -0.046878 -0.025837 -0.009401  0.035255  0.057057

   Coefficients:
   Estimate Std. Error t value Pr(>|t|)
   (Intercept) -0.678790    0.062513   -10.86 4.57e-06 ***
   dbh          0.145796    0.001612    90.46 2.49e-13 ***
   ---
   Signif. codes:  0 '***' 0.001 '**' 0.01 '*' 0.05 '.' 0.1 ' ' 1

   Residual standard error: 0.03984 on 8 degrees of freedom
   Multiple R-squared: 0.999,  Adjusted R-squared: 0.9989
   F-statistic:  8183 on 1 and 8 DF,  p-value: 2.489e-13
```

Line 1 gives the code of the linear regression and the following lines are the result of the summary() command. The R package MASS again provides methods for robust linear regression.

Fig. C.7 Example of a
scatterplot with a
superimposed linear trend
curve

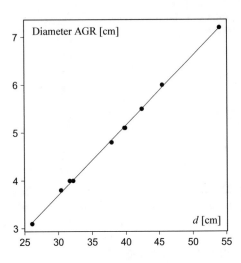

Incidentally, intercept (a), slope (b) parameters and coefficient of determination, R^2, can also be calculated "manually" in the following way:

```
> (b <- cov(dbh, id) / var(dbh))
[1] 0.145796
> (a <- mean(id) - b * mean(dbh))
[1] -0.6787903
> cor(dbh, id)^2
[1] 0.9990233
```

We can now use the regression results again to plot a trend line. Consider the following code.

```
1  par(mar = c(2, 2, 0.5, 0.8))
2  > plot(dbh, id, ylab = "", xlab = "", pch = 16, cex = 1.7,
3  + las = 1, cex.axis = 1.7, lwd = 2)
4  > lines(dbh, fitted(lm.inc), col = "black")
5  > box(lwd = 2)
```

The lines() command adds the actual regression line as shown in Fig. C.7. The command abline(lm.inc, col = "black") would produce a similar trend line.

For examining the normality of the residuals graphically we can, for example, employ the QQ plot (quantile quantile plot). It draws the sample quantiles against the quantiles of a normal distribution, see Fig. C.8.

```
> qqnorm(lm.inc$residuals)
> qqline(lm.inc$residuals)
```

Without going into detail, the data points should ideally lie on or near a straight line. In our case, there are too few observations to make this a worthwhile exercise.

Incidentally, it sometimes makes sense to assume that a regression line passes through the origin, (0, 0), i.e. the intercept of the regression line is zero. This can be specified in the model formula by adding the term -1 ("minus intercept") on the

Fig. C.8 Normal quantile plot of residuals

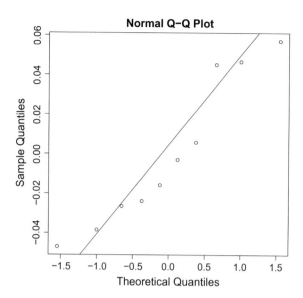

right-hand side (Dalgaard 2008, p. 198): `id ~ dbh - 1`. Alternatively you can also write `id ~ 0 + dbh`. Again, Dalgaard (2008, p. 109ff.) has prepared a chapter on simple linear regression in R, which is recommended for further reading.

C.5   Functions and Flow Control

As previously discussed, `min()`, `max()` and `sum()` are functions that are part of the standard libraries of R. The user has, of course, also the possibility to define his own function. To write functions is a way to extend R and to reduce complexity by writing certain elements of code that are frequently used only once. Functions are self-contained units. They take inputs, do calculations and produce outputs (Braun and Murdoch 2007). As an example we use the calculation of the quadratic mean diameter:

$$d_g = \sqrt{\frac{\sum_{i=1}^{N} d_i^2}{N}} = 200 \cdot \sqrt{\frac{\sum_{i=1}^{N} g_i}{\pi \cdot N}} \tag{C.1}$$

Here d_i and g_i are stem diameter and basal area of tree i and N is the total number of trees accounted for. The R syntax is simple. The word `function` followed by the list of arguments in round brackets, `()`, is assigned to the function name.

```
> calcQuadraticMean <- function(myVector) {
+ x <- sqrt(sum(myVector^2) / length(myVector))
+ return(x)
+ }
```

In a next step, the quadratic mean is calculated and assigned to the local variable x. Local variables are not known outside a function unless their values are explicitly returned by a return statement. This is the case in our function and the value of x is then finally returned to the calling instance with the statement return(x). The whole function body is wrapped in curly braces, {} demarcating the beginning and the end of the function. The location of the first, opening curly brace can be at the end of the first line or at the beginning of the second, this is a matter of taste.

Prior to using the new function you need once to highlight the whole function code and to execute the run command (Ctrl–R or Cmd–Enter). Possible errors in the code will be identified by R at this stage. Afterwards you can apply your own function in all possible contexts, e.g.

```
> calcQuadraticMean(myData$dbh)
[1] 34.7506
```

Since the calculations in the function calcQuadraticMean are simple and consist only of a single line, the function code can be simplified to

```
> calcQuadraticMean <- function(myVector)
+ return(sqrt(sum(myVector^2) / length(myVector)))
```

However, it is important that every user adopts a programming style that best works for him or her. Above all any code has to be correct in the first place.

Structures of flow control are useful for repetitive tasks. Often such code can be avoided by pre-defined functions and implicit loops in R. In case they are really necessary for a given task, a brief introduction is given here by continuing the work with the data frame used in this section and the mean function. Applied to the data set that we have imported earlier from an ASCII file the following code can be employed.

```
> mean(myData$dbh)
[1] 33.34107
```

Since an R function is available, there is no need for programming the calculation of arithmetic means from scratch. However, expressing the same calculation by means of loops helps to understand how they work and how they can be implemented. The following listing shows how the mean function can be simulated with a for loop.

```
1  > mean.xfor <- 0
2  > for (i in 1 : length(myData$dbh)) {
3  + mean.xfor <- mean.xfor + myData$dbh[i]
4  + }
5  > mean.xfor <- mean.xfor / length(myData$dbh)
6  > mean.xfor
7  [1] 33.34107
```

In line 1, the variable collecting the summed stem diameter values is set to zero for initialisation. The loop statement defining the beginning and the end of the loop is given in line 2. In line 3, all stem diameter values are summed up. Note that individual dbh values are accessed by putting the running variable i in square brackets. The loop is executed exactly length(myData$dbh) times. Finally the sum is divided by the number of observations. Since only one line of code is included in the for loop, the above listing can be simplified by omitting the curly braces.

The arithmetic mean can also be implemented with a `while` loop. A little more effort is required as the running variable i needs to be initialised (line 2) and incremented (line 5). The `while` loop is particularly useful where the number of repetitions is difficult to determine beforehand.

```
1  > mean.xwhile <- 0
2  > i <- 1
3  > while (i < length(myData$dbh) + 1) {
4  + mean.xwhile <- mean.xwhile + myData$dbh[i]
5  + i <- i + 1
6  + }
7  > mean.xwhile <- mean.xwhile / (i - 1)
8  > mean.xwhile
9  [1] 33.34107
```

Another option in R is the `repeat` loop, where the abort condition is at the bottom of the loop introduced by an `if` statement.

```
1  > mean.xrepeat <- 0
2  > i <- 1
3  > repeat {
4  + mean.xrepeat <- mean.xrepeat + myData$dbh[i]
5  + i <- i + 1
6  + if(i == length(myData$dbh) + 1)
7  + break
8  + }
9  > mean.xrepeat <- mean.xrepeat / (i - 1)
10 > mean.xrepeat
11 [1] 33.34107
```

The `repeat` loop is not frequently used in R. However, the `if` statement is quite common, mostly in connection with loops and could also include an `else` statement for alternative pathways.

Many loops can be and should be avoided in R, as they require much computation time. In the following code snippet, one of three height bands is assigned to each tree depending on the maximum tree height in a forest stand, `maxh`, and on the total height `myData$ht` of each tree.

```
> myData$band <- 1
> myData$band[myData$ht > max(myData$ht) * 0.8] <- 3
> myData$band[myData$ht > max(myData$ht) * 0.5 &
+ myData$ht <= max(myData$ht) * 0.8] <- 2
```

Instead of using a `for` loop and `if` statements it is possible to exploit the strengths of R. In this case, a default value of 1 is assigned to all trees and then the two other values are assigned using conditional statements in square brackets. This strategy makes use of the vector philosophy of R and conditional statements replace the traditional `if` statements.

Another example illustrating how to replace `for` loops by using the `diff()` function is shown in Sect. 6.2.3.

C.6   Extending R with C++

In some situations, loops are unavoidable and in that case it is recommended to program them externally in C++ or Fortran. R can then utilise compiled or uncompiled external code. This is a kind of 'outsourcing', i.e. the strengths of both R and higher programming languages are combined. Complex loops run much faster in C++ or Fortran and considerable time savings can be achieved with this strategy.

A simple way of combining C++ and R is using, for example, the Rcpp package (Eddelbuettel and François 2011; Eddelbuettel 2013). Using the R Package Installer the package Rcpp first needs to be installed in R. When working with Mac OS Xcode needs to be installed from the Apple Developer site (https://developer.a-pple.com/xcode/). In MS Windows, you need to download and install Rtools (http://cran.r-project.org/bin/windows/Rtools/).

To illustrate the use of combined C++ and R code we continue with the theoretical example of the previous section. In a higher programming language, calculating an arithmetic mean usually involves using a loop. Therefore we program this part in C++ and the corresponding code is given below and saved as meanVector.cpp in ASCII format.

```
1   #include <Rcpp.h>
2
3   using namespace Rcpp;
4
5   // [[Rcpp::export]]
6   double meanVector(NumericVector a) {
7
8   int n = a.size();
9   double xsum = 0;
10
11  for (int i = 0; i < n; i++)
12  xsum += a[i];
13
14  return xsum / n;
15  }
```

In lines 1 and 3, reference to the Rcpp package is made. The code in line 5 is necessary in order to be able to access the function meanVector from within R. The algorithmic structure is essentially the same that we already know from the previous section, only the programming language and the syntax that comes with it is different. Also the Rcpp package provides a number of variable types that otherwise do not exist in C++, e.g. NumericVector in line 6. These additional types allow a smoother cooperation with R, because they resemble R data structure.

The C++ function meanVector is now ready for use in R. In line 1 of the code below all pre-existing R objects are deleted from memory. Then the Rcpp library is loaded in line 3. The code in line 5 is crucial, as the C++ code is loaded and compiled "on the fly". This may take a few seconds. Potential C++ programming errors can now be viewed in the R console.

```
1   > rm(list = ls())
```

```
2  >
3  > library(Rcpp)
4  >
5  > sourceCpp("/MyDataAnalysis/TreeData/
6  + meanVector.cpp")
7  > v <- c(1.5, 2.9, 3.2, 4.1, 5.5)
8  > mean(v)
9  [1] 3.44
10 > meanVector(v)
11 [1] 3.44
```

If the compilation was successful, it is now possible to use the C++ function meanVector from within R. For this purpose we first construct a vector v in line 7. Then we use the R function mean to compute the arithmetic mean of the vector values. In a final step, the self-made function meanVector is applied to calculate the same mean of vector values in line 10 and the results in lines 9 and 11 are the same. Should anything be the matter in this process, it is sometimes helpful to check whether Rcpp is fully functioning by using the code Rcpp::evalCpp("2 + 2").

In analogy to this simple example, more complex (simulation) code can be programmed in C++ and afterwards called from within R. It is for example possible to implement a whole individual tree model (see Sect. 5.2) in C++/R. For this purpose all detailed core model functions are implemented in C++ and then called in R where the simulation results are then statistically analysed and visualised in graphs.

For details of the C and C++ languages please refer to the books and manuals on that language, which exist in great abundance. Also note that the syntax of Java and C# is quite similar so that existing code can easily and quickly be modified for use in Rcpp/R.

References

Bolker BM (2008) Ecological models and data in R. Princeton University Press, Princeton, 396 p

Braun WJ, Murdoch DJ (2007) A first course in statistical programming with R. Cambridge University Press, Cambridge, 163 p

Dalgaard P (2008) Introductory statistics with R. Statistics and computing, 2nd edn. Springer, New York, 363 p

Eddelbuettel D (2013) Seamless R and C++ integration with Rcpp. Springer, New York, 220 p

Eddelbuettel D, François R (2011) Rcpp: seamless R and C++ integration. J Stat Softw 28:1–18

Hamilton GJ, Christie JM (1973) Construction and application of stand yield models. For Comm Res Dev Pap (Edinburgh) 96:120 p

Jones O, Maillardet R, Robinson A (2009) Introduction to scientific programming and simulation using R. Chapman & Hall/CRC, Boca Raton, 453 p

Pienaar LV, Turnbull KJ (1973) The Chapman-Richards generalization of von Bertalanffy's growth model for basal area growth and yield in even-aged stands. For Sci 19:2–22

Porkress R (2004) Collins dictionary statistics. Harper Collins Publishers, Glasgow, 316 p

Robinson AP, Hamann JD (2010) Forest analytics with R. An introduction. Use R! Springer, New York, 339 p

Index

© Springer Nature Switzerland AG 2019
A. Pommerening and P. Grabarnik, *Individual-based Methods*
in Forest Ecology and Management, https://doi.org/10.1007/978-3-030-24528-3

in point process statistics, 202, 203, 231
  dependent, 204
intensity, 4, 67, 80, 82, 93, 306, 319, 320,
  334, 341, 348
intervention, 65–67
law, 26
local, 4, 5, 67, 71, 77, 79, 82, 317, 329
low, 79, 313, 327, 331, 335, 349
mechanical, 67
method of nature, 69
model, 310
natural, 108
pre-commercial, 66, 91, 93
random, 333
regime, 30, 307
release, 80
respacing, 66, 87, 91, 93
schematic, 4
selection, 93
selective, 8, 59, 67, 75, 170, 320
self-, 8, 26, 28, 33, 34, 65, 69, 155, 170,
  171, 202, 204, 244
self-thinning rule, 26, 30
situative, *see* Thinning, local
structural, 77

systematic, 67
type, 4, 67, 70, 80, 82, 94, 313, 334, 337,
  339
urgency, 37, 313, 361
variable-density (VDT), 70
Tipping point, 32, 240, 241
Torus, *see* Periodic boundary conditions
Twin plots, 313, 345, 366

V
Variability between people, 309
Variability within people, 309
VDT, *see* Thinning, variable-density (VDT)
Vorobyov mean, 322–324

W
Wisdom of crowd, 321, 324, 335

Z
ZOI, *see* Zone of influence (ZOI)
Zone of influence (ZOI), 72, 73, 79, 114–
  116, 226–228

Printed in the United States
By Bookmasters